HEALTH ECONOMICS

Health Economics

EFFICIENCY, QUALITY, AND EQUITY

Steven R. Eastaugh

AUBURN HOUSE
Westport, Connecticut • London

Library of Congress Cataloging-in-Publication Data

Eastaugh, Steven R.
    Health economics : efficiency, quality, and equity / Steven R.
Eastaugh.
      p. cm.
    Companion v. to: Health care finance. 1992.
    Includes bibliographical references.
    ISBN 0–86569–196–7 (HC : alk. paper).—ISBN 0–86569–197–5 (PB :
alk. paper)
    1. Medical economics. I. Eastaugh, Steven R. Health
care finance. II. Title.
    [DNLM: 1. Economics, Medical—United States. W 74 E135h]
RA410.E28 1992
338.4′33621—dc20
DNLM/DLC
for Library of Congress   91–26275

British Library Cataloguing in Publication Data is available.

Library of Congress Catalog Card Number: 91–26275
ISBN: 0–86569–196–7
     0–86569–197–5 (pbk.)

First published in 1992

Auburn House, 88 Post Road West, Westport, CT 06881
An imprint of Greenwood Publishing Group, Inc.

Printed in the United States of America

∞™

The paper used in this book complies with the
Permanent Paper Standard issued by the National
Information Standards Organization (Z39.48–1984).

10 9 8 7 6 5 4 3 2 1

This book is dedicated to my wife,
Janet A. Eastaugh, M.D.

Contents

Figures and Tables

FIGURES

TABLES

Preface

In preparing this book I have intentionally cast a wide net to include policy makers, providers, managers, and students. I anticipate that this wide audience is more interested in a synthesis of currently available study results and possible policy implications than in new econometric methods. This book and its antecedent, my text *Medical Economics*, parallel the development of the field of health economics. Our focus has shifted from medicine to health care, and balancing efficiency and quality are now paramount issues for public policy. Almost 50 percent of this new text centers on the topics of cost-benefit, cost-effectiveness, quality enhancement, and technology assessment. By contrast, most health economics texts spend very little time on these four critical topics. In this text major emphasis is placed on concepts and their applications, as opposed to dry standard presentation of microeconomic theory. Many faculty members in this discipline teach both economics and finance and might utilize the companion volume to this text, *Health Care Finance: Economic Incentives and Productivity Enhancement*.

Part 1 presents a basic overview of the overtilled and recently developed fields of cost analysis, production functions, and provider cost behavior (chapters 1 and 2). Part 2 considers economic models of physician and hospital behavior and recent changes in methods for paying physicians (chapters 3 and 4). In Part 3 (chapters 5 and 6) the focus shifts to employee cost sharing, health maintenance organizations (HMOs), gatekeepers to contain utilization, and the use of case managers in long-term care.

Part 4 involves a discussion of equity, social welfare, and the unique problems of the urban medical center; chapter 7 considers access and the uninsured population, and chapter 8 presents cost studies for teaching hospitals and outlines a number of patient-severity systems. Part 5 (chapters 9 and 10) focuses on consumer information, quality measurement, and health manpower policies for nonphysician providers. In Part 6 (chapters 11–13) we discuss cost-effectiveness, hypothetical willingness-to-pay surveys, and cost-benefit analysis. One cannot help but observe that the prospective payment system (PPS) for Medicare furnished a regulatory language, diagnostic related groups (DRGs), that brought into the picture a key group of players: the doctors. We survey physician concerns for quality and cost analysis throughout the second half of the text. As an alumnus of two graduate schools of public health, I cannot resist pointing out that health care can be conceived of as either a final output of our industry or an intermediate input in the production of "good health." Consequently, health finance could have been misinterpreted by some readers as the study of how society finances improved health in the population. However, many studies reviewed in this text have posed the tougher basic question regarding the minimal marginal impact that increased hospital-services delivery has had on improving the health status of Americans. We end chapter 13 with a discussion of the need to justify AIDS care and AIDS research by willingness-to-pay surveys that shadow-price subtle intangible benefits. Providers can do more to establish preferred practice guidelines, maintain quality, and assist in cost-effectiveness analysis. Part 7 summarizes a number of future policy options and concludes that no single cost-containment strategy will be sufficient. Rather, a number of mixed strategies are suggested, including capitation (chapter 14).

This book contains 1,300 published references. However, since not everything worth knowing is published in the journals, a second source of information is utilized. For two decades I have sought to accumulate, through management consulting work, firsthand accounts of ways to improve economic efficiency, productivity, quality, and access. As an economist I grew tired of sterile econometric measurement of a cost function and wanted to jump into the tougher task of cutting costs while enhancing service quality. Such real-world experience helps improve the text by reporting success and failure (authors seldom advertise failures in the journals). Under the coming era of barebones reimbursement, learning from our failures and the failures of the competition will become increasingly important for managers.

ACKNOWLEDGMENTS

I acknowledge, first of all, my wife Janet, who provided me with a provider perspective and the life-sustaining critical review of this book during the long preparation period. I have depended on the ideas and assistance of others in writing this book, including Professors Philip Reeves, Warren Greenberg, Richard Riegelman, Ruth Hanft, Duncan Neuhauser, Jim Begun, and former student David Dranove. A number of research assistants over the years deserve special thanks for their help: Susan Labovich, Ascanio Terracciano, Bonnie Horvath, Susan Clark, Juan Acevedo, Janet Nuggent, Carolyn Lankford, Jay Higham, Tina Kao, Tom Caldwell, Michael Jernigan, Steven Klapmeier, Gary Selmeczi, Susan Cosgrove, and Nancy Bohn. I acknowledge the invaluable help of the two editors Charles Eberline and Lynn Flint. For any errors that remain in the book I am responsible.

COST BEHAVIOR AND COST FUNCTIONS

1 Cost Inflation: Overtilled and Undertilled Fields

The need for reform in the health care system is widely accepted. We may not agree on the methods, but we do agree on the outcomes of assuring access to quality services, stopping cost escalation, preserving the best aspects of our present system, compensating providers fairly, and maintaining freedom of choice and private initiatives.

—Sye Berki

The health care system is what we make it for good or ill, both a charity and a business, because the quality of American medical care is indeed an index of American civilization.

—Rosemary Stevens

Change is already here, like it or not. More change is in view. Change breeds doubt. Doubt kindles choice. Choice is opportunity, opportunity to do better or worse.

—Steven Muller

Health care has priced itself into the public eye and has assumed an increasing fraction of the general economy. In the quarter century from 1966 to 1991 health care has grown from 5.8 to 12.4 percent of the gross national product (GNP). This book will cover a number of segments of the health economy, from hospital care to physician services. We shall begin with the largest segment, the hospital sector, representing 4.7 percent of GNP. Prior to beginning a discussion of hospital cost inflation, it is essential first to explain how it is known that costs are in fact increasing each year. In other words, it is necessary to identify the indexes of cost inflation being used and to understand their implications. One broad indicator of the *relative* quantity of resources devoted to health care is the percentage of the GNP devoted to health expenditures. National health expenditures rose from 4.5 percent of the GNP in 1950 to 7.2 percent in 1970, 10.7

percent in 1983, 11.8 percent in 1990, and an estimated 12.7 percent by 1992 (see table 1.1).

INSURANCE AND THE DEMAND FOR CARE

How does the tremendous increase in expenditures on hospital care relate to the out-of-pocket costs borne by the consumer of hospital care at the time of illness? In other words, how is it that consumers are willing to bear the costs of such an increase in the intensity of hospital care without an equivalent return in the form of better health? Part of the answer lies in the fact that although there has been a great increase in the amount of national resources devoted to hospital care, there has been very little change in the cost of hospital care to the consumer at the time of illness.

In 1950 approximately 50 percent of the cost of hospital care (short-term, nonfederal) was paid directly by the consumer and 50 percent was paid by third parties, including government and private insurance. By 1983 the proportion of costs paid directly by the consumer had dropped to 13.9 percent, and by 1987 to a record low of 12.9 percent. However, since 1988 this figure has increased, reaching an estimated 16.3 percent in 1991 because of the hikes in cost-sharing provisions outlined in Chapter 6. (Out-of-pocket consumer payments as a percentage of hospital revenues are two-thirds lower because of the fraction of consumer copayments, deductibles, and coinsurance channeled through third parties.) The result of the deep insurance coverage of hospital services is summarized as follows: The average cost of a patient day to the consumer has doubled in constant dollars since 1950, whereas the 1991 average cost per patient day (ACPPD) was 579 percent what it was in constant dollar terms in 1950. In this context it is not surprising that our health care sector could grow to $1.5 trillion (15.2 percent of GNP) by the year 2000 (Ginzberg 1990). Ideally one should not use hospital list price per diem, even if it is a component of the Consumer Price Index (CPI) as an index of inflation. List price inflation has greatly exceeded actual inflation (Dranove et al.,1991) as more patients receive discount prices, and the negotiated discounts are larger in recent years. However measured, the inflation in health care costs is more substantial than any other sector of the American economy.

There is substantial evidence to indicate that when a large proportion of medical costs are offset by insurance, doctors will recommend more services, and consumers in turn will demand more and better services. Thus as insurance increases, a higher quantity and quality of care are demanded. At this juncture, it is important to make the point that the increase in demand is for greater intensity of care per diem, rather than for more bed days. This is not to say that there was not a dramatic expansion in the demand for days of hospitalization prior to 1975, but the demand for days abated in the 1970s (Table 1.2) and declined in the 1980s. Hospitals, as they work to fill the demand for increased services, raise prices in order to raise revenue that can be used to provide the more

Table 1.1
National Health Expenditures (Aggregate and per Capita)

Year	GNP (in billions)	Health Expenditures (in millions)	Health Expenses per Capita	Health as a Percentage of GNP	Hospital Care as a Percentage of GNP[a]
1929	$ 101.3	$ 3,589	$ 29	3.5	0.7
1935	68.9	2,846	22	4.1	0.9
1940	95.4	3,883	29	4.1	0.9
1950	264.8	12,027	78	4.5	1.0
1955	381.0	17,330	104	4.5	1.1
1960	498.3	25,856	142	5.2	1.5
1965	688.0	38,892	198	5.9	1.9
1966	722.4	42,109	212	5.8	1.9
1967	773.5	47,897	238	6.2	2.2
1968	830.2	53,765	264	6.5	2.3
1969	904.2	60,617	295	6.7	2.4
1970	960.2	69,201	333	7.2	2.7
1971	1,019.8	77,162	368	7.6	2.9
1972	1,111.8	86,687	410	7.8	3.0
1973	1,238.6	95,383	447	7.7	3.0
1974	1,361.2	106,321	495	7.8	3.1
1975	1,487.1	127,719	588	8.6	3.4
1976	1,667.4	145,102	663	8.7	3.5
1977	1,838.0	162,627	737	8.8	3.5
1978	2,107.6	192,400	863	9.1	3.6
1979	2,346.5	216,500	964	9.3	3.7
1980	2,631.7	247,500	1,049	9.4	3.7
1981	2,957.8	285,200	1,197	9.6	3.9
1982	3,069.2	321,200	1,334	10.5	4.2
1983	3,304.8	355,100	1,461	10.7	4.3
1984	3,662.8	387,400	1,580	10.6	4.1
1985	4,015.1	420,100	1,701	10.6	4.1
1986	4,232.0	450,500	1,806	10.7	4.1
1987	4,524.0	488,800	1,941	10.8	4.2
1988	4,881.1	544,000	2,124	11.1	4.3
1989	5,209.0	604,400	2,398	11.6	4.5
1990	5,455.3	633,000	2,488	11.8	4.5
1992 est.	5,764.0	735,000	2,820	12.7	4.9
1995 est.	6,753.0	934,000	3,285	13.9	5.4
2000 est.	8,779.0	1,334,000	4,212	15.2	6.0

Sources: Health Care Financing Review 12:4 (Fall) 1991; author estimates for 1992, 1995, and 2000.

[a]This is an underestimate of the hospital sector's share of GNP because the figure does not include services provided by nonsalaried physicians within hospitals. Because physicians have increasingly pursued subspecialty careers that demand increased reliance on the hospital, the magnitude of the hospital-sector underestimation bias has undoubtedly increased since the 1950s.

Table 1.2
Growth Rates in the Demand and Supply of Nonfederal Short-Term Hospitals, Selected Years, 1950–1991

Year	FTE Personnel per Adjusted Patient Day[a]	Patient Days (millions)	Admissions per 1,000 Citizens	Number of Hospitals	Number of Beds	Bed Occupancy (percent)	Outpatient Visits (millions)
1950	1.62	136	111.4	5,031	505,000	73.7	
1955	1.85	149	117.3	5,237	568,000	71.5	
1960	2.06	174	129.2	5,407	639,000	74.7	
1965	2.24	205	138.8	5,736	741,000	76.0	93
1966	2.37	215	138.9	5,812	768,000	76.5	96
1967	2.41	223	139.0	5,850	788,000	77.6	103
1970	2.65	242	145.6	5,859	848,000	78.0	134
1974	2.89	256	157.8	5,977	931,000	75.3	195
1978	3.23	263	161.1	5,935	980,000	73.5	204
1979	3.28	267	162.4	5,923	988,000	73.8	204
1980	3.34	279	165.8	5,905	992,000	75.4	207
1981	3.47	281	161.9	5,879	986,000	75.9	207
1982	3.52	284	156.7	5,863	982,000	75.2	214
1983	3.59	277	154.4	5,843	988,000	73.4	231
1984	3.67	254	147.1	5,814	961,000	66.8	232
1985	3.85	236	139.0	5,774	940,000	64.0	234
1986	3.92	229	133.7	5,720	920,000	63.4	245
1987	4.00	226	131.7	5,650	909,000	64.2	268
1988	4.04	225	130.0	5,570	897,000	64.7	287
1989	4.11	223	127.7	5,487	884,000	65.5	301
1990	4.18	221	126.4	5,408[b]	873,000	65.7	319
1991	4.33	213	124.0	5,358	863,000	63.9	333

Source: American Hospital Association panel survey, includes over 1,270 hospitals each year.
[a]Full-time-equivalent (FTE) personnel adjusted for outpatient visits rendered.
[b]If figures include specialty hospitals and federal and state hospitals, 698 closed in the period 1980-90.

expensive form of care demanded. Since most consumers do not pay out-of-pocket for hospital care because they are heavily insured, they are shielded from the resulting increase in prices and do not respond in the normal way by curtailing demand. On the contrary, as consumers observe the higher prices, or cost, of medical care, their desire for insurance increases and likewise the demand for medical care increases, so the inflationary cycle continues. This six-step medical cost inflationary cycle is illustrated in figure 1.1. The rate-limiting step, the stage in the cycle at which intervention is most effective, is between A and B, the point at which insurance stimulates demand.

It is easy to see why individuals would want to insure themselves against the risk of a very large medical bill; it is not so readily apparent why they are willing to pay the additional actuarial charges associated with insurance for small bills when these extra charges could be avoided if the small bills were paid out-of-pocket. The reasons for the proliferation of comprehensive "first-dollar" insurance policies are twofold. First, the present tax structure encourages such policies. Second, these insurance policies can be seen as a form of precommitment on the part of policyholders.

The current tax structure encourages comprehensive health insurance in the following way. Employer-paid health insurance may be deducted from the employing company's taxable income. At the same time, employees need not include the value of health insurance policies in their taxable income, nor are the premiums subject to Social Security or state income tax. Thus health insurance can be considered to be a form of tax-exempt extra income. In addition, approximately one-half of the amount an individual pays for health insurance is tax deductible. The "tax break" amounted to some $7 billion for individuals and $37 billion for businesses in 1986, and a net $64 billion in 1991 ($600 per insured employee). Department of Health and Human Services (DHHS) Secretary Dr. Louis Sullivan has asked for some policy options in 1992 to target the incentive to purchase insurance. For example, one could means test (exclude the rich) for both the tax exemption and the Medicare program, thus concentrating federal resources where they are most needed. Another approach would be to give the working poor tax credits to enable them to buy their health insurance (Butler 1990) and to federalize and limit the scope of Medicaid. Medicaid expenses increased 18 percent in 1990 and 24.3 percent in 1991.

Havighurst and Hackbarth (1979) argued that when individuals select the lower-cost insurance plan, they should be given the savings tax free. By eliminating the practice of requiring the employer to pay the entire premium, society can end the forced subsidy of traditional solo-practice fee-for-service medicine at the expense of the more efficient modes of practice. The Federal Employees Health Benefits Program is the oldest prototype of a consumer-choice health plan with a fixed dollar contribution on behalf of the employer. This program was originally promoted in 1959 by public officials in the name of fair market competition and has served both the taxpayer and federal employees well.

Health insurance can also be viewed as a form of "precommitment" on the

Figure 1.1
The Six-Step Medical Cost Inflation Cycle

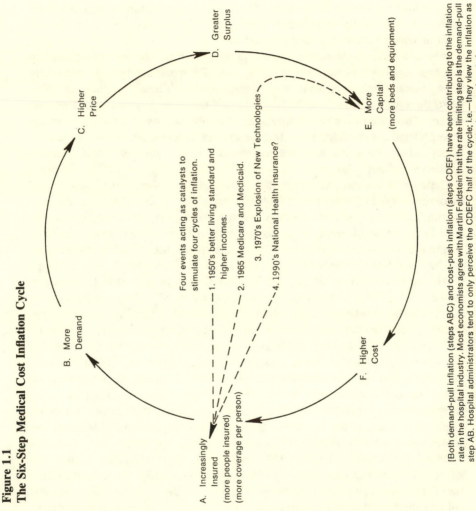

Four events acting as catalysts to
stimulate four cycles of inflation.

1. 1950's better living standard and
   higher incomes.
2. 1965 Medicare and Medicaid.
3. 1970's Explosion of New Technologies
4. 1990's National Health Insurance?

A. Increasingly
   Insured
   (more people insured)
   (more coverage per person)

B. More
   Demand

C. Higher
   Price

D. Greater
   Surplus

E. More
   Capital
   (more beds and equipment)

F. Higher
   Cost

[Both demand-pull inflation (steps ABC) and cost-push inflation (steps CDEF) have been contributing to the inflation rate in the hospital industry. Most economists agree with Martin Feldstein that the rate limiting step is the demand-pull step AB. Hospital administrators tend to only perceive the CDEFC half of the cycle; i.e.—they view the inflation as cost-push, with the various production costs forcing their prices to rise to meet the increased costs.]

part of individuals who do not want monetary costs to influence their choice of medical care. By precommitting themselves through insurance, individuals do not have to make the choice between expensive, highly intensive care and cheaper, less intensive care (Fuchs 1986). In addition, insurance is a form of self-control for individuals who feel that they might spend all their money now, in the short term, and not have it in the long term when they need it for medical care; it therefore acts to relieve some of the tension in the conflict between long-term and short-term goals.

The underlying causes of the inflation in overall expenditures on hospital care can be divided into four categories: (1) increased demand (demand-pull); (2) increases in the cost of producing care; (3) increases in the prices of inputs used to produce care; and (4) changes in the markets that supply inputs, particularly the labor market (supply-push). When a product is demanded at a rate faster than it can be produced, the product is considered scarce and its price rises. At the same time, the demand rises for factors used in its production, and so the prices of the factors rise. This form of inflation has been labeled "demand-pull" and is considered a major cause of inflation in medical costs (Salkever 1975; Eastaugh 1987).

The past three decades of medical cost inflation can be divided into two basic periods: 1950–81 and 1983 to the present. The demand-pull theory attracted a surplus of scholarly labor from 1950 to 1981. Health expenditures increased 2,270 percent during this period, with a marked increase in hospital usage. Analytical studies of medical cost inflation are important because such increases reflect a serious misallocation of resources toward expensive medical practice and a basic failure of the health care system to reflect individual consumer preferences (Feldstein 1977; Eastaugh 1983).

The current demand-pull inflation manifests itself through the escalation of expensive procedures. For example, the number of coronary artery bypass operations performed annually increased 372 percent from 1983 to 1990. The number of magnetic resonance imaging (MRI) scans done annually has increased 590 percent since 1985 (see chapters 11–13).

The two major ingredients to understanding this inflation in health care costs are obvious: the growth in health insurance and the changing nature of the hospital. Medicare and private payers began to reverse this demand-pull incentive structure in the period 1982–83. This is not to say that the demand-pull for lifesaving technology has abated, but rather that the demand-pull is not manifest in terms of increasing admissions, patient days, and hospital-bed construction. All three measures of output and capacity have declined since 1982. Competition is even more cost-decreasing—nothing new for private industry but quite a revolutionary development in the health care industry. The American public is relying less on hospital beds and more on lower-cost care settings.

Just because more Americans have been channeled into more low-cost channels of service distribution does not mean that health care spending has been curtailed. A treatment alternative like ambulatory surgery might be a cost add-on rather than a substitute for expensive inpatient surgery. In the next section we shall consider the expansion in hospital outpatient surgery, which rose from 4.2 million operations a year in 1982–83 to 10 million in 1989 and 11.1 million in 1991. Policy makers should ask: Has this trend been cost-effective? For whom?

AMBULATORY SURGERY

When ambulatory surgery was first proposed as a health care cost-containment strategy, it was thought that this alternative surgical setting would result in an equivalent or improved clinical outcome at a lower cost. The true costs must be calculated. Unless operating rooms and hospital beds are closed, staffing patterns reduced, and overhead costs diminished, hospital costs remain relatively unchanged. Ambulatory centers will then only add to total health care expenditures by aggravating preexisting hospital capacity. The literature states that savings derived from ambulatory-surgery sites in the early 1970s have now all but dissipated (Evans 1990).

Hospitals to date have had no economic incentive to utilize outpatient surgery as a substitute rather than a new-business-generating technique. Their goal has been to utilize ambulatory surgery as an addition to their services that increases utilization and staff and thus produces a larger volume of work. Will hospital beds made available from the shift to ambulatory surgery actually result in increased admissions? Wennberg, Freeman and Culp (1987) indicated that hospitals with low occupancy rates have actually increased their volume of admissions as a response to bed-reduction threats. Furthermore, as the surgical caseload expanded to compensate for the increased available capacity, net costs also increased (Pro PAC 1991).

PITFALLS AND FADS THAT FAIL

One basic axiom in the business world is the "strategic advantage of being first," being the first entrant or the first to move into a new product line. This idea does not always work in the business world, and it sometimes does not work in the health field. Consider the example of urgent-care centers, which grew in number from 300 in 1982 to 1,380 in 1986. Very few urgent-care centers have been initiated since 1986 because the prospector advantage of being a first mover did not exist. Urgent-care centers are an idea that can be easily imitated at low cost by competitors. Therefore, unless the center can differentiate on the basis of quality and promote a product with a quality label (brand name), it is hard to retain market share and profit margins in the long run. Some hospitals produced redesigned emergency-department walk-in services that competed with the hospital's own urgent-care center. This sort of service cannibalism, competing with oneself, is a very poor strategy. Bigelow (1991) reports that ambulatory centers do not improve marketshare or financial position of the sponsor hospital.

If entry cost is low, and skills and experience can be easily transferred to the competition by ex-employees or consultants, first-entrant advantages do not exist. But if a hospital can be one of only 80 hospitals in the country with a positron emission tomography (PET) machine, the strategic advantage of being a first mover into this product line was high in 1991 (even if it cost the facility $2.2 million). On the other hand, the strategic advantage of being the sixth entrant into the market with the single photon emission computed tomography (SPECT) machine, a faster and cheaper technology than a PET scanner, may be low. Over 1,300 SPECT machines existed in hospitals and physician offices in 1991. Reimbursement is another concern in adopting a new product line or keeping an existing service. If a hospital's market has too high a share of cheap payers that refuse to pay break-even prices of $510 for a SPECT brain scan or $820 for a heart study, the smart manager may act as a defender and avoid (or drop) this technology.

Charges, the prices set by the provider, are a less important concern for the most highly regulated health services with few patients paying price. But some services are more price sensitive and offer the consumer time to shop for a better price, like maternity care or sports medicine. For price-sensitive services, volume building on low prices (and package pricing including aftercare) can be a good strategy. Other services are more physician driven and receive biomedical research dollars, like AIDS care, oncology, and cardiology. Price deals for these services are not a good business strategy. In any case, if the product line is a major source of prestige to the hospital, the board can designate the department a center of excellence, for example, in AIDS, cancer care, heart surgery, cholesterol control and lipid research, family medicine, sports medicine, arthritis, or long-term care (vintage caring).

DISTRIBUTIONS OF HEALTH CARE EXPENDITURES

Hospital expenditures, excluding physician billings for services performed in the hospital, represented 39.5 percent of health care spending in 1991. In 1992 hospitals will receive an estimated $290 billion in revenue. Public funds finance 55.2 percent of all hospital care: Medicare represents 29.8 percent, Medicaid 10.8 percent, state and local tax subsidies represent 6.8 percent, and the Department of Defense and the Veterans Administration provide 7.3 percent. Private funds finance 44.8 percent of hospital services: Employer-based health insurance represents 32.3 percent, consumer cost-sharing and individual-insurance plans represent 7.9 percent, and 4.7 percent of revenues comes from nonpatient sources (philanthropy, gift shops, office space rental, educational programs, and so on).

An estimated 12.66 percent of GNP ($735 billion) will go to health care expenditures in 1992. Hospital services represent 39.5 percent of the total, and physician services represent 20.3 percent ($149 billion). Nursing home expenditures are estimated at 8.45 percent of the health budget ($62 billion) in 1992 (financed 47 percent by Medicaid, 1.8 percent by Medicare, 1.4 percent by private insurance, and 49.8 percent by out-of-pocket spending). In 1992 home health care should exceed $7.1 billion (financed 45 percent from Medicare and 35 percent from Medicaid). Prescription drug spending will reach $36 billion, and nonprescription drugs and other medical nondurables should cost $19.5 billion. Commercial research expenditures should exceed $10 billion, while government-sponsored research and other noncommercial research should exceed $17 billion. Dental services will represent $39.5 billion, vision care products $10.1 billion, and other durable medical products $4.4 billion in 1992.

Although the explosion in health insurance during the past 40 years is the single most important factor in the increased demand for medical care, other factors have had an influence as well. Growth in population and increases in the average life span have contributed to the demand for medical care. The fastest-growing age group is the 65-and-older category, whose per capita expenditures on health care are four times those of adults 19 to 64. In addition, many innovations in medical technology are extremely expensive and increase the demand for medical care in a multiplicative fashion. Although the development of antibiotics and other drugs has been cost-effective in saving lives, new developments in medical technology, such as chemotherapy and organ transplantation, require expensive equipment and skilled personnel; by prolonging life instead of curing illness, such technology can be radically cost-increasing (Eastaugh 1990a). The cost-increasing nature of medical technology will be discussed in Chapters 11–13.

MALPRACTICE COST INFLATION SLOWS

Several factors, aside from nationwide inflation and excess aggregate demand, have contributed to an increase in the cost of producing medical care. Malpractice insurance, a negligible problem 20 years ago, increased an average of 29 percent a year from 1970 to 1978 (Freeland, Anderson, and Schendler 1979). The rate of increase has slowed since 1988. The threat of malpractice suits has caused an increase in the number of tests ordered by physicians. Some groups would like to explain the cost-control problems in terms of defensive medicine (estimated by a 1990 Harvard study team at costing at least $15 billion annually). The American Medical Association (AMA) in Chicago provided a rather high estimate of $30 billion in 1991 for such unnecessary tests. We shall see in chapter 12 that much unnecessary testing may be taking place, but not all of it is attributable to the malpractice crisis. Of the $1,820 spent on health care by the average American in 1986, $19 went toward malpractice insurance (Arnett et al. 1986). Some doctors may spend $100,000 a year in malpractice premiums, but the average doctor spends only 6.8 percent of gross income on such premiums (Office of National Cost Estimates [ONCE] 1991). In fact, the average doctor pays more for an automobile than for malpractice premiums. Those who blame the "terrible for-profit insurance companies" for the malpractice crisis will be dismayed to discover that the 32 nonprofit, physician-owned companies have premiums that have been rising since 1978 at the same annual rate as those of the for-profit companies because of comparable claims experience. Providers should do a careful cost-benefit comparison between various claims-made coverage plans and occurrence coverage.

Many physicians have argued that the best form of malpractice prevention is through the sharing of uncertainty (with the patient) and better-informed consent (Gutheil, Bursztajn, and Brodsky 1984). Malpractice will continue to be a problem in certain towns that cannot find enough doctors (e.g., obstetricians), but the self-serving anecdotal reports of "early retirement" forced by malpractice problems represent an ice cube floating on the surface of a lake, not the tip-of-an-iceberg "crisis." Steps to moderate the liability crisis in the 1990s by federal and state governments across the entire nation may reduce the level of "crisis" rhetoric.

Rising physician expenditures also play a major role in the inflation of medical care costs (see chapter 12). However, in some sense, hospitals have grown "richer" than physicians, especially following the passage of Medicare and Medicaid. From 1950 to 1983 the rate of physician price inflation was less than the rate of hospital price inflation (in table 1.3, column 2-C is less than column 3 until 1983 to 1990), although both the hospital industry and the physician service industry are outperforming (inflating faster than) the general economy. Physician price inflation was a problem of both consumer demand-pull (increased per capita usage) and pure price effects from 1955 to 1982. However, the demand-pull impact of increased consumer demand was lacking from 1983 to 1986, as evidenced by the negative figure in column 2-B in table 1.3. The AMA's Socioeconomic Monitoring System reported a 16 percent decline in the number of outpatient visits per physician per week between the first half of 1982 and the first half of 1986. Physician price expansion was as much a problem in 1985–86 as it was following the Nixon price-control program—the so-called five-year "catch-up" period of 1974–79. Annual cost inflation for physician services averaged 13.2 percent in the period 1986–90, a rate that was exceeded only by the inflation during the "catch-up era" (1974–77) following the lifting of the Nixon price-control program.

COST CONTAINMENT

One may approach the problem of containing rising hospital costs from two directions. First, attempts could be made to lower the cost of production of hospital care at any level of intensity by improving efficiency, by achieving greater economies of scale through building larger hospitals, or by redesigning the market to encourage competition. Second, the current trend toward more intensive care could be curtailed through programs designed to limit supply expansion (for example, the certificate-of-need program), through preventive medicine, or through attempts to decrease the demand for medical care by encouraging greater cost consciousness on the part of consumers (Whitted and Torrens 1989).

Table 1.3
Physician Services: Annual Rates of Increase in Expenditures, Allocation of Cost Inflation to Price, per Capita Use, and Population Shifts

Time Period	(1) Annual Increase in Total Expenses for Physician Services	Sources of Physician Cost Inflation			(3) Annual Increase in Hospital Price
		(2-A) Population	(2-B) Per Capita Use	(2-C) Price	
1950-1955	6.0%	1.7%	0.9%	3.5%	6.3%
1955-1960	9.1	1.7	4.1	3.3	6.5
1960-1965	9.0	1.5	4.9	2.6	6.6
1965-1968	9.8	1.1	2.5	6.2	11.3
1968-1971	10.9	0.9	2.9	7.1	14.6
1971-1974b	10.0	0.8	5.2	4.0	11.0
1974-1977	17.6	0.8	5.8	11.0	15.2
1977-1980	13.2	0.8	3.5	8.9	14.0
1980-1983	9.3	0.8	2.9	5.6	9.6
1983-1986	6.0	0.8	-3.4	8.6	5.8
1986-1990	13.2	0.9	2.1	10.1	6.2

Sources: Health Care Financing Administration; Eastaugh (1991).
aCharges per inpatient day.
bThe Economic Stabilization Program was in effect 8/15/71 to 4/30/74.

Essentially, any attempt to lower costs while not reducing the quality or intensity of care is an attempt to improve efficiency. Efficiency can be identified in three forms: technical, economic, and allocative. *Technical efficiency* refers to the relationship between input and output, irrespective of cost. If one cannot reduce the amount of input and still produce the same amount of output, then maximum technical efficiency has been achieved. In a hospital context, for example, inputs might be full-time-equivalent employees, and outputs would be days of care. *Economic efficiency* refers to the relationship between inputs and cost. When a day of care is provided at the minimum possible cost, there is economic efficiency. *Allocative efficiency* in health care involves determining from among which inputs the allocation of resources would be least costly for achieving an improved level of output (health status). A health production function is necessary to describe the relationship between combinations of inputs and the resulting output. Fuchs (1986) reviewed the findings and limitations of a number of studies whereby improved levels of health output were produced using different combinations of inputs. The reader should be careful to differentiate production functions from a closely similarly labeled concept—the production possibility curve—which describes the trade-off between different outputs from a given set of resources. We shall consider in the coming sections the impact of pricing policies and capacity (size, equipment) decisions on efficiency.

The advent of federal and private prospective pricing has placed hospitals at risk for their cost behavior and has created a revolution in two senses. First, and for the first time, hospitals that are the most successful in holding down costs receive the advantages of higher operating margins and retained earnings for future capital replacement and growth. Second, the term ''price'' no longer refers to the old friendly concept of ''charges'' set by the hospital or in negotiation. Price has been exogenously thrust upon the sellers—in this case hospitals—by third-party payers interested in price competition. However, the seller could rightfully complain that the Health Care Financing Administration (HCFA) has offered something other than a free-market-determined price. HCFA has utilized its monopsony power to administer a form of price controls and to act as a ''prudent buyer'' on the taxpayers' behalf.

Many clinicians and hospital managers have found that the transition from reimbursement to payment and from cost-based to price-based financing has been far from smooth. The past two decades of blank-check, pay-hospitals-what-they-spend financing arrangements have done little to control costs. In fact, under cost payment, voluntary efforts to cut costs became a voluntary suicide program to shrink the assets and prestige of the hospital. In the 1990s era of unilateral price payment and price controls, cost containment has become a virtue.

A number of hospitals are experiencing financial downturns (Schwartz and Stone 1991). The public may be misled into undersupplying debt or equity funds to hospitals if it continues to read doom-and-gloom rhetoric about the hospital industry. The popular press often produces doom-and-gloom statistics as if the end of the world is at hand for American hospitals. For example, the *Washington*

Post listed 698 fewer hospitals in the 1980–90 period as if "698 hospitals closed" (Eastaugh 1990b), but in fact only 107 hospitals closed, 84 restructured into long-term-care facilities, 118 mergers swallowed 123 hospitals, 262 hospitals consolidated with other hospitals, and 127 restructured into specialty hospitals (e.g., psychiatric facilities). Young health care managers need not fear an insufficient future job market, and the public need not avoid purchasing hospital bonds, because "hospitals do not always go bankrupt." A consolidation occurs when two or more hospitals join to form an entirely new hospital (with a new name). Mergers involve separate firms that combine, with one hospital absorbing the other facility.

Akin to the airlines and banking industries, hospitals are overstaffed and overbuilt. Closures are a healthy sign because they get some of the pathology out of the system, eliminate fixed costs, and stimulate control over the total health care bill. As Egdahl (1984) observed, in the labor-intensive hospital business, bringing about significant cost savings without reducing staff and closing facilities is no easy task. Layoffs, or "managed attrition" that avoids firing people, are necessary to draw staffing into line with declining workloads. Hospitals, like airlines and banks, will continue to adapt to deregulation, trim their staffs, and close unnecessary service sites. At the same time, they will be diversifying into newly identified service product lines (Eastaugh 1987, 1984).

CHANGES IN THE INSURANCE INDUSTRY

Nearly 60 percent of the American public is covered by employer-based health insurance. Over 72 million Americans use Blue Cross/Blue Shield, and 77 million Americans used commercial insurance contracts in 1991. The annual premium hikes averaged 17.6 percent over the period 1987–91. The lowest premium hikes were for group-model HMOs, 11.3 percent over the period 1987–91 (37.7 million Americans subscribe to the four basic HMO types; see chapter 5).

Two basic trends dominate the insurance business. Almost 52 percent of companies self-insured in 1991, up from 5.7 percent in 1980. Under self-insurance the employer utilizes the insurance carriers simply to process medical claims and not to act as an insurance conduit of funds (the employer carries all the risk). The second major trend is the movement away from community rating to experience rating. Under community rating in the 1960s the insurance carrier with 900 people and $360,000 of annual expenses would simply charge each person a $400 annual premium. Community rating depended on a large number of younger, healthier people using less than $200 of services per year to subsidize a smaller number of older or sicker people consuming an above-average amount of health services each year. However, faced with rapidly rising medical costs, employers and employees began to insist that this kind of subsidy was inappropriate, and they demanded community rating of insurance premiums. Nobody wanted to "be their brother's keeper anymore" and subsidize the employed older or sicker individuals. Under experience rating the premiums are calculated from a company's own health care bills. Over 89 percent of the insurance carriers for small business firms and 65 percent of commercial insurers for large employers screen applicants for risk conditions that might be excluded (or priced higher) because of the associated risk factors, like kidney or liver conditions, diabetes, or cardiovascular disease. The special problems of small companies facing high risk-related premiums is discussed in chapter 6.

Insurance companies in search of cost-effective business have gone so far as to place ads stating "You don't take risks, why should you pay for someone else's risks?" This practice has drawn criticism from state lawmakers. Connecticut and Massachusetts, along with a dozen other states, have risk pools, force insurers to take all groups, and limit the maximum premiums that can be charged to high-risk groups. The insurance company can transfer responsibility for patients experiencing high expenses onto the state risk pool. Vertical equity may be compromised if the large employers can avoid the insurance companies, self-insure, and avoid paying into the state risk pools. But the large self-insured companies defend their exemption from state insurance laws in the name of actuarial fairness; contributions to the health insurance system should be in proportion to cost experience. Moreover, we as taxpayers act as our brother's keeper by paying taxes that support services for 26 percent of the population under Medicare, Medicaid, and other public programs. Self-insured industries say that they should not make a second contribution or subsidy by paying excess health insurance premiums to cross-subsidize expenses in high-risk employer groups (such as mining, gas stations, construction, and restaurants).

UNNECESSARY UTILIZATION INTENSITY?

Insurance companies go beyond experience rating and demand side strategies (like higher coinsurance; see chapter 6) to constrain health care costs. Insurance companies use utilization review and preadmission certification to trim annual premium increases by one-eighth (Gabel et al. 1990), but premiums still grow by more than double the rate of inflation in the general economy. According to the Lewin/ICF study (1987), about 40 percent of admissions to hospitals were avoidable. While nonhospital care was probably necessary, the hospital admissions would have been avoidable if the system had offered (1) gatekeepers to prevent unnecessary care, (2) consumer education, and (3) preventive care and access so conditions could be treated soon (prior to the need for hospitalization). Two important points seem clear: (1) Declines in admission rates predated PPS, and (2) we appear to have returned to 1960 admission rates (with more ambulatory care, compensating for the increased demands of a more aged population). If admission rates continue to decline, there are no easy, reliable answers to the questions "Are we saving much money?" and "Is any harm being done to patient health status?" We shall consider these issues in subsequent chapters.

Ginsburg and Hackbarth (1986) concluded that professional review organizations (PROs) may also contribute to continued declines in admission rates, but they will not be as cost-effective as those HMOs and preferred provider organizations (PPOs) facing the immediate threat of financial failure. PROs face the less immediate threat that they will lose their federal contracts. However, well-managed HMOs, PPOs, and the full spectrum of managed-care alternatives (discussed in chapter 5) could produce further declines in admission rates.

Inpatient costs are down, but much of the forgone costs may have simply been shifted to outpatient settings. Many of these alternative care sites are owned by diversified and restructured hospitals and may be providing a healthy contribution to total operating profit margin of the parent companies. Also, the credit for much of this decline in inpatient expenses may rest with the fall in the basic national inflation rate—that is, the consumer price index (CPI).

THEORIES OF REGULATION

The capture theory of regulatory behavior is the most prevalent regulatory model among American economic theorists (Eastaugh 1982). According to the capture notion, the regulated group gradually comes to dominate the decisions of the regulators until the watchdog agency is converted to an ally, or even a subsidiary, of the private-sector group. Truman (1951) was one of the first to point out that capture is a natural process in the life of any federal agency. Truman argued that the regulated have more cohesion than the bureaucrats, that they keep closest track of the agency, that they are sure to reveal any malfeasance by the agency at the annual budget hearings, and that consequently, little will be done by the agency beyond what is desired by the regulated group.

Bernstein (1955) carried the Truman argument further and suggested that all agencies pass through a life cycle from early zeal to a period of debility and decline in which the regulators become the captive of the regulated. Capture is not necessarily bad if efficient decision making requires cooperation between industry and government. Effective cooperation must be a two-way street, rather than a one-way dominance of the industry by regulators. Social reformers who often get carried away by the one-way-street view of regulation should pause to reconsider the value of regulators as adversaries (Eastaugh 1990a). The social and economic cost of an antagonistic relationship between regulators and the industry may be much higher than society is willing to bear. If you destroy the motive of the regulated to cooperate, what is the result? More regulation and lower productivity?

Three new variants of the capture theory have appeared in the literature. One moderate variant of the capture concept advanced by Peltzman (1976) postulated "bureaucratic survival through politics" in observing that agencies respond primarily to the politicians in control of their budget. Maintaining the proper balance in the relationship is not always easy. There is a danger that the regulated can become the determining voice at the budgetary hearing, especially in the current era of antiregulatory spirit. In this regard, Cohen (1975) suggested a second variant to the capture theory. He postulated that after initial popular support for regulation has waned, the regulated become the only substantive and ongoing interest group concerned with the agency. Thus, over time, some degree of capture is inevitable if the industry exercises its monopoly power. A third theory of regulatory behavior as advanced by Hilton (1972) is "minimal squawk," or, in other words, the "squeaky wheel gets the grease." The key idea is that the regulator acts to minimize complaints. Bureaucrats are viewed as rational economic individuals operating in a complex political environment and attempting to minimize the sum total of government-consumer-industry dissatisfaction with regulatory policies. According to this view, the regulatory agencies and staff that experience the longest tenure pursue the most purely reactive policy possible. Agencies that follow the path of least resistance are destined to become less combative and avoid the ire of politicians on whom their survival depends.

Gutterman, Altman, and Young (1990) outlined the financial strain within the hospital industry. If the financial pressures on hospitals are sufficient, perhaps we shall experience a rebirth in shared services in the 1990s. If many institutions bind together as a cooperative group, duplication of marketing research efforts is avoided. To achieve the best allocation of resources, the group can divide the service area among its members and develop a vertically integrated sharing agreement where each institution provides the service at which it is the most proficient. However, even if the financial pressure to share services is strong, in a highly competitive market, with low occupancy rates and rampant fears of patients being "stolen," the prevalence of shared service arrangements may actually decline over time.

UNCERTAINTY AND MEDICARE PAYMENT RATES

The existence of "DRG creep"—that is, the deliberate and systematic labeling of case mix so as to maximize reimbursement—was first postulated by Simborg (1981) in the context of the New Jersey all-payers system. Carter and Ginsburg (1986) studied the evidence of DRG creep and concluded that it explained 70 to 75 percent of the increase in case-mix index in 1981–84. In the initial three years of PPS, we observed some significant shifts in popularity (prevalence) of certain DRGs. Cases of pneumonia DRG 89 increased to 274,538 in 1985, in contrast to DRG 182 cases, which declined from the second to the fourth most popular DRG in 1984–85. Attributing cause and effect in assessing these shifts is hard, except in a few obvious cases (DRG 39 lens procedures are increasingly done more profitably on an outpatient basis). The industry argues that most DRG creep represents honest improvement in coding practices. Furthermore, better coding of medical records is done if hospitals are paid on the basis of this coding. Needless to say, for Medicare patients the medical record determines payment (by determining the patient's DRG), not the amount collected on charge routing slips.

During the spring of 1986 the Medicare actuaries and the Prospective Payment Assessment Commission disagreed by 0.8 percent over the size of the offset for the following year's DRG rates. The issue was not trivial to the hospital industry, as a 0.8-point disagreement represented about $405 million. The more restrictive (high estimates of DRG creep) offset by the actuaries won the policy debate, and Congress confirmed a mere 1.15 percent price increase for 1987. Since 1987 DRG creep has been less substantial, but the rate increases have been equally low (Soderstrom 1990; Eastaugh 1990a).

Why the inability to differentiate among patient types threatens to undermine the per case payment system can best be illustrated by an example. A patient with a peptic ulcer can be treated nonsurgically under DRG 176 and receive a payment of $4,800 or be treated with endoscopic therapy as DRG 155 and receive a payment in excess of $9,000. The hospital earns an easy windfall profit for this minimally invasive, well-established diagnostic procedure. The endoscopic approach to therapy earns a $6,600 premium if bleeding esophageal varices are scoped (DRG 201) and not just treated medically. Sometimes the drift to a more profitable DRG pigeonhole (category) may be a completely paper exercise, without any real shifts in treatment patterns. We need better models to analyze the shifts in case mix (Gustafson, Catsbaril, and Alemi 1992).

LOCAL STATE HOSPITAL RATE-SETTING PROGRAMS

A practical rate-setting system should try to limit regulatory costs (1) by limiting the cost of compliance for small, less sophisticated hospitals and (2) by limiting costly detailed review only to the hospitals asking for big rate increases. Some rate regulators assume a presumption of economic efficiency within peer groups of providers and only red-flag the inefficient 25 percent of each peer group. Those facilities with greater than average efficiency may be allowed to keep 50 to 100 percent of the gains from their internal cost-reduction efforts (incentive carrots); but the 25 percent of highest-cost, least efficient facilities in a peer group are offered "sticks" (low rate increases) to penalize inefficiency. Rate-setting methods range from annual review of budgets to formula or formula with appeals.

To be fair, a rate-setting system should pay for outlier cases and also adjust for appropriate changes in patient volume. Some states pay for volume changes at marginal costs (60 percent of average costs in the cost studies referenced in this chapter), while other states are less generous (paying for marginal additional patient volume at 40 percent of average costs); and some states mimic Medicare high-cost outlier payment rules and reimburse for additional patient volume above the baseline period at 80 percent of average cost.

Some state rate-setting programs are an arm of state government, while others function as independent commissions. Many state rate-setting programs have very limited budgets and low salaries (and thus inexperienced staff). The style of the rate-setting program varies from cooperative (e.g., Maryland) to adversarial (e.g., New York and Massachusetts). Cleverley (1991) outlined the need for hospitals to preserve their capital position. As a rule of thumb, the price-level-adjusted return on investment (ROI) should at minimum be 10 percent for an urban teaching hospital and 6.5 to 7.0 percent for a small rural hospital.

The rate-setting program with the highest level of stability and effectiveness is the Maryland Health Services Cost Review Commission. The Maryland system promotes performance (cost control) without capital erosion because it offers a sufficient ROI to assure financial viability. Effectiveness is measured in two dimensions in this context: (1) long-run cost control (percentage increase in cost per adjusted admission, 1977–91), and (2) payer equity (percentage markup of charges over costs). Over the years 1985–91 Maryland had the lowest percentage markup of charges over costs (8.4 percent) in the nation, followed by New Jersey (11.3 percent), New York (14.9 percent), Washington (15.8 percent), and Massachusetts and Maine (19 percent). Maryland also had the best rate of long-run cost control, that is, the lowest percentage increase in cost per adjusted admission during the period 1977–91 (176 percent), followed by New York and New Jersey (198 percent), Massachusetts (200 percent), and Maine and California (255 percent).

The Maryland rate-setting process may not remain an all-payer system. Maryland has only maintained its Medicare waiver to operate the only single-payer (all-payer) rate-setting system by counting pre–1985 savings for the Medicare program to offset slightly higher than average absolute dollar costs per admission in 1991. New York, New Jersey, and Massachusetts all lost their Medicare waiver and capacity to operate a single-payer statewide system in the 1980s. The demise of the single-payer system in Maryland in 1992–93 would be sad in two basic ways. First, the state commission could no longer redistribute $270 million of funds (1991) from the wealthy areas to the 23 hospitals with the highest charity-care patient volume. Second, the demise of the last experimental all-payer state program would be a setback for policy advocates offering reform proposals that focus on a unified payment system (see chapter 7). However, Maryland will probably not retain its Medicare waiver, given that the state's average length of stay is 0.8 days higher than the national average. If Maryland Medicare patients are thrust onto the national DRG system, the incentive to trim length of stay will become much stronger (see chapter 12).

HEALTH PLANNING BY EXTERNAL AGENCIES: DID IT SAVE MONEY?

All the multiple regression studies of certificate-of-need (CON) programs suggest that health planning did not reduce the supply of hospital beds, plant assets, or total assets per bed (Eastaugh 1987, 1982; Sloan and Steinwald 1980; Salkever and Bice 1976). For this reason, corporate planning has replaced community-based health planning as a topic in the literature; and 23 states have dropped the CON process for hospitals since 1984.

Planners might have had some limited effect of increasing the cost of a capital project by delaying the date of project initiation with paper roadblocks. However, the investor community largely determines the size of a firm's debt capacity (and net available capital stock), and the firms simply bombard the planners with spending proposals until the funds are exhausted. Health planning may still prove cost-effective in a cost-reimbursed market (e.g., nursing homes), but in a price-payment hospital market the business risk associated with a proposal will determine whether the capital venture is good or bad for the institution. Corporate planning imperatives have essentially replaced community-based planning. Moreover, as many hospital chain managers can attest, only an idiot builds financially unnecessary bed capacity and equipment.

Eastaugh (1987) reported some adaptive responses that hospitals might pursue in highly regulated situations. Hospital administrators have three methods of co-opting the regulatory process. First, they can purchase equipment that is below the CON program review ceiling (figure 1.2, section D). Depending on the state, these are items costing less than $100,000 to $200,000. Second, if the administrators cannot spend money on new bed construction or modernization, they can bombard the CON agency with a number of capital equipment requests (figure 1.2, section F). Failing at either of these strategies, the administrator can hire an excessive number of LPNs or grant above-average wage increases (figure 1.2, section G). This third phenomenon is consistent with all nonprofit models of hospital behavior and has been observed in a sample of 1,228 hospitals by Sloan and Steinwald (1980). In summary, the compensatory response to regulation can occur on both the capital and wage sides of the patient-care production process.

THE THEORY OF RATIONAL EXPECTATIONS

The theory of rational expectations has been widely heralded in the popular press as one of the most exciting advances in economic theory. However, older economists have always considered anticipatory behavior and announcement effects as being key hypotheses within the classical theory of the firm. Social scientists will find this "new" theory of the firm entitled "rational expectations" to be similar to the more familiar concept of the self-fulfilling prophecy (Eastaugh 1979). Simply stated, the theory of rational expectations postulates that people and institutions will take action based on how they expect outsiders, including government, to behave. In the process of attempting to predict or foresee the timing and details of new regulations, medical staff and hospital administrators, commensurate with the theory, are believed to behave with anticipatory actions (Relman 1991). Administrators who rush into new purchases of hospital equipment are eschewed as "irrational" by regulators, but if their behavior stems from anticipatory actions designed to increase the reimbursement base, such behavior may be considered a rational measure of self-protection. The smart administrator learns to anticipate future edicts from the rule makers and merely devises a new set of games for co-optation of future rules. One rational response

Figure 1.2
Conceptual Framework for the Hospital Investment Decision-making Process

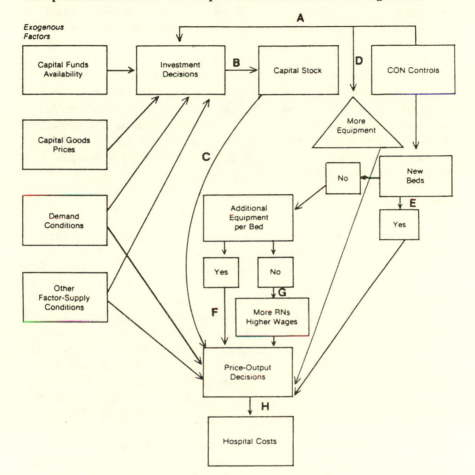

to the implementation of DRGs and other price-control schemes was the trend toward specialization in the hospital sector.

With increased competition and discounting, hospitals may react like department stores in earlier times. In the 1950s every department store tried to operate with 450 product lines, from food to men's formal wear. The surviving department stores now specialize in 50 to 90 percent fewer product lines (Eastaugh 1992). Consider a second analogy. The national association of gas station owners in 1972 suggested that every gas station must be full service and have a mechanic on duty. Contrary to this viewpoint, the successful gas stations now sell self-service gas and food. Specialization and modest diversification may be an optimal strategy for American hospitals that are not sole community providers. A hospital with poor cardiac surgery or oncology might drop these services and acquire narrow specialized services like in vitro fertilization. A small sole community provider with 25 to 75 beds has a monopoly hold on the market and lacks the opportunity to specialize and reap economies of scale in high-volume specialty departments.

Specialization should never be achieved by dumping market segments of people (e.g., the uninsured), but rather by dropping product lines better served by the competition and by recommitting resources to what a provider does best. Hospitals are not alone in the 1980s tendency to specialize. General Motors might be a better company if it became Specific Motors. Specialization has been the key to survival for business. In a decade where automakers and hospitals are experiencing fiscal troubles, no point of differentiation is likely to prove more powerful than quality.

SPECIALIZE OR OFFER WIDE SCOPE OF PRODUCT LINES?

Finkler (1983) offered the traditional argument for avoiding specialization: Hospitals with a broad product scope attract more physicians. Many hospitals offer a broad range of prestige-maximizing high-technology services, often at low volume, and consequently do not financially benefit from the wide scope of product lines offered. Trustees and other interested individuals might accrue intangible benefits (e.g., pride) from being associated with a hospital that offers so many product lines. However, in the current climate of prospective payment many hospitals miss the era of cost reimbursement, where low-volume departments could be maintained. Low-volume departments with high unit costs do not get their inefficiency reimbursed under prospective payment. Hospitals operating small HMOs have a limited ability to dump low-volume departments. Other hospitals can more easily specialize. The Graduate Hospital in Philadelphia dropped maternity. A hospital on Long Island went from being a general community hospital to a facility that only does open-heart surgery.

To maintain an equally high patient census, a hospital that specializes must open up the geographic range of its marketing effort. For example, when the 990-bed Memorial Medical Center of Long Beach decided to market its specialized advanced cancer treatment program, it began to admit patients from a wider array of zip codes. The impact of consumer behavior is more obvious for smaller hospitals. As more hospitals specialize in fewer than 200 DRGs, patients will have to drive by a number of hospitals to get to "the hospitals right for them." The patient is increasingly going to the specialized hospital that creates a point of differentiation in his or her mind, rather than stopping at a full-service hospital offering every DRG.

The demise of cost reimbursement means that underspecialized hospitals are no longer protected from close scrutiny. Low-volume departments are under scrutiny for economic reasons (poor profit margins, poor productivity) and for quality reasons. It is difficult to establish cause and effect on the quality issue, given two alternative explanations. One is that volume is too low to maintain sufficient quality. Competition is a factor; that is, if some hospitals closed the service, market share and volume of those keeping this product line would rise. The other is that low-quality providers discourage doctors from sending patient referrals and so keep the volume low (Eastaugh and Eastaugh 1986). Irrespective of the cause-and-effect dynamics, specialization is associated with maintaining or enhancing the quality of patient care. Luft et al. (1990) indicated that specialization allows nurses and physicians to develop more expertise with respect to a specific category of patients.

Rational Behavior in the Hospital Marketplace

Robinson and Luft (1987) speculated that hospitals refuse to specialize because they would rather engage in a cost-raising "medical arms race." The authors admitted that this speculation was more relevant in the bygone era of cost reimbursement. Farley and Hogan (1990) reported that hospitals specialized 9.8 percent in DRG-weighted terms during the initial two years of the Medicare prospective payment system. They found a higher level of specialization (13.9 percent) during the same two years if the specialization was measured in terms of major diagnostic categories (MDCs, fewer in number than DRGs). Herrmann (1990) reported that 35 percent of chief executive officers (CEOs) in a survey of hospitals were considering product-line reductions in their facilities.

Quality and marketing are becoming increasingly important topics for hospital managers. Developing areas of specialization can bring prestige to a hospital and serve as a magnet for bringing in more patients. Special centers also assist hospitals in gaining access to capital (donors like giving to centers for treatment of a particular disease or ailment). Few hospitals have sufficient resources to add specialized services without cutting budgets in other areas.

In addition to potential quality improvements, the benefits of hospital specialization for society include eliminating expensive duplication of services and underused technology. Internal corporate planning to cut duplication of departments and equipment in a marketplace can trim costs better than community-based health-planning regulations (Eastaugh 1982). External government planning does not prove effective in the American context because regulation operates at the periphery of the resource decision-making process. Internal cost control within the hospital is more effective than government planning guideposts, especially when the rise in discount payers and quality competition creates the need to trim product lines. Some demographic variables will be included in the analysis to assess the nature of the marketplace (competition and physician supply).

Sample and Study Methodology

The sample hospitals represent a 20 percent sample of short-term nongovernmental hospitals with more than 75 beds. Only 58 percent of the hospitals were willing and able to provide data for the two study years. The sample is explained in more detail elsewhere (Eastaugh 1991), but there was no statistically significant bias present in the sample based on seven variables (urbanicity, teaching status, size, ownership control, disproportionate share of patient volume, Medicare case-mix index, and length-of-stay index).

An unbiased information-theory measure of specialization has to be a scalar measure of output that is independent of scale (Barer 1982), so that the analyst can measure any nonlinear impact of economies of scale by including beds and beds squared in the equation. Utilizing the Farley and Hogan (1990) measure of specialization, let B_c be defined as the baseline proportion of cases in the category c, and let F_{cn} be the fraction of cases in the nth hospital observed in category c. The categories for inpatient specialization will be DRGs and MDCs, creating two alternative measures for specialization (DRG-based and MDC-based). The information-theory index I of specialization for hospital n collapses information about differences between B_c and F_{cn} as follows:

$$I_n = \sum_{c=1} F_{cn} \times \ln(F_{cn}/B_c),$$

where ln is the natural logarithm. This index equals zero when $F_c = B_c$ for all patient categories, and the index increases as case-mix fractions move away from one another. National case-mix fractions serve as the baseline. In each year (1983 and 1990) the specialization index was over 10 percent higher in western states and over 13 percent lower in two northeastern states. The results in table 1.4 suggest that specialization has been highest in competitive West Coast markets and lowest in the rate-regulated states (New York and Massachusetts). Hospitals have less incentive to contain costs by decreasing the array of services offered in stringent rate-setting states, like New York and Massachusetts, than in flexible rate-setting states (e.g., Maryland) that let the management reap the gains from any resulting cost savings. Because the MDCs are more heterogeneous categories and fewer in number than the DRGs, their information-theory index values are lower than the DRG index in table 1.4. For example, MDC 5, the circulatory system, is a grab bag of cardiac surgery (DRG numbers 103–9), pediatrics (137), vascular surgery (110–12, 119, 128, 130, 131), general surgery (113, 114, 120), and cardiology (115–18, 121–27, 129, 132–36, 138–45). The DRG-based measure of specialization increased 26.9 percent in the period 1983–90. The MDC-based measure of specialization increased 37.6 percent in the period 1983–90.

What Drives Specialization?

A number of factors are hypothesized to impact specialization, including bed size, rate regulation, and ownership. For-profit hospitals have been found to

Table 1.4
**Information-Theory Index of Case-Mix Specialization by Geographic Location,
1983 and 1990**

	Sample	1983	1990	Percentage Increase, 1983 to 1990
Index I DRG-based				
1. New York, Massachusetts	N = 26	.299	.371	24.1
2. Western United States	N = 50	.414	.508	22.7
3. Other 39 states	N = 156	.359	.458	27.6
4. United States	N = 232	.362	.459	26.9
Index I MDC-based				
1. New York, Massachusetts	N = 26	.102	.143	40.2
2. Western United States	N = 50	.158	.197	24.7
3. Other 39 states	N = 156	.107	.153	43.0
4. United States	N = 232	.117	.161	37.6

specialize somewhat more (Eastaugh 1987; Farley and Hogan 1990), as have
large teaching hospitals (those in the Council of Teaching Hospitals [COTH];
Eastaugh 1984; Farley and Hogan 1990). Melnick and Zwanziger (1988) reported
that in the state of California inpatient costs, adjusted for inflation, decreased
11 percent in hospitals located in highly competitive markets. They used the
Herfindahl index (Eastaugh 1984) by summing the squares of market shares for
all the competitors in an area. If specialization is a reaction to competitive
pressures, the index I should be lower in markets with a high Herfindahl index
(in a monopoly single-hospital area the Herfindahl index is at the maximum
value of 1.0). All else equal, specialization has been found to be higher in
markets with a higher density of HMOs, hospital beds, physicians, and long-
term-care units (Farley and Hogan 1990).

The DRG-based specialization index was regressed on the 13 variables outlined
in table 1.5 to account for cross-sectional variations in case-mix proportions.
The results in table 1.5 agree with the hypothesized signs from previous studies
and support the DRG I-index as a measure of specialization. Specialization was
high in moderately sized hospitals (100 to 300 beds) and declined up to 760
beds. Beyond 760 beds it appears that the scale of financial reserves or institutional slack enabled big hospitals to increase specialization for a wider scope
of services (consistent with Dranove 1987 and Farley and Hogan 1990).

Does Specialization Reduce Cost per Admission?

To find out whether specialization can trim unit cost, one has to adjust for
case mix in greater detail. One does not have sufficient sample size to introduce

Table 1.5
Variables Impacting Inpatient Case-Mix Specialization, 1983 and 1990

Variable[a]	Hypothesized Sign	Coefficient Estimate	Standard Error
A. Capacity (number of beds in 100s)			
1. Acute-care beds[b]	-	-.0984**	.0199
2. Acute-care beds squared	+	.0082*	.0040
B. Management focus (ownership, teaching status)			
3. For-profit hospital	+	.0703*	.0295
4. Member, COTH	+	.0961**	.0302
5. Affiliated with a medical school	?	-.0074	.0118
C. Competitive location and alternatives			
6. Herfindahl index bed concentration	-	-.1261**	.0292
7. In a metropolitan SMSA	+	.0329	.0204
8. Number of HMOs in the county	+	.0128*	.0047
9. Hospital beds/100 pop. in county	+	.0852	.0049
10. Physicians/100 pop. in county	+	.2596*	.1003
11. Fraction beds in long-term care units	+	.0464*	.0214
D. State regulatory pressures			
12. Located in New York or Massachusetts	-	-.0409*	.0076
13. Located in western state	+	.0230*	.0080
E. Control for bias in index of specialization			
14. Inverse of the number of patient records	+	192.4**	49.8

[a]Ordinary least squares regression estimate with DRG-based information theory index of specialization as the dependent variable.
[b]National sample of 232 hospitals with more than 75 beds.
*$p < 0.05$, two-tailed test; ** $p < 0.01$, two-tailed test.
R^2-adjusted = .628; F-ratio (14 d.f./216 d.f.) = 19.83.

one variable for each product in the multiproduct firm, so the analyst does the second-best thing, which is to build a hedonic cost function (Eastaugh 1987; Barer 1982). The hedonic proxy measures for case mix include our DRG-based specialization index, a length-of-stay-weighted case-mix index, and three measures of emergency-department and outpatient-surgery volume. In building the cost function in table 1.6, one must include three measures of factor prices (if labor and debt are more expensive, then cost per admission will be more expensive) and admissions (as a measure for economies of scale in line 12, rather than bed capacity). The results in table 1.6 indicate that a 26.9 percent rise in specialization yielded a 6.9 percent reduction in cost per admission in the period 1983–90. Reducing costs 1 percent per year over seven years is a small, but not inconsequential, improvement in efficiency. The capacity for generating cost savings is one rationale for the rise in specialization. A second rationale for specialization involves shifts in technology and physician preference for certain procedures and product lines (Farley and Friedman 1991). From these regression equations one cannot ascertain how much of the specialization is provider/physician driven, management driven (by selection of product lines), or payment driven (either the reimbursement rates are too low or the inefficient departments have unusually high average cost).

The coefficients of the within-hospital regression equation explaining shifts in specialization over the period 1983–90 are given in table 1.7. The signs are consistent with the cross-sectional results in table 1.5, except that the fifth variable (affiliation with a medical school) and the ninth variable (bed density) have different signs. One cannot conclude much from the observation that the HMO density variable is more significant (0.01 level) but the Herfindahl index is slightly less significant (0.05 level) in table 1.7 than in table 1.5. Not surprisingly, the western states appear to be associated with more specialization, and the environment in New York and Massachusetts tends to retard specialization. The most substantial finding in table 1.7 is the large highly significant coefficient for cost per admission in line 7, suggesting that hospitals facing higher costs per DRG specialize more. One caveat should be introduced: It is difficult to assess the reliability in going from such cross-sectional data to a comparison over time.

Policy Discussion

Not so long ago there lived a happy paradigm that said that hospitals that specialized were too internally focused because they turned away patients and doctors in areas outside their limited product lines. Today the reduction of product lines in a more specialized hospital can reduce the inefficiency (unjustified costs) in individual hospitals (Kusserow 1991; Eastaugh 1991). The new paradigm for the 1990s is that specialization breeds quality, and this section has offered evidence that efficiency is improved. The hospital offering every DRG is too internally focused and provides care at a higher unit cost (with less service quality). The obvious exception to this broad generalization is the few huge academic medical centers (AMCs) with departments already large enough to reap any possible economies of scale. About half of the 122 academic medical centers fall into this category (15 of the 232 hospitals in this study are AMCs). In the future the other 1,100 teaching hospitals may have to specialize or pool

Table 1.6
Impact of Case-Mix Specialization on Inpatient Hospital Costs per Admission Based on a Within-Hospital Regression Equation

Variable[a]	Hypothesized Sign	Coefficient Estimate	Standard Error
A. Hedonic descriptors for case mix[b]			
1. ln (DRG-based I index)	-	-.1309**	.0285
2. ln (LOS-weighted case-mix index)	+	.7043**	.0920
3. Emergency-dept. visits/total visits	+	.0009	.0086
4. Outpatient-surgery visits/tot. visits	+	.0273**	.0072
5. Fraction of surgery done outpatient	+	.0601*	.0242
B. Competitive location and alternatives			
6. Herfindahl index bed concentration	-	-.1107*	.0429
7. Fraction of revenue not from operations	+	.1968*	.0857
8. Number of HMOs in the county	-	.0192**	.0037
9. Hospital beds/100 pop. in county	-	-.0684*	.0300
10. Physicians/100 pop. in county	?	-.0315*	.1798
11. Nonpatient care revenue/total revenue	+	.1689	.0995
C. Economies of scale (impact of volume)			
12. ln (acute-care admissions)	-	-.2034**	.0462
D. Management focus (ownership, teaching status)			
13. For-profit hospital	-	.0612	.0352
14. Member, COTH	+	.0810*	.0345
15. Affiliated with a medical school	?	-.0036	.0129
E. Input factor prices (labor, debt)			
16. Ratio of long-term debt/total assets	+	.2070**	.0387
17. ln (total interest expense/long-term debt)	+	.0192**	.0051
18. ln (average payroll expense per FTE)	+	.1849**	.0220

[a]Least squares estimate with ln (average cost per admission) as dependent variable and instruments used for ln (I) and ln (admissions).
[b]LOS = length of stay; I = Information-theory case-mix index.
*$p < 0.05$, two-tailed test
**$p < 0.01$, two-tailed test
R^2-adjusted = .397; F-ratio (18 d.f./444 d.f.) = 26.69

Table 1.7
Variables Impacting Within-Hospital Variance in Hospital Case-Mix
Specialization, 1983–1990 (n = 232 hospitals)

Variable[a]	Hypothesized Sign	Coefficient Estimate	Standard Error
A. Capacity (number of beds in 100s)			
1. Acute-care beds[b]	-	-.0815**	.0217
2. Acute-care beds squared	+	.0059*	.0025
B. Management focus (ownership, teaching status)			
3. For-profit hospital	+	.0509	.0314
4. Member, COTH	+	.0702*	.0333
5. Affiliated with a medical school	?	.0058	.0118
C. Competitive location and alternatives			
6. Herfindahl index bed concentration	-	-.0652*	.0278
7. 1n (average cost per inpatient admit)	+	.1873**	.0319
8. Number of HMOs in the county	+	.0065**	.0016
9. Hospital beds/100 pop. in county	+	-.0369	.0208
10. Physicians/100 pop. in county	+	.2701*	.1144
11. Fraction of beds in long-term care units	+	.0824*	.0292
D. State regulatory pressures			
12. Located in New York or Massachusetts	-	-.0641**	.0053
13. Located in western state	+	.0358**	.0051
E. Control for bias in index of specialization			
14. Inverse of the number of patient records	+	221.6**	35.7

[a]Ordinary least squares estimate with DRG-based index as dependent variable using an instrument for 1n (average cost per admission).
[b]National sample of 232 hospitals with more than 75 beds.
*$p < 0.05$, two-tailed test
**$p < 0.01$, two-tailed test
R^2-adjusted = .285; F-ratio (15 d.f./444 d.f.) = 21.06

resources and become less full service (offering over 400 DRGs) but better positioned to survive in an era of cost competition and quality competition.

Studies of specialization should consider the direction in which the specialization is planned or driven. No current evidence exists to suggest that specialization has harmed access (Eastaugh 1991), but in the future specialization might produce less product differentiation, with every hospital moving in the same direction. Under such conditions, all hospitals in a market area might vacate a necessary product line and perhaps harm the health of the population.

Future trends are hard to project from retrospective analysis. The observed 26.9 percent rise in specialization was associated with a 6.9 percent decline in unit cost (per admission) from 1983 to 1990. However, this does not mean that an additional 26.9 percent rise in specialization will yield a further 6.9 percent decline in cost per admission. One must not forget the role of the consumer. Travel time and search time to find that "right hospital" for a given condition will rise if the average hospital offers only 150 DRGs. Future research should consider whether the cost to consumers and physicians in the search process is worth the benefits in terms of (1) rising levels of quality and (2) declining unit cost per admission. With a good public information network and rising interest in value shopping (Eastaugh 1987), specialization may continue to be a bargain for providers and consumers. However, physicians may not like the fact that they have practice privileges to admit patients at a smaller number of specialized hospitals. On the upside for hospitals, they may have the economic power to charge a high fee (like a condo fee or rent) to doctors in search of admitting privileges. The political power of some physicians within a given hospital may lead to underspecialization, the inability of some hospital managers to selectively prune out some product lines.

To maintain an equally high patient census, a hospital that specializes must open up the geographic range of their marketing effort. For example, as the 990 bed Memorial Medical Center of Long Beach decided to market their specialized advanced cancer treatment program, they began to admit patients from a wider array of zip codes. The impact of consumer behavior is more obvious for smaller hospitals. As more hospitals specialize in less than 200 DRGs, patients will have to drive by a number of hospitals to get to "the hospitals right for them." Patients are increasingly going to the specialized hospitals that create a point of differentiation in their minds, rather than stopping at a full service hospital offering every DRG.

Future research should consider whether any future improvement in cost efficiency per admission outweighs the cost to patients. If patients have to spend more time (travel time, lost wages) driving to fewer specialized providers, the monetary savings for payers may not be worth the resulting costs to the households. However, one recent study suggests that patients are increasingly willing to travel. Bronstein and Morrisey (1991) report that 50 percent of rural pregnant women bypassed the nearest rural hospital still providing obstetrics services. If mean travel distance increased by just a few miles, hospital specialization may yield net gains for society that outweigh the costs to consumers (but this generality may not be true in some unstudied rural areas where the opportunity costs for longer distances are more substantial).

THE ROAD AHEAD

In the following chapters we shall consider in detail various aspects of efficiency, equity, and service quality. In chapter 2 we outline a number of recent examples of hospital cost functions and nursing production functions. Economic models of physician and hospital behavior (chapter 3) and recent changes in methods for paying physicians (chapter 4) set the context for discussing competition health plans and business efforts for containing expenses (chapters 5 and 6). Some chapters have a consumer focus (chapter 7, equity and the uninsured; chapter 9, value shopping; chapter 13, consumer surveys), while other chapters have a provider focus (chapter 8, teaching hospitals; chapter 10, health manpower; chapters 11 and 12, technology assessment). The concluding chapter 14 offers an international comparative systems approach to interrelate the disparate economic and social issues raised in the text. Perhaps the nation will soon consider a systematic reform of the health care system that offers universal coverage, universal access, cost control, and sufficient flexibility to allow steady quality-of-care improvements.

REFERENCES

Arnett, R., McKusick, D., Sonnefeld, S., and Cowell, C. (1986). "Projections of Health Care Spending to 1990." *Health Care Financing Review* 7:3 (Spring), 1–36.

Atkinson, G., and Eastaugh, S. (1991). "State Rate Setting Programs." Working paper, Department of Health Services Management and Policy, George Washington University, Washington, D.C.

Barer, M. (1982). "Case Mix Adjustment in Hospital Cost Analysis: Information Theory Revisited." *Journal of Health Economics* 1:1, 53–80.

Berki, S. (1990). "Approaches to Financing Care for the Uninsured." *Henry Ford Hospital Medical Journal* 38:3 (Fall), 119–122.

Bernstein, M. (1955). *Regulating Business by Independent Commission*. Princeton: Princeton University Press.

Bigelow, B. (1991). "Ambulatory Care Centers: Are They a Competitive Advantage?" *Hospital and Health Services Administration* 36:3 (Fall), 351–63.

Bronstein, J., and Morrisey, M. (1991). "Bypassing Rural Hospitals for Obstetrics Care." *Journal of Health Politics, Policy and Law* 16:1 (Spring), 87–118.

Broyles, R. (1990). "Efficiency, Costs, and Quality: The New Jersey Experience Revisited." *Inquiry* 27:1 (Spring), 86–96.

Butler, S. (1990). *Is Tax Reform the Key to Health Care Reform?* Washington, D.C.: Heritage Foundation.

Carter, G., and Ginsburg, P. (1986). *The Medicare Case Mix Index Increase: Medical Practice Changes, Aging, and DRG Creep*. Rand Corporation Report R–3292 (June). Santa Monica, Calif.: Rand Corporation.

Cleverley, W. (1990). "Improving Financial Performance: A Study of 50 Hospitals." *Hospital and Health Service Administration* 35:2 (Summer), 173–187.

Cleverley, W., and Harvey, R. (1992). "Competitive Strategy for Hospital Management." *Hospital and Health Services Administration* 37:1 (Spring), 53–69.

Coddington, D., Keen, D., and Moore, K. (1991). *The Crisis in Health Care*. San Francisco: Jossey-Bass.

Cohen, H. (1975). "Regulatory Politics and American Medicine." *American Behavioral Scientist* 19:1 (September/October), 122–136.

Dranove, D., Shanley, M., and White, W. (1991). "How Fast Are Hospital Prices Really Rising?" *Medical Care* 29:8 (August), 690–697.

Dranove, D. (1987). "Rate-setting by DRGs and Hospital Specialization." *Rand Journal of Economics* 18:3 (Autumn), 417–427.

Eastaugh, S. (1992). "Hospital Specialization and Cost-efficiency: Benefits of Trimming Product-lines." *Hospital and Health Services Administration* 37:2 (Summer), forthcoming.

——. (1991). "Improvements in Hospital Cost Accounting." *Hospital Topics* 71:1, 10–22.

——. (1990a). "Financing the Correct Rate of Growth of Medical Technology." *Quarterly Review of Economics and Business* 30:4 (Winter), 34–60.

——. (1990b). "Defining Rates of Hospital Closure." *Washington Post*, September 18, p. H2.

——. (1987). *Financing Health Care*. Dover, Mass.: Auburn House, 657–683.

——. (1984). "Hospital Diversification and Financial Management." *Medical Care* 22:8 (August), 704–723.

——. (1983). "Placing a Value on Life and Limb." *Health Matrix* 1:1 (Winter), 5–21.

——. (1982). "Effectiveness of Community-Based Hospital Planning: Some Recent Evidence." *Applied Economics* 14:5 (October), 475–490.

——. (1979). "President's Hospital Cost Containment Proposal." Subcommittee on Health Hearings, Committee on Ways and Means, 96th U.S. Congress, First Session, April 2, 1979, Part 2, Serial 96–19, 396–418. Washington, D.C.

Eastaugh, S., and Eastaugh, J. (1990). "Putting the Squeeze on Emergency Medicine: Pressures on Emergency Medicine." *Hospital Topics* 68:4 (Fall), 21–26.

——. (1986). "Prospective Payment Systems: Further Steps to Enhance Quality, Efficiency, and Regionalization." *Health Care Management Review* 11:4 (Fall), 37–52.

Egdahl, R. (1984). "Should We Shrink the Health Care System?" *Harvard Business Review* 62:1 (January–February), 125–132.

Evans, R. (1990). "Surgical Day Care: Measurements of the Economic Payoff." *Canadian Medical Association Journal* 123:11 (November), 874–877.

Farley, D., and Friedman, B. (1991). "Hospital Operating Margins: Noisy Equilibrium and Risk." Agency for Health Care Policy and Research, U.S. Department of Health and Human Services, Rockville, Maryland.

Farley, D., and Hogan, C. (1990). "Case-Mix Specialization in the Market for Hospital Services." *Health Services Research* 25:5 (December), 757–783.

Feldstein, M. (1977). "The High Cost of Hospitals and What to Do About It." *Public Interest* 12:48 (Summer), 40–54.

Feldstein, M., and Taylor, A. (1981). "The Rapid Rise of Hospital Costs." In M. Feldstein (ed.), *Hospital Costs and Health Insurance*, chap. 1. Cambridge, Mass.: Harvard University Press.

Fetter, R. (1991). *DRGs: Their Design and Development*. Ann Arbor, Mich.: Health Administration Press.

Finkler, S. (1983). "The Hospital as a Sales-maximizing Entity." *Health Services Research* 18:2 (Summer), 117–133.

——. (1979). "On the Shape of the Long Run Average Cost Curve." *Health Services Research* 14:4 (Winter), 281–289.

Fisher, E., Welch, H., and Wennberg, J. (1992). "Prioritizing Oregon's Hospital Resources." *JAMA* 267:14 (April 8), 1925–1931.

Freeland, M., Anderson, G., and Schendler, C. (1979). "National Hospital Input Price Index." *Health Care Financing Review* 1:4 (Summer), 37–52.

Freeland, M., and Schendler, C. (1984). "Health Spending in the 1980s: Integration of Clinical Practice Patterns with Management." *Health Care Financing Review* 5:3 (Spring), 1–68.

Fuchs, V. (1986). *The Health Economy*. Cambridge, Mass.: Harvard University Press.

Gabel, J., DiCarlo, S., Sullivan, C., and Rice, T. (1990). "Employer Sponsored Health Insurance." *Health Affairs* 9:3 (Fall), 161–175.

Ginsburg, P., and Hackbarth, G. (1986). "Alternative Delivery Systems and Medicare." *Health Affairs* 5:1 (Spring), 6–22.

Ginzberg, E. (1990). *The Medical Triangle: Physicians, Politicians, and the Public*. Cambridge, Mass.: Harvard University Press.

Gray, B. (1992). "Why Nonprofits? Hospitals and the Future." *Frontiers of Health Services Management* 8:4 (summer), 3–26.

Gustafson, D., Catsbaril, W., and Alemi, F. (1992). *Systems to Support Health Policy Analysis: Theory, Models, and Uses*, Ann Arbor: Health Administration Press.

Gutheil, T., Bursztajn, H., and Brodsky, A. (1984). "Malpractice Prevention through the Sharing of Uncertainty: Informed Consent and the Therapeutic Alliance." *New England Journal of Medicine* 311:1 (July 5), 49–51.

Gutterman, S., Altman, S., and Young, D. (1990). "Hospital Financial Performance in the First Five years of PPS." *Health Affairs* 9:1 (Spring), 125–133.

Havighurst, C., and Hackbarth, J. (1979). "Private Cost Containment." *New England Journal of Medicine* 300:23 (June 7), 1298–1305.

Health Insurance Association of America (HIAA) (1991). *Source Book of Health Insurance Data, 1991*. Washington, D.C.: Health Insurance Association of America.

Herrmann, J. (1990). "New Strategies—Managing Hospitals in the 1990s." *Federation of American Health Systems Review* 23:4 (July/August), 14–23.

Hilton, G. (1972). "The Basic Behavior of Regulatory Commissions." *American Economic Review* 62:2 (May), 47–54.

Keating, B. (1984). "Cost Shifting: An Empirical Examination of Hospital Bureaucracy." *Applied Economics* 16:3 (July), 279–289.

Kellermann, A., and Ackerman, T. (1988). "Interhospital Patient Transfer: The Case for Informed Consent." *New England Journal of Medicine* 319:8 (August 29) 643–647.

Kusserow, R. (1991). "Report of the HHS Inspector General: Performance under the Prospective Payment System, Results from Hospitals," Department of Health and Human Services, Washington, D.C.

Latta, V., and Helbing, C. (1991). "Medicare Short-stay Hospital Services by DRGs." *Health Care Financing Review* 12:4 (Summer), 105–139.

Lewin/ICF (1987). "Medically Preventable Hospital Admissions." Report to the DHHS. Washington, D.C.: Lewin/ICF Inc.

Luft, H., Garnick, D., Mark, D., and McPhee, S. (1990). *Hospital Volume, Physician Volume, and Patient Outcome: Assessing the Evidence*. Ann Arbor, Mich.: Health Administration Press.

Maryland Hospital Association. (1991). *A Guide to Rate Review in Maryland Hospitals*. Lutherville, Md.: Maryland Hospital Institute.

Melnick, G., and Zwanziger, J. (1988). "Hospital Behavior under Competition and Cost-

Containment Policies: The California Experience." *Journal of the American Medical Association* 260:18 (November 11), 2669–2675.

Office of National Cost Estimates (ONCE). (1991). "National Health Expenditures." *Health Care Financing Review* 13:4 (Fall) 1–35.

Peltzman, S. (1976). "Toward a More General Theory of Regulation." *Journal of Law and Economics* 19:3 (August), 211–248.

Pope, G. (1991). "Measuring Geographic Variations in Hospitals' Capital Costs." *Health Care Financing Review* 12:4 (Summer) 75–85.

Prospective Payment Assessment Commission (ProPAC). (1991). *Medicare Prospective Payment and the American Health Care System: Report to Congress.* Washington, D.C.: ProPAC.

Relman, A. (1991). "The Health Care Industry: Where Is It Taking Us?" *New England Journal of Medicine* 325:12 (September 19), 854–59.

Robinson, J., and Luft, H. (1987). "Competition and the Cost of Hospital Care, 1972 to 1982." *Journal of the American Medical Association* 257:23 (19 June), 3241–3245.

Rosko, M. (1989). "Impact of the New Jersey All-Payer Rate-setting System: An Analysis of Financial Ratios." *Hospital and Health Services Administration* 34:1 (Spring), 53–69.

Salkever, D. (1975). "Hospital Wage Inflation: Supply-Push or Demand-Pull?" *Quarterly Review of Economics and Business* 15:33 (Autumn), 33–48.

Salkever, D., and Bice, T. (1976). "The Impact of Certificate-of-Need Controls on Hospital Investment." *Milbank Memorial Fund Quarterly* 54:2 (Spring), 195–214.

Samuels, S., Cunningham, P., and Choi, C. (1991). "Impact of Hospital Closures on Travel Time to Hospitals" *Inquiry* 28:2 (Spring), 194–199.

Schaafsma, J. (1986). "Average Hospital Size and the Total Operating Expenditures for Beds Distributed Over H Hospitals." *Applied Economics* 18:1 (April), 279–290.

Schwartz, G., and Stone, C. (1991). "Strategic Acquisitions by Academic Medical Centers." *Health Care Management Review* 16:2 (Spring), 39–47.

Sherman, D. (1988). *The Effect of State Certificate of Need Laws on Hospital Costs.* Washington, D.C.: Federal Trade Commission.

Siegel, J. (1989). "Interhospital Patient Transfer." *New England Journal of Medicine* 320:3 (January 19) 258–259.

Silverman, H. (1991). "Medicare Covered Home Health Services." *Health Care Financing Review* 12:2 (February), 113–125.

Simborg, D. (1981). "DRG Creep." *New England Journal of Medicine* 304:26 (June 25) 1602–1604.

Sloan F., and Steinwald, B. (1980). "Effects of Regulation on Hospital Costs and Input Use." *Journal of Law and Economics* 23:1 (April), 81–109.

Soderstrom, N. (1990). "Are Reporting Errors under PPS Random or Systematic?" *Inquiry* 27:3 (Fall), 234–241.

Steinwald, B., and Dummit, L. (1989). "Hospital Case-Mix Change: sicker patients or DRG Creep?" *Health Affairs* 8:2 (Summer), 35–47.

Stern, R., Weissman, J., and Epstein, A. (1991). "Emergency Department as a Pathway to Admissions for Poor and High-cost Patients." *Journal of the American Medical Association* 266:16 (October 30), 2238–2243.

Stevens, R. (1989). *In Sickness and in Wealth: American Hospitals in the Twentieth Century*. New York: Basic Books.

Stockwell, S. (1991). "One Step Forward, Two Steps Back: Labor Issues." *Emergency Medicine News* 13:6, 8–11.

Thorpe, K. (1988). "Why Are Urban Hospital Costs So High? The Relative Importance of Patient Source of Admission, Teaching, Competition, and Case Mix." *Health Services Research* 22:6 (February), 821–836.

Truman, D. (1951). *The Governmental Process: Political Interests and Public Opinion*. New York: Alfred Knopf.

Tuckman, H., and Chang, C. (1992). "Nonprofit Equity: A Behavioral Model and Its Policy Implications." *Journal of Policy Analysis and Management* 11:1 (Winter), 76–87.

Wennberg, J., Freeman, J., and Culp, W. (1987). "Are Hospital Services Rationed in New Haven or Over-utilized in Boston?" *Lancet* 1:8543, 1185–1187.

Whitted, G., and Torrens, P. (1989). *Managing Corporate Health Care Expenses: A Primer for Executives*. New York: Praeger.

Wilensky, G. (1990). "Technology as Culprit and Benefactor." *Quarterly Review of Economics and Business* 30:4 (Winter), 45–49.

Williams, B., Mackay, S., and Torner, J. (1991). "Home Health Care: Comparison of Patients and Services among Three Types of Agencies." *Medical Care* 29:6 (June), 583–587.

Williams, D., Hadley, J., and Pettengill, J. (1992). "Profits, Community Role, and Hospital Closure: An Urban and Rural Analysis." *Medical Care* 30:2 (February), 174–186.

2 Cost Functions and Production Functions

> One should strive to trim unnecessary costs and achieve the greatest output for the least input effort, better balancing all factors of service delivery to achieve the most with the smallest resource effort. Trim costs and enhance productivity.
>
> —Peter F. Drucker

> When you are through improving, you are through.
>
> —Bo Schembechler

Applied economists make a living performing two basic tasks: estimating production functions (Eastaugh 1990) and estimating cost functions (e.g., chapter 8). Sometimes these estimates have applications in the rate-setting context: paying teaching hospitals (Thorpe 1988) or setting inpatient payment rates for Medicaid patients. Since passage of the 1981 Boren Amendment in Congress, inpatient Medicaid must be "reasonable and adequate to meet costs that must be incurred by efficiently and economically operated providers" (42 U.S.C. SS1396a [a] [13] A). This language is ambiguous, because the phrase "incurred by efficiently and economically operated" hospitals could refer to short-run marginal cost or long-run marginal cost. The word "incurred" implies the cost to serving Medicaid patients compared to the cost of not serving Medicaid patients at the margin. If this decision is a one-shot annual contract, then perhaps the short-run marginal cost equation is best. But is this fair to the hospital sector if a short-run focus like the California MediCal contracting rates of 1983 receive insufficient annual updates because Medicaid is taking unfair advantage of its market power (Pauly 1988; however, Medicaid is not a monopsony single buyer, because it represents under 11 percent of inpatients)? Alternatively, contracting with Medicaid may be permanent and not temporary. States like Oregon take a long-run focus, as if the Medicaid block of business is recurring, and pay in excess of long-run marginal cost (Eastaugh 1991).

FAIR PAYMENT RATES

There is a wide difference of opinion as to whether rates are fair and adequate. Noneconomists do not understand that a long-run marginal cost (LRMC) curve is an idealist minimum average cost and that no single hospital may reside on the curve. LRMC only equals the average cost when no economies of scale exist (but 3 to 10 percent scale economies do exist in many states). Therefore, an efficiently and economically operated hospital might have average costs that are 60 to 85 percent of actual average costs, because actual cost is typically 13 to 30 percent above the theoretical minimum cost curve. The state Medicaid program need only show that it is paying above some fraction of average cost to demonstrate payment in excess of the LRMC. A state paying short-run marginal cost often need only show that it pays more than 40 to 60 percent of average actual cost.

Different professions measure costs in different ways. Accountants like to take a short-run budget-year focus and add up all the fixed and semifixed costs to tabulate a marginal cost estimate that is 40 to 60 percent of average cost (Eastaugh 1991), whereas economists like to estimate LRMC curves that have the explicit assumption that all costs are 100 percent variable (one could rebuild a new wing at any moment, or, to paraphrase Lord John Maynard Keynes, ''In the long run we are all dead,'' so everything is variable). For an economist the semifixed-cost item or the fixed-cost debt service is really variable (one could decide not to pay it or change careers or the building's mission statement). Economists claim that accountants are equally arbitrary in guessing what cost items are fixed or semivariable or variable. There is merit to both points of view. Cost behavior varies as a function of the market. Those analysts studying inner-city hospitals will report that short-run marginal cost spikes upward in a hospital with an increasing, very high occupancy rate. Why? Because the urban hospital under stress has to pay more employee overtime and make more emergency repairs of outdated equipment and facilities. On the other hand, the inefficient hospital in the overbedded area may face a short-run marginal cost that is only 40 percent of average cost. What you experience depends on where you sit.

Is this state of affairs an example of regulatory unfairness or of the state government acting as a prudent buyer for the taxpaying public? There will always be some tension between the regulators and the regulated. The regulated industry will always claim that it does not receive enough money for its value. Consumer groups and regulators will worry that they are not receiving enough value for their money. Regulators worry that they will offer no incentive to promote efficiency if they pay de facto cost reimbursement of every dollar spent. Does paying 60 percent of average cost (or 80 percent) present some risk for society? Two basic risks are present. If nongovernmental patients are not picking up the full share of fixed costs, insufficient government payment to the hospital will not cover total financial requirements, and in the long run the hospital may close. (However, some regulators would like to debed their marketplace, close excess capacity, and then improve payment rates to surviving hospitals.) Hospitals may debase the quality of care from Mercedes quality to compact quality of amenities in response to the lower payment rates (Friedman and Pauly 1981; Eastaugh 1991). Hospital Z may differentiate quality of care between Medicaid and private patients, whereas ethical hospital A may work to enhance productivity and cut needless amenities (comfort frills) rather than debase the technical quality of care (quality will be discussed in chapter 9).

Many hospitals complaining about low payment rates are willing to volunteer for even lower Medicaid payment rates by joining a selective contracting plan. Is the fact that they voluntarily sign a contract prima facie evidence that the rates cover their marginal costs? Perhaps. Hospital managers may sign a financially inferior contract under the belief that "anything beats cold sheets" and hope that they will avoid adverse media publicity (if they refuse to take Medicaid cases). In a sense the marginal cost rate a price setter tags makes an implicit statement on the desired level of quality and an explicit statement on the need to trim inefficiency and cut costs (Eastaugh 1990; Pauly and Wilson 1986). Discounts breed efficiency, but some providers operating as efficiently as they can under their current workload (case mix) will not be able to survive.

A third type of cost function frequently reported in the literature is average incremental costs. Average incremental costs (AIC) are relevant in starting a new product line, referring in the multiproduct institution to the additional cost incurred if it starts a new product or service. This new product was formerly not produced, and its AIC equals the combination of the specific new (start-up) fixed costs plus the marginal costs associated with the new product.

Cost functions can be calculated for a number of reasons: to identify variable costs to be trimmed (McClain and Eastaugh 1983), to assess profitability (Salmon 1991; Health Care Investment Analysis [HCIA] 1991), or to set government payment policies. This chapter will present four examples of cost functions and will offer an example of a hospital production function. We shall first review hospital economies of scale.

HOSPITAL ECONOMIES OF SCALE

In considering what happens to the level of output as the level of input increases, we are addressing the issue of economies of scale. If output grows at the same rate as inputs are increased, then there are constant returns to scale (per unit costs are the same at any given level of output). If output increases at a rate greater than inputs are increased, then there are increasing returns to scale (per unit costs decrease at high levels of output). If output grows at a rate less than the corresponding increase in inputs, then there are decreasing returns to scale (per unit costs increase as output rises).

Hospitalwide economies of scale are typically small. Within individual hospital departments and product lines there are substantial economies of scale to be observed. The most common problem faced by the analysts is that of comingling case-mix effects with unit cost; there tends to be a correlation between more difficult case mix and size (Keating 1984). Schaafsma (1986) studied 40 hospitals and concluded that in medium-size hospitals (60 to 293 beds) the economies-of-scale effect (12 percent) was more than offset by a case-mix effect, and hence costs increased slightly with volume. However, in hospitals with over 300 beds the economies-of-scale effect was sufficiently powerful to swamp any case-mix effect.

Economies of scale are generally illustrated by the long-run average cost curve (LRACC) in figure 2.1. Hospital size is measured either by number of beds or by average daily patient census. Output is typically measured by patient days and in some cases by patient discharges or admissions. The classic configuration of the LRACC is the U-shape illustrated in figure 2.1A, case 2. Generally, average costs are expected to decrease as output increases up to a point of minimum average costs, after which diseconomies of scale may take over. This point of minimum average costs is the optimal size for a firm or hospital (or the optimal level of output). Diseconomies beyond a certain point may be the result of inefficient management in large-scale facilities, or they may reflect the costs of increased travel time for physicians and patients (Fuchs 1986; Eastaugh 1987).

The central problem with applying the concept of economies of scale to hospital size is that hospitals do not produce a uniform product. Generally, the larger hospitals tend to treat more complex cases and to provide a much broader spectrum of care; thus a patient day in a small hospital is not equivalent to a patient day in a large hospital. Accordingly, any study of economies of scale must take case mix into account.

Research studies on economies of scale in the hospital sector have found five different shapes of the LRACC (see table 2.1). Failure to account for case mix results in a U-shaped LRACC. When adjustment for case mix is made, the LRACC is found to be slightly downward-sloping or flat for larger hospitals, indicating that economies of scale may exist, although the economies may not be great enough to justify much larger hospitals. An additional criticism of studies of the LRACC is that highly aggregated cost data make it impossible to separate the diseconomies due to size from those due to inefficiency, thus potentially leading to wrong conclusions regarding the optimal hospital size (Finkler 1979).

Much more significant economies of scale have been found on a departmental basis, under conditions where the product is homogeneous, by Hospital Administrative Services (HAS) researchers. Consequently, one would presuppose that if we could perform a perfect study adjusting for heterogeneous product mix of patient cases, then economies of scale would be more significant than the 16 percent difference between the smallest and largest hospitals in figure 2.1B, case 4. In summary, the data on economies of scale are not persuasive enough to suggest that we close all hospitals below a certain size. The increased travel time

Figure 2.1
Relationships between Hospital Size and Cost

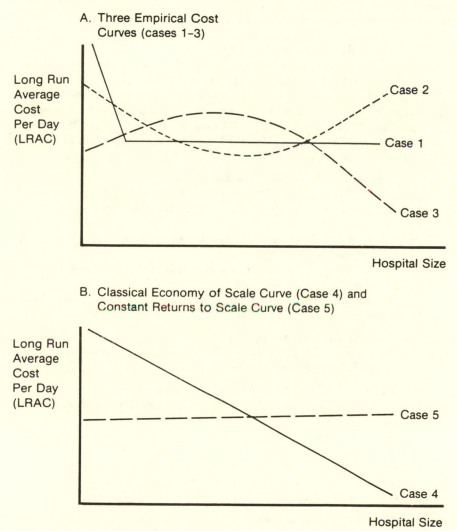

A. Three Empirical Cost
   Curves (cases 1–3)

Long Run
Average
Cost
Per Day
(LRAC)

Case 2

Case 1

Case 3

Hospital Size

B. Classical Economy of Scale Curve (Case 4) and
   Constant Returns to Scale Curve (Case 5)

Long Run
Average
Cost
Per Day
(LRAC)

Case 5

Case 4

Hospital Size

Note: Case numbers are referred to in Table 2.1.

to consumers and staff associated with closing all below-average-size hospitals would probably outweigh the benefits accrued in increasing returns to scale.

In a study for the Federal Trade Commission Bureau of Economics, Sherman (1988) reproduced the Grannemann, Brown and Pauly (1986) study for a sample of hospitals. Updating the Sherman study, including some regulatory variables (Eastaugh 1982), table 2.2 reports the scale economies and marginal costs for

Table 2.1
Survey of Studies Concerning Economies of Scale in the Hospital Sector

Case 1.   L-Shaped Average Cost Curve Found:
Feldstein, M. S., and J. Schuttinga. "Hospital Costs in Massachusetts: A Methodological Study." *Inquiry* 14:1 (March 1977), 22–31.
Francisco, E. W. "Analysis of Cost Variations Among Short-Term General Hospitals." In H. E. Klarman (ed.), *Empirical Studies in Health Economics*. Baltimore, Maryland: Johns Hopkins University Press, 1970, pp. 321–332.
Lave, J. R., and L. B. Lave. "Hospital Cost Functions." *American Economic Review* 60 (June 1970), 379–395.

Case 2.   U-Shaped Average Cost Curve Found:
Schaafsma, J. "Average Hospital Size and the Total Operating Expenditures for Beds Distributed over H Hospitals." *Applied Economics* 18:1 (April 1986), 279–290.
Carr, W. J., and P. J. Feldstein. "The Relationship of Cost to Hospital Size." *Inquiry* 4:2 (June 1967), 45–65.
Cohen, H. A. "Variations in Cost Among Hospitals of Different Sizes." *Southern Economic Journal* 33 (January 1967), 355–366.
Feldstein, M. S. *Economic Analysis for Health Service Efficiency*. Amsterdam: North-Holland Publishing Co., 1968.

Case 3.   Inverted U-Shaped Average Cost Curve Found:
Ingbar, M. L., and L. D. Taylor. *Hospital Costs in Massachusetts*. Cambridge, Mass.: Harvard University Press, 1968.

Case 4.   Downward Sloping Average Cost Curve Throughout:
Baron, D. P. "A Study of Hospital Cost Inflation." *Journal of Human Resources* 9 (Winter 1974), 33–49.
Berry, R. E., Jr. "Returns to Scale in the Production of Hospital Services." *Health Service Research* 2 (Summer 1967), 123–139.
Feldstein, P. J. *An Empirical Investigation of the Marginal Cost of Hospital Services*. Chicago, Illinois: University of Chicago, Center for Health Administration Studies, 1961.

Case 5.   Constant Returns to Scale:
Bays, C. "Specification Error in the Estimation of Hospital Cost Functions." *Review of Economics and Statistics* 42:2 (February 1980), 302–305.
Evans, R. G. "Behavioral Cost Functions for Hospitals." *Canadian Journal of Economics* 4 (May 1971), 198–215.
Lipscomb, J., I. E. Raskin, and J. Eichenholz. "The Use of Marginal Cost Estimates in Hospital Cost Containment Policy." In M. Zubkoff, I. E. Raskin, and R. S. Hanft (eds.), *Hospital Cost Containment: Selected Notes for Future Policy*. New York: Prodist Press, 1978, pp. 514–537.

Table 2.2
Estimated Long-Run and Short-Run Cost Equations and Economies of Scale for a Sample of 232 Hospitals

Output	Long-Run Cost Equations, 1970-90			Short-Run (1 year) Equations		
	Marginal Costs	Average Incremental Costs	Scale Economies[a]	Marginal Costs	Average Incremental Costs	Scale Economies
Emergency-department visits	390.29	476.18	1.22	116.02	142.73	1.23
Other outpatient visits	81.64	88.96	1.09	50.19	54.72	1.09
Subacute inpatient days	528.53	539.10	1.02[b]	126.02	124.80	.99[b]
Acute inpatient days	819.93	844.56	1.03	108.98	121.01	1.11
Intensive-care days	1,175.26	1,267.48	1.07	297.60	328.25	1.10

[a] If this number exceeds 1.0, economies of scale exist.
[b] Not significant at the 0.05 level; other variables significant at the 0.01 level.

two equations on a random sample of 232 hospitals with more than 75 beds. The long-run cost equation is the better specification; that is, it is more reasonable because the weighted cost estimates obtained from a full cost specification are much closer to the actual revenue figures for the 232 hospitals. Short-run equations are always lower estimates and represent only a fraction of total revenue and the expense of operating a facility. Marginal cost is the increase in total costs of producing an extra unit of output (the five hospital outputs listed in table 2.2), holding other outputs constant. As a rule of thumb, marginal costs equal 0.6 to 0.66 of average total cost in the studies in table 2.1. However, average total cost differs from the average incremental costs listed in table 1.6. The incremental costs of producing output 5 is the difference between the costs of producing all outputs and all the other outputs listed (table 2.2, 1 through 4). Dividing the average incremental costs by the marginal costs yields the product-specific economies-of-scale factor listed in table 2.2, columns 3 and 6. In agreement with previous studies, shallow economies of scale exist (under 12 percent), except for one output—emergency-department visits.

DEMAND-PULL IN EMERGENCY-DEPARTMENT VISITS

The fact that substantial scale economies exist for emergency departments may be a by-product of the stressed urban hospital. In many urban areas the emergency department functions as the only available clinician for the poor. From 1983 to 1990 the number of emergency departments in the nation declined by 6.1 percent (from 5,406 to 5,077), and yet the number of annual visits increased by 19.6 percent (from 77.5 million to 92.7 million).

A number of complex factors have contributed to emergency-department (ED) overcrowding. With 15,000 beds closing each year, fewer beds translate into a lowered capability to shift sick ED patients into inpatient beds. A more complex patient mix, including an increased number of AIDS patients utilizing the ED department for primary care, is a major problem in urban hospitals. In 1985 people with AIDS accounted for 2.0 percent of patient ED workload in New York City hospitals. By 1991 this figure surged to 60 percent in New York City and 20 percent in Washington, D.C. Why do patients without AIDS use the ED for primary care? The answer is that the number of persons eligible for Medicaid shrank to 31 percent of poor citizens in the 1980s (Eastaugh and Eastaugh 1990). Inappropriate low staffing levels, due to a shortage of ED-qualified health care professionals, adds to the problem of overcrowding. Low Medicaid reimbursement policies contribute to all four of these problems.

EMERGENCY OVERCROWDING: A GROWING PROBLEM

Managed-care plans and barebones hospital reimbursement systems are changing the practice of emergency medicine and ambulatory care. Prior to 1984 cost reimbursement allowed emergency physicians to test, transfer, and admit patients without any concern for the price tag. Economic transfers of patients are on the rise even while socially responsible physicians cry out that care of the poor is incumbent upon society (Thorpe 1988). The pressures to transfer come jointly from medical staff and a hospital concerned with its own profit margins. Federal legislation and Joint Commission on Accreditation of Healthcare Organizations (JCAHO) regulations concerning transfers, mixed with declining government payment rates and more stringent utilization review, amplify the difficulties with emergency care of the uninsured and the underinsured patients (Kellermann and Ackerman 1988).

Emergency physicians as a group enjoy the luxury of an interesting clinical practice with limited paperwork and billing hassles and with the resources of the entire hospital available for diagnosing and treating patients. The motivation of the emergency physician, who is most often paid by salary or hourly wage, is less profit oriented than that of the typical private physician or the hospital. The private admitting physician wants a paying patient, and the hospital desires to minimize losses (if it is not capable of generating a profit). Financially distressed hospitals increasingly report that the emergency department is the first to be cut when requests are made for staffing increases, equipment expenditures, or costly renovations (Eastaugh and Eastaugh 1990). While inpatient-care volume has declined 5 to 10 percent since 1984, the ED volume has increased 40 to 60 percent in the typical inner-city hospital. In New York City the inpatient volume has increased, while the ED volume is up more than 60 percent. The ED gets the short end of the stick: more AIDS patients, more severely ill elderly patients, and a smaller share of the hospital budget.

Hospital managers rightly argue that emergency care is too expensive. Emergency physicians sometimes overutilize costly lab tests and radiology studies in the name of defensive medicine. The ED is an inefficient setting for primary care of chronic stable patients. Do not blame the patients: Those lacking access to private care only have EDs. However, EDs are making plans to do harm to access. Hospitals in California and a number of other states have implemented incentive-pay plans for emergency physicians that stimulate maximum practice revenue and discourage the provision of uncompensated care. One should not conclude that all incentive-pay plans set up a system of two-tiered medicine: Overtreat the rich when billings will not be overturned by the utilization reviewers, and undertreat the poor. One 937-bed inner-city Detroit hospital has run an incentive-pay program that promotes productivity without discrimination against the uninsured patients.

Alternative delivery systems and new criteria for reimbursement are needed to provide efficient care for nonurgent ED patients so that optimal resources are available to treat truly urgent patients. Emergency physicians should be able to "do what is best for the patient" and still be a partner in maintaining the economic viability of their hospital. Before offering one case example, we shall outline the current legal context.

FEDERAL LAWS: SAY NO TO DUMPING THE POOR

The Consolidated Omnibus Budget Reconciliation Act (COBRA) of 1986 required all hospitals to examine and treat all patients presenting for emergency services regardless of ability to pay. The law further specified stringent requirements for patient transfers and imposed fines and penalties on hospitals for inappropriate transfers. The punitive possibilities were increased by the Omnibus Budget Reconciliation Act (OBRA) of 1987. Hospitals can now be fined $50,000 and physicians $25,000 per violation of federal patient-transfer laws. In addition, the secretary of the DHHS can terminate physician participation in Medicare for up to five years. The transferring physician is legally bound to ensure that the medical benefits outweigh the potential risks from the transfer, that the patient is stable, and that the accepting facility agrees to the transfer. Patients in active labor are by definition unstable for transfer.

Laws can discourage economic transfers, but they do not eliminate the problem. When a transfer is considered primarily for economic reasons, there are no expected medical benefits to justify the risks to the patient. Patients may decompensate or even die in transfer; delays in treatment occur; tests and radiology are frequently repeated at the receiving institution (even when all records are sent). Yet it can be argued that those indigent patients who are truly "stable" yet in need of hospitalization are better served in facilities given public funds to care for them, with a system (however underfunded) for follow-up care in the outpatient setting that can provide primary care and preventive care (Siegel 1989).

The world of practice is often different from the world of the Trauma 101 classroom. The constant pressure on emergency physicians to transfer nonpaying patients is exemplified when a young diabetic arrives in the ED by ambulance. He is lethargic and febrile, with a pH of 7.14 and a glucose of 732. His mother names a certain doctor as his private physician. That physician is contacted, and when the patient's clinical status is described, the emergency physician is instructed to transfer the patient across town to the city public hospital. "He's not my patient anymore. Last time he was admitted he stayed in the hospital three weeks and didn't pay my bill." When the emergency physician insists that the patient is too sick to transfer, the private internist instructs: "Give him some insulin and an amp of bicarbonate, call him stable, and send him to the city hospital." This example is not an atypical case. The COBRA laws give ammunition to emergency physicians who may be pressured to transfer indigent patients. The threat of legal and monetary sanction makes good care economically desirable even for those patients who do not pay. The next section will survey the production process for hospital nursing, another highly stressed profession.

HOSPITAL NURSING PRODUCTIVITY

The hospital nursing profession is undergoing a major transformation. Task delegation and the allocation of nurses within the hospital have become major medical economics issues for the 1990s (Aiken 1990). Nursing-department employees represent 62 percent of the hospital employees and 36 percent of hospital expenses (Eastaugh 1990). Hospitals increased their employment of full-time registered nurses (RNs) per 100 patient days by 56 percent in the period 1982–88. The report of the Secretary's Commission on Nursing (1988) indicated that the hospitals reporting the most severe RN shortages have been the leaders in replacing licensed practical nurses (LPNs) with more expensive RNs. Alternative labor input in the form of the technician nurse extender (NE) is an increasingly popular approach to alleviating the problem of inadequate nurse staffing levels (Klein 1989). While careful empirical study has not yet been done to assess the degree to which employment of NEs and efficient task delegation to clerks (or LPNs) can enhance department productivity and free nurses to perform their unique clinical activities, in theory, NEs can intensify the marginal value product of the most educated nurses when RNs are able to concentrate their workday around the most severely ill patients.

Hospital nursing has undergone a number of major organizational shifts, from functional nursing in the 1940s to team nursing in the 1960s and primary nursing in the 1970s. The 1960s' innovation of team nursing set the experienced RN as the team leader, working with nursing aides and LPNs. The team leader delegated much of the patient care to the team members and planned the care for each patient during that specific shift (Shukla 1983a). Team nursing had the financial benefits of cost-effectiveness and the positive and negative aspects of any task-oriented system. Hospital administrators liked team nursing's focus on centralization of control while nurse educators desired a new system that would focus on the autonomy of the BSN-trained RN (and would maximize reliance on RNs while decreasing employment of LPNs).

Primary nursing became popular in the 1970s as nursing focused on the need for autonomy and the evolution of a knowledge-based professional practice (Aiken and Mullinix 1987). Primary nursing involves decentralization of the nursing unit and the establishment of a responsibility relationship between a nurse and the patient. The primary nurse writes a 24-hour-care plan for each patient, and the associate nurse implements the plan when the primary nurse is not working. Primary nursing has the advantage of improved continuity of care but carries the cost of a smaller number of patients per RN (Shukla 1983b)

The nurse extender concept, as a substitute or complement to primary-care nursing, has become increasingly popular since 1985 (Eastaugh and Regan 1990). The NE technologist label is an attempt to rid the profession of any sexist bent and recruit men (NEs are typically two-thirds male and earn 20 to 45 percent less per hour than RNs).

Nurse extender technicians became popular because the hospital sector experienced difficulty in finding a sufficient supply of RNs for primary nursing staffs (Eastaugh 1985). Some nursing groups were not receptive to the NE concept because of fears that it represented a return to team nursing and undertrained LPNs with a new job title (Lenehan 1988). However, task delegation to NEs by itself does not undermine the standardization of nurse education. In fact, the realization that the nation needs more caregivers and that NEs would still be under the control of the nursing department prompted the nursing literature to became less militant. Now the NE is referred to in the literature as a "technical assistant to an experienced RN in a primary partnership" or an "executive administrative assistant assisting the executive nurse (Manthey 1989; McCarthy 1989). Such glowing titles may seem unimportant to economists, but in the workplace it is important for job retention that NEs not be labeled reborn LPNs who do "scutwork" or "menial tasks." One profession's menial task is another profession's vital activity, so NEs spend most of their workday performing a "noninterpretive" collection of vital signs, EKGs, lab slips, and paperwork.

The Production-Function Approach

Production-function studies of technical efficiency (productivity) have been done by economists since the 1930s. Production functions are useful to understand how resources are combined by the department or firm (hospital) to produce some particular level of output and to ascertain how these resources complement or substitute for one another in the service-production process (Arthur Young and Policy Analysis Inc. 1987).

A number of studies have analyzed production functions in business and in the hospital sector (Arthur Young and Policy Analysis Inc. 1986; Kalirajan and Shand 1989). The first major study of American hospital production functions involved a sample of 60 Ohio nonteaching hospitals in 1975. Hellinger (1975) utilized a translog (transcendental logarithmic) production function, which attenuates or eliminates restrictions on the functional form, thereby leaving as much generality and flexibility as possible in the service-production-estimation process (in contrast to the traditional Cobb-Douglas model). The translog form used in this study involves two basic assumptions. First, managers monitor nursing costs when deciding the appropriate staff mix and range or level of hospital output and nurse workload. This assumption does not mean that nurse managers are perfect cost minimizers operating at the production possibility frontier of 100 percent technical efficiency. The second assumption is that nursing departments exhibit constant returns to scale in producing their output; that is, a fourfold increase in inputs leads to a fourfold increase in output. Consequently, there is no reason to presuppose that nurses are any more productive in a 1,022-bed hospital than in a 260-bed hospital. (Previous hospital cost studies, not focused on the nursing department, reported very shallow economies of scale of only 11 percent [Eastaugh 1987]).

In comparing isoquants—curves producing the same output for different quantities of inputs—two extreme situations can exist. Under perfect complementary production between inputs, no substitution at all is possible between inputs A and B, and inputs A and B must always be used in fixed proportions (isoquants are straight downward-sloping lines) (Feldstein 1989). Under the opposite extreme, perfect substitutability between inputs defines the isoquants as perfect right angles. In the first step in the data analysis to follow, a translog production function will be estimated from data at 29 hospitals. The second step measures the curvature of the nursing isoquants and thereby the substitution among inputs (the elasticity of substitution).

Since nursing is a complex production process, we will be assessing a production process with five inputs and thus five-dimensional isoquants. Between each pair of inputs partial elasticities of substitution will be measured (e.g., NE substitution for RNs). The five basic inputs studied include (1) NEs (nurse extenders), (2) RNs, (3) H (house-staff residents and interns performing some nursing activities while nursing is understaffed), (4) A (clerks, LPNs, and nurse aides), and (5) E (capital).

Sample Framework and Data Analysis

Collection of data on labor inputs is straightforward and has been done in a number of previous studies. Nursing output is specified by a point-scoring system sold by the largest proprietary vendor of nurse-workload and nurse-scheduling systems (Medicus System Corporation 1989). This same system tracks work hours to measure the contribution of nonphysician inputs (input factors 1, 2, and 4). House-staff resident and intern input was measured not on an annual basis, but only on a one-shot, two-month sampling basis in one year, 1985. However, we have no reason to presuppose that house-staff input to nursing activities should exhibit any major change in 1986–88. Filled residency slots have been largely time-invariant for the 14 sample teaching hospitals, and physician labor in nursing activities only ranges from 0.1 to 1.2 percent of nursing activities. To omit this measured work input in the analysis would slightly overstate the productivity of nursing departments in certain hospitals.

One last caveat must be presented concerning measurement error in this study: Measurement of capital inputs must avoid the pitfalls of using depreciation charges to more accurately reflect differences in the age and productivity of the capital stock. I have used the same index I employed in the Arthur Young study (1987) to adjust the capital expenses for differences across the 29 sample hospitals in the average age of their capital stocks. For each hospital the ratio of accumulated depreciation to total assets is taken as a measure of age. Age-adjusted capital input was calculated as follows:

$$E = UA \times \mathrm{Exp}(M - R), \tag{2.1}$$

where UA is the unadjusted capital expenses, R is the ratio of accumulated depreciation to total assets, M is the mean value of R for the sample, and Exp is the inverse natural logarithm.

The sample is a convenience sample of hospitals with active nursing-activity-research programs: 15 of 17 hospitals in a previous study by Eastaugh and Regan (1990) and 14 of 45 hospitals in an earlier study by Arthur Young and Policy Analysis Inc (1987). Obviously, the sample is not generalizable to all American hospitals. The more progressive hospitals, with active support for health-services research, may have production technologies (scheduling and staff education; Eastaugh 1985) that are ten years more advanced than those of the average American hospital. Each of the sample hospitals had subscribed to the same nurse-workload system since 1985, and the hospitals ranged in size from 194 to 1,092 beds. The hypothetical frontier production function can be expressed as

$$y_{ij} = \prod_k (x_{ijk})^{\beta_k} e^{u_{ij}} \tag{2.2}$$

where y_{ij} is the nurse output of the jth hospital in the ith period for periods 1–4 (1985, . . . ,1988) and x_{ijk} is the kth input applied by the jth hospital in the ith period. If the jth hospital realizes its full technical efficiency at 100 percent, then inefficiency u_j takes the value zero, and if not, u_j takes a value less than zero depending on the extent of the lost productivity. The $e^{u_{ij}}$ term provides a measure of hospital-specific productivity, and improvement in $e^{u_{ij}}$ will be reflected in higher mean productivity over time. Inefficiency can be expressed as

$$u_j = \ln y_{ij} - (\Sigma \, \beta_k \ln x_{ijk} + v_{ij}). \tag{2.3}$$

Estimation of u_j and then e^{u_j} is possible once density functions for u and v are assumed. Let u follow a half-normal distribution and v follow the full normal distribution. (The validity of the half-normal distribution was verified at the end of the analysis by plotting the combined residual ($u + v$), the hospital's technical efficiency and the output levels.) Equation (2.2) can be rewritten as

$$y_{ij} = \prod_k (\chi_{ijk})^{\beta_k} e^{\epsilon_{ij}}$$

where $\epsilon_{ij} = u_j + v_{ij}$ \hfill (2.4)

The estimation of the maximum possible stochastic output, had the hospital realized its full technical efficiency, is carried out by applying maximum-likelihood methods (Johnston 1989) to equation (2.4). With this model one can estimate individual hospital technical efficiencies together with the mean technical efficiency using four years of panel data (dummy variable D [0,1] for each of the last three years 1986, 1987, 1988). One can hopefully also target some factors causing variation in technical efficiencies in nursing among the 29 sample hospitals.

Maximum-likelihood methods of estimation (Chambers 1988) were applied to equation (2.4), and the parameter estimates of the translog model are presented

Table 2.3
Translog Production Function for Medical/Surgical Nursing Service Delivery in a Sample of 29 Hospitals, 1985–1988

Variable[a]	Parameter Estimate[b] (Maximum Likelihood)
D_1, 1986	0.002 (9.4)
D_2, 1987	0.013 (28.1)
D_3, 1988	0.022 (50.4)
$\beta NE,E$	0.082 (7.5)
$\beta H,E$	0.098 (18.2)
$\beta H,NE$	0.137 (29.3)
$\beta RN,H$	-0.059 (9.6)
$\beta RN,E$	0.102 (19.4)
$\beta RN,NE$	-0.098 (24.1)
$\beta A,NE$	0.089 (17.0)
$\beta A,H$	-0.006 (1.4)
$\beta A,RN$	-0.047 (8.3)
$\beta A,E$	0.119 (16.8)
Constant α	0.038 (7.7)

Source: Eastaugh (1990).

[a]NE = nurse extenders, RNs, H = house staff residents and interns doing some nursing activities while understaffed, A = clerks, LPNs, and nurse aides, E = capital.
[b]T-values in parentheses. Log likelihood = -42.075.

in table 2.3. The ratio of hospital-specific variability in productivity was significant at the 0.01 level, indicating that productivity dominates in explaining the total variability of nurse output produced. Judging by the significance of the four dummy variables, we can reject the hypothesis that productivity was time-invariant over the four years. Most of the parameters not involving the two weakest variables (*H* and *E*) are significant at the 0.05 level.

A second alternative partial elasticity can also be derived. The Allen elasticity of substitution holds constant the quantities of all other inputs in addition to the level of nurse output. The Allen elasticities are related econometrically to the cross-price elasticity of demand for factor inputs (Johnston 1989), for example, the demand for input 1 (nurse extenders) to change in the price of input 2 (RNs). The sign of a cross-price elasticity of demand (column 3 of table 2.4) by itself is an indicator of gross substitution—a negative sign indicating complementary factors, a positive sign indicating substitution. As line 11 of table 2.4 reveals, a negative sign on the elasticity of demand for NE labor with respect to the price of RN labor indicates that as RN labor becomes more costly, the labor of NEs is used less extensively in place of RNs. On the positive side, this suggests that NEs and RNs are complementary team members, not in competition with each

Table 2.4
Allen Partial Elasticities of Substitution for the Input Factors of Medical/Surgical Nursing Productivity

Lines 1-5: own price partial elasticities negative (as expected).

1.	NE/NE[a]	-0.234	Complements
2.	RN/RN	-0.157	Complements
3.	H/H	-0.140	Complements
4.	A/A	-0.079	Complements
5.	E/E	-0.388	Complements
6.	NE/E	0.353	Substitutes
7.	H/E	0.796	Substitutes
8.	H/NE	0.907	Substitutes
9.	RN/H	-0.231	Complements
10.	RN/E	0.519	Substitutes
11.	RN/NE	-0.448	Complements
12.	A/NE	0.586	Substitutes
13.	A/H	-0.026	Complements
14.	A/RN	-0.230	Complements
15.	A/E	0.372	Substitutes

Source: Eastaugh (1990).

[a]NE= nurse extenders, RNs, H = house-staff residents and interns doing some nursing activities while understaffed, A = clerks, LPNs, and nurse aides, E = capital.

other. On the other hand, this suggests that a rapidly inflating costly all-RN nursing staff trades away efficiency by avoiding the opportunity for NE-induced productivity gains. Moreover, using nonemployee RNs, the temporary agency nurses can cost many urban hospitals as much as $55 to $75 per hour.

The NEs substitute fairly well and fluidly for clerks and LPNs (line 12) while complementing RNs. A positive sign in line 8 on the elasticity of demand for NE labor with respect to the price of house-staff (resident) labor indicates that as house-staff labor (*H*) becomes more costly per hour, the labor of NEs is used more extensively in place of residents. As some state regulators and hospital managers have moved to restrict the house-staff workweek—fewer hours at the same fixed annual wage—this raises the hourly wage of the house staff and raises the employment level of NEs. However, the negative sign in line 9 of table 2.4 reveals that no increase in RN employment can be expected as New York and other states implement a maximum hourly workweek for residents and interns.

Lines 6, 7, 10, and 15 in table 2.4 have the expected positive signs, indicating that labor can substitute for capital (0.01 level of significance). Line 7 has the highest observed elasticity, suggesting that the highly skilled M.D. members of house staff, with their technical diagnostic skill as doctors, partially substitute

Table 2.5
Frequency Distribution of Nursing Departments' Productivity and Nurse Extender Staffing Mix

Productivity Level (Range)	Number of Hospitals	Percentage of Hospitals	Ratio of NEs to RNs
0.55-0.60	3	10.34	0.0
0.60-0.65	4	13.79	0.0
0.66-0.70	4	13.79	0.16
0.71-0.75	8	27.59	0.37
0.76-0.80	5	17.24	0.54
0.81-0.85	3	10.34	0.79
0.86-0.90	2	6.90	0.71
Total	29	100.0	mean = 0.35
0.72 = mean Productivity			

Source: Eastaugh (1990).

for more equipment and physical capital. This generalization may be increasingly true in the future as more residents benefit from economic grand rounds, think-before-testing education programs, and the cost-effective clinical decision-making ethic.

Improving Nurse Productivity

The three dummy variables at the top of table 2.3 indicate that nurse productivity for this sample of 29 hospitals was not time-invariant over the four-year period. Mean nurse productivity for each cross-sectional equation improved from 0.696 to 0.741 from 1985 to 1988, but in 1988 nursing departments were still realizing only 74.1 percent of their technical efficiency (productivity). While averages are interesting, distributions are more policy relevant. Table 2.5 lists the average productivity level across the 29 nursing departments and the factor input (nurse extenders) with the two highest t-values (from table 2.3). Individual nurse productivity ratings ranged from 0.56 to 0.89. Table 2.5 suggests discrete differences in production technologies as well as differences in input mix. This wide range could in theory reflect differences in organizational efficiency (Kalirajan and Shand 1989) or differences in the availability and use of factor inputs (e.g., a shortage of nurses; Eastaugh 1987). However, the 7 hospitals with the worst nursing productivity at the top of table 2.5 employed no nurse extender technicians, operated a 100 percent RN primary-care nursing organization, and exhibited productivity 9 to 16 percent below average. The 5 hospitals in table 2.5 with the highest levels of nurse productivity made heavy use of nurse extenders: 2 used the team-nursing organizational concept, but 3 employed primary-care nursing with a 57 to 62 percent BSN RN staff.

In summary, the results suggest that (1) primary-care nursing can be either highly productive or inefficient; (2) the all-RN nursing staff, used in only 8 of the 29 hospitals, reported the worst productivity performance; (3) a shortage of nurses did not drag down productivity levels in table 2.5 as the four cities with the tightest nursing markets contained the 5 hospitals with the highest levels of productivity; and (4) employment of nurse extenders reduces wasted labor and enhances productivity.

The last of these four conclusions indicates a number of avenues for future research. For example, the results at the end of the last column in table 2.5 weakly indicate that nurse extenders, as with any labor input, may approach a level of diminishing returns. Does having 8 to 10 NEs per 10 RNs constitute a zone of diminishing returns? Does a primary-care nursing staff with greater than 80 percent BSN RNs constitute an inefficient staff mix of diminishing returns? Does deploying 5 to 8 NEs per 10 RNs harm patient-care quality? Judging from the deployment of NEs at prestigious hospitals (e.g., Johns Hopkins Hospital; Eastaugh and Regan 1990), task delegation can enhance the quality of patient care.

Last, what additional tasks can be delegated to NEs beyond obtaining vital signs and EKG results, patient transport, procuring supplies and equipment, procedural assistance, and paperwork (e.g., lab slips)? Some of the 21 hospitals utilizing NEs have begun to utilize specialist technicians to dress wounds and do other nursing functions. Other activities performed by nurse extenders are outlined in table 2.6. Progressive nurse managers will participate in careful studies to set standards, study task-delegation feasibility, and circumscribe the job descriptions for two to three levels of NE technicians (Powers 1990; Bennett and Hylton 1990).

With future funding limitations, barebones reimbursement dictates that the recent tradition of 100 percent RN primary-care nursing must be abandoned. Development of an efficient staff-mix criterion in nursing should enhance nursing's rising sense of professionalism. In this regard Manthey (1988, 1970), one of the initial founders of primary-care nursing, has recently subscribed to the idea that the 100 percent RN concept is not a necessary component for primary-care nursing. Maximizing RN hospital employment levels is hardly a desirable or economical goal unless America has a gross oversupply of nurses. Since no such oversupply exists, increased reliance on nurse extenders is good economics, good nursing, and good medicine. The validity of this assertion will be retested, utilizing 1991 data, in the next section.

Alternatives to Production Functions

The production functions in the previous section are helpful in assessing nurse productivity. For line managers there is a simpler technique called data-

Table 2.6
Selective Examples of Nonnursing Menial Tasks versus Important Nursing Tasks

Nonnursing Tasks to Delegate to Nurse Extenders (NE)[a]	Important Nursing Tasks
1. Obtaining vital signs	Interpreting vital signs
2. Patient transport	Physical assessment and condition monitoring
3. Housekeeping and bedmaking	Technological monitoring, Infusion pumps, Swan-Ganz catheters
4. Meal trays	Tube and IV feedings
5. Physician procedural assistance (pelvic exam)	IV Therapy: nitroglycerine, insulin, TPA drips
6. Venipuncture	Evaluation/outcome documentation
7. Getting supplies and equipment	Discharge planning
8. Secretarial (e.g., lab slips)	Special tube placements: NGs, foleys, oxygen therapy
9. Obtaining EKGs	Narcotic count

Source: Eastaugh (1990).
[a]Nonnursing tasks, often called "scutwork," are activities easily delegated to NEs in a high-productivity unit.

envelopment analysis (DEA) for considering relative labor productivity between hospitals. DEA is a mathematical programming technique that optimizes the relative technical efficiency (productivity) ratio of current inputs over current outputs for each nursing department. DEA has the advantage of neatly dividing departments into two classes (efficient and inefficient) and producing a summary scalar efficiency ratio for each nursing department. DEA has been used in the health care field since publication of the Charns, Cooper, and Rhodes (1981) study. The data are for 1991, and the sample has been expanded from 29 to 39 hospitals (with the inclusion of 2 public hospitals, 6 voluntary tax-exempt hospitals, and 2 for-profit hospitals).

The data-envelopment analysis sums up all nursing services and takes RN, NE, and other-nurse (e.g., LPN) labor input into account separately, assessing the overall performance of the inpatient nursing department. The DEA model generates a scalar efficiency categorization using nonparametric deterministic mathematical programming to optimize the technical efficiency ratio in each department. One generic advantage of DEA analysis is that each input and each output variable can be measured independently in a useful unit without being transformed into a single metric. One advantage of the DEA analysis in tables 2.7, 2.8 and 2.9 is that in contrast to previous DEA studies of nursing (Nunamaker

Table 2.7
A Data-Envelopment Analysis of the Relationship between Productivity and Nursing Organization (N = 39 Hospital Inpatient Nursing Departments, 1991)

	Efficient Departments	Inefficient Departments
Primary-care nursing (all-RN staff)	0	7
Team nursing (limited use of nurse extenders)[a]	3	9
Primary-care nursing (limited use of nurse extenders)[a]	3	6
Heavy reliance on 0.56-0.8 nurse extenders per RN	11	0
	—	—
	17	22

[a]Ratio of nurse extenders to RNs in the 0.17 to 0.41 range.

1983), output measures are not simply inpatient days, but rather the DRG-adjusted Medicus-standardized nurse workload (Medicus 1989; Eastaugh 1990).

The sample of 39 hospitals divides into two categories in table 2.7. The 17 efficient nursing departments are not necessarily efficient in the absolute sense (compared to an updated production function like that in table 2.5 their productivity is 9 to 21 percent less than perfect), but in the DEA analysis they represent "best-performance" departments compared to the 22 inefficient departments. The inefficient departments have productivity levels that are 28 to 44 percent less than perfect. The chi-squared value of table 2.7 is significant at the 0.05 level with two degrees of freedom. It is interesting to note that 3 of 16 primary-care nursing departments achieved the DEA label of efficient by employing a staffing ratio of NEs to RNs in the 0.30–0.41 range, whereas all 100 percent RN nursing departments were found to be inefficient. The 11 departments with heavy reliance on NEs were all judged efficient by 1991.

To validate the DEA results, a logistic regression equation was run, and the results are reported in table 2.8. Primary-care nursing in itself was not a statistically significant drag on productivity, given that by 1991, 9 of 16 primary-care nursing departments had begun to make use of task delegation to nurse extenders. The more interesting question is what the 22 inefficient hospitals can

Table 2.8
Logistic Regression Analysis of the Relationship between Nursing Organization, Nurse Extenders, and Efficiency (N = 39 Hospital Inpatient Nursing Departments, 1991)

Independent Variables[a]	BETA	Standard Error	R
Nurse extenders high[b]	3.16*	1.37	.291
Nurse extenders low[c]	1.43*	1.14	.128
Primary nursing	-.89	1.03	-.006
Team nursing	-.92	1.01	-.004

[a]Dependent variable efficiency classification of DEA (table 2.7). Only 2 of the 3 variables need be included in each category.
[b]Ratio of nurse extenders to RNs in the 0.56 to 0.80 range.
[c]Ratio of nurse extenders to RNs in the 0.17 to 0.41 range.
*Chi-square test significant at 0.05 level.

Table 2.9
A Data-Envelopment Analysis of Average Inefficiency (N = 39 Hospitals, 1991)

Factor (Workload/Input)	Current Value *Value If Efficient in 1991*
•Workload per Case-Mix-Adjusted Admission	
1. General nursing administration	18.6% inefficient
2. Assessing and monitoring physical condition	17.4% inefficient
3. Planning for patient discharge	14.9% inefficient
4. Completing evaluation/outcome documentation	14.8% inefficient
5. Administering tube or IV feedings	9.5% inefficient
6. Placing special tubes (NGs, Foleys, O_2)	8.2% inefficient
7. Monitoring tech equipment (Swan-Ganz catheter)	7.9% inefficient
•Labor Input	
1. Nursing administration	21.3% oversupply
2. Nurse extender (technicians)	24.7% undersupply
•Uncontrollable (Ownership)	
1. Hospital is for-profit (n = 2)	output/input 2.4% above mean
2. Hospital is public facility (n = 2)	output/input 4.9% above mean

do differently to improve productivity. The DEA output of the average inefficient department divided by the guidepost value if efficient in 1991 is presented in table 2.9. The values-if-efficient denominators (bottom of the fraction in the last column of Table 2.9) are obtained by multiplying the peak technical efficiency ratio of 0.91 by the current values, then subtracting the slack (Grosskopf and

Valdmanis 1987). Nursing departments should work to trim the inefficiency associated with the seven top tasks in table 2.9 and should especially target ways to trim unneeded bureaucratic tasks. Judging by the results for labor inputs, the 22 inefficient nursing departments could trim administrative activities by 21.3 percent and expand the supply of NE employees by 24.7 percent. The one uncontrollable variable in table 2.9 is hospital ownership type (not under the control of the nursing department). One would not want to generalize much from a sample of only two for-profit hospitals and two public hospitals, but it is interesting to note that the efficiency levels were 2.4 percent better for "inefficient for-profit" hospitals than for peer hospitals and 4.9 percent lower for the two public hospitals. In the Valdmanis (1990) study Michigan public hospitals in 1982 had slightly higher levels of productivity than tax-exempt voluntary hospitals.

Task delegation to nurse extenders, a leaner nursing administration bureaucracy, and nurse-scheduling systems using optimizer linear programming software (Shorr 1991) appear to be the three keys to enhancing nursing productivity. Nurse productivity is important because nurses represent over 60 percent of hospital employees. However, other departments have need for productivity improvement. Better scheduling systems for staff and patients can enhance productivity in radiology, respiratory therapy, and a number of other departments. Staffing standards for efficient (good, 70th percentile) hospital departments and very good (top 10 percent) departments are given in table 2.10. Data-envelopment analysis can also be used on smaller-scale health care facilities, like rural primary-care centers and community health centers (Huang and McLaughlin 1989).

A total quality-management program should focus on both external customers (patients, employers) and internal customers. Frequently one department does not understand how its work product is utilized by the next department; for example, quality and productivity may be enhanced if a hospital lab stops skimping on hiring a $7.50 per hour technician without which the talents of a $75 per hour emergency-room doctor are being wasted waiting for lab results. The concept of internal customers (Deming 1986), fostering respect and efficient interdependency between departments, can help morale in the total organization. Doctors are a "customer" of the nursing department, the medical floor is a "customer" of the recovery room, and the recovery room is a "customer" of the operating room. Sometimes certain departments can be inappropriate or excessive customers of another department. In the typical hospital the patient-transport department should have its work done by nurses for 0.3 to 0.4 percent of the workweek. For example, in one hospital the nurses were spending 8.1 percent of their time doing patient transport. Was the patient-transport department understaffed (so it needed nurses to do their work)? No. Patient transport was overstaffed 90 percent and would typically fill up its day by creating unnecessary meetings and calling up nurses to transport patients to radiology (where three or four idle patient-transport employees would talk to the nurse on line). Overstaffing is seldom a self-diagnosing problem. Departments fill up the idle time with makework activity while other departments go understaffed.

Table 2.10
Productivity Standards for Performance in Select Departments, 1991

Department	Performance Target Standards per Unit of Service (UOS)	
	Good 70th Percentile	Very Good 90th Percentile
Radiation oncology	1.16	0.73
Respiratory therapy (RT)	0.25	0.20
Pulmonary (in dept. RT)	0.57	0.46
EEG (in dept. RT)	1.42	1.25
EKG (in heart center, HC)	0.60	0.51
Echocardiology (in dept. HC)	1.63	1.47
Emergency department (ED)	1.77	1.50
Behavioral services (M.H. & S.W.)	7.30	6.40
Laundry (linen per diem)[a]	16 lbs/patient day	14 lbs/patient day

Source: Eastaugh Consulting Services, N = 199 hospitals.
[a]Productivity enhancement can also involve decreasing unnecessary units of activity or unneeded output, for example, minimizing linen consumption per patient per day.

Consider an example of doctors as customers of the nursing department. Attending physicians at one hospital often complained that they seldom saw the same faces twice. A team was formed to study the problem and provide solutions. The problem was caused by an insufficient supply of RNs to recruit and a nursing department that believed in 100 percent RN primary-care nursing. Rather than continue the expensive habit of hiring agency nurses that were new to the department and unknown to the doctors, the solution involved maximizing use of existing RNs' clinical skills by employing NEs to do the 43 percent of nurses' work that the law dictated that a nonnurse could perform. Morale among nurses improved because their time was no longer wasted doing menial work. Morale among attending physicians improved because they could identify specific RNs in connection with their individual patients. A good hospital does not need a sign Our Nurses Care; the RNs, NEs, managers, and physicians just know it. Improvements in efficiency of labor utilization should also be supplemented by a reduction in excess supply (capacity).

CLOSING ACUTE-CARE BEDS: WHERE ARE THE SAVINGS?

The American Hospital Association (AHA) has taken the position that national occupancy rates indicating that hospitals are one-third empty are a ''clear'' sign that hospitals are efficiently managed. Under the AHA logic, only patients who require inpatient care are admitted to hospitals, and inpatient stays in the expensive hospital bed are as short as medically appropriate. Services previously performed on an inpatient basis are done at alternative sites (e.g., home care or outpatient care), which helps explain why outpatient services rose to 30 percent of hospital revenues in 1991. However, patients, third-party payers, and employers have one difficult question to ask the hospital industry: Where is the piece dividend from using a smaller piece of the inpatient hospital-bed supply? Estimates of how many acute-care beds are empty for 100 percent of the year—never used for any outpatient service or inpatient case—vary from 100,000 to 176,000 beds. How can we as a nation reap the benefits of closing excess beds in order to finance the extra services provided for the elderly, for outpatients of all ages, and for home care and long-term care?

The intent of this section is not to play the health-planning game and set a normative estimate on benefits to society from having an additional reserve supply of empty beds weighed against the cost of adding to that reserve pool. There will always be people who will claim that some influx of patients will fill those beds in a few years, even if each "excess" bed has remained empty for the past decade. Rather, we shall ask the more practical question: What does it cost to maintain a fully empty excess acute-care hospital bed? Estimates vary from a low of $29,000 in 1991 dollars (Pauly and Wilson 1986) to a high estimate of $65,000 by Anderson (1991).

Anderson (1991) offered the better estimate because he included the recent rise in outpatient demand at the hospitals as a variable in the analysis, and he had department estimates over the budget year for safety margins against surges in demand for a sample of 39 Maryland hospitals. This last point is clearly more refined than simply having a hospitalwide estimate of the fluctuation in occupancy rates over the year (Pauly and Wilson 1986; Friedman and Pauly 1981). Pauly's concept (1990) of a subjective need to overbuild (to avoid the crowding costs of having a hospital too full) does not offer a rate regulator any guideposts to constrain capital payments to overbuilt, overcapitalized hospitals. The theoretical model of asserting that 100 percent of hospitals are efficient and that in the long run no excess capacity exists offers a poor description of the world.

Anderson (1991) calculated the cost of an excess hospital bed with a three-year standard hospital cost function for a national sample of 5,068 hospitals. An excess bed cost 29 percent of the average cost of an occupied bed ($224,000), or $65,000 in 1991 dollars. The definition of a bed was the AHA statistical bed, a bed set up and staffed for use (regularly maintained). The average cost of an occupied bed was only $177,500 in 1985.

Pauly and Wilson (1986) used a sample of Michigan hospitals and concluded that the cost of an excess bed was 13 percent (or less) of the average cost of an occupied bed, or $29,000 in 1991 dollars. However, they distinguished unforeseen empty beds from planned excess capacity (foreseen empty beds). In their cost function, short-run marginal cost was 57 percent of average cost; therefore, the residual, or 43 percent of the average cost of an occupied bed, was the cost of an unforeseen empty bed, but the cost of a foreseen empty bed was 13 percent of the average cost of an occupied bed.

Politicians may be surprised to discover that closing beds at hospitals that remain in business or bankrupting entire hospitals will only save 13 to 29 percent of the average cost of an occupied bed (or $29,000 to $65,000 per bed). The high estimate is probably more reliable because the data base was larger, was more recent, included higher capital spending patterns in recent years, and incorporated day-to-day department variations in workload.

Many noneconomists were under the false impression that closing a bed would save 100 percent of the average cost of an occupied bed. The marginal benefit (cost savings) of closing a bed is under 30 percent of the average cost. The optimal statewide occupancy rate may range from 75 percent for a rural state with many small hospitals to above 85 percent for a highly urbanized state. By 1992–93 the average capital cost per bed, occupied or empty, will exceed $25,000. The average annual variable cost of maintaining an empty bed, including light, heat, and labor expenses (maintenance, cleaning, and security) will exceed $50,000.

MEDICARE PROSPECTIVE PAYMENT FOR CAPITAL

In January 1992 the Medicare program began to phase in $6.4 billion of prospective payment for capital. "Old" (preexisting) hospital capital will continue to be partially cost reimbursed, but at a 10 percent discount. This phase-in schedule allows hospitals to adjust their capital spending patterns in line with the new limited revenue stream. Over the past three decades capital spending as a fraction of operating expenses increased from 5.1 to 9.13 percent of costs. This inflation was largely fueled by cost reimbursement and expanding medical technology. When Congress began to phase in DRGs in 1983, it deliberately ducked the issue of capital payments and continued to pay for capital on a cost-reimbursement basis. However, each year the federal government tightened the reimbursement formula, paying only 85 percent of Medicare's fair share (market share) in the late 1980s. Starting in 1992, the average hospital will receive $692 per case in capital payments. A low-cost hospital that spends less than its capital allowance will be allowed to keep the difference and spend it in other areas (e.g., enhanced labor productivity or quality assurance). However, a high-cost hospital spending too much on capital (exceeding its allowance) will have to either defer expensive capital expenses or find the extra dollars elsewhere (from non-Medicare patients).

MERGERS, COMPETITION, AND COST CONTROL

Recent evaluations of mergers suggest that cost control for society, in terms of lower costs for the community, will not be a primary benefit of the organizational marriage. Greene (1990) surveyed the result of a Health Care Investment

Analysts (HCIA) study of financial results two years before and after mergers. The results suggest that mergers slightly improved profitability by reducing expenses and increasing gross and net patient revenues. The results contradict any claim that mergers save patients money, because the rise in billed charges more than makes up for any cost cuts; that is, cost reductions are not partially passed on to consumers through reduced patient expenses. Most of the 36 merging facilities realized that one cannot merge a little bit; a merger is all or nothing. Some hospitals also experience marginal cost increases in overhead due to the Noah's ark effect, the urge to keep two of everything, such as two department heads in too many areas of each hospital after the merger. Such lack of cost cutting does not make sense, unless one thinks that the hospital exists as an employment program for hospital employees. In a competitive world, cost control and product enhancement (quality) are keys to success. Merger participants must also consider Department of Justice antitrust concerns (Guthrie 1990). Recently cost functions have been used to analyze spatial competition and cooperation (Luke 1991).

For the traditional economist, nonprice competition is to competition what noncontact sex is to sex, a poor approximation at best. Friedman and Shortell (1988) reported that price competition for HMO business kicked in during the early 1980s. Robinson and Luft (1988) did a good job of studying nonprice competition or rivalry behavior to maximize prestige and acquisition of hospital technology. Noneconomic competition for prestige creates higher costs. Robinson and Luft also reported from a sample of 5,490 hospitals in 1986 that investor-owned hospitals experienced rates of cost increase 11.6 percent higher than those of tax-exempt private hospitals and 15 percent higher than those of public hospitals. They indicated that in the period 1983–85 the average inflation-adjusted cost per nonelderly patient declined 0.71 percent in high-competition markets and increased 2.82 percent in low-competition markets. Market failure may be prevalent in the hospital industry, but competition does have the expected impact on hospital costs (contrary to the results of their previous studies in an era of cost reimbursement; Robinson and Luft 1987).

EVOLVING A LEANER ORGANIZATION

Hospitals should annually reevaluate their workload-driven staffing ratio in line with fiscal goals and shifts in payment rates. Managers should use "best-cost" standards from engineering studies. Staff need to realize that downstaffing usually correlates with better-quality care (Walton 1990) and that staff-to-patient ratios can be cut by over 15 percent in many cases (e.g., Emanuel Hospital in Portland in 1990 and Beloit Hospital in Wisconsin in 1987). White Memorial Medical Center in East Los Angeles reduced nursing hours per patient day from 10 in 1988 to 7.1 by September 1990, while total FTEs per adjusted patient day declined from 4.94 to 4.0. Redundant staffing in a fat organization leads to low-quality care (Ahmadi 1989; Caldwell, McEachern, and Davis 1990).

In direct-patient-care departments bureaucracy, paperwork, and other useless units of activity should be eliminated. One hospital had six patient charting forms until this process was replaced by a single flow sheet in 1991. Lab results should be reported to the floor and the emergency department by computer, and medication orders should be either faxed to the pharmacy or sent by computer systems to eliminate the need to transcribe orders. The modern hospital should realize that its employees are increasingly members of the MTV television generation and should communicate productivity messages and Deming-method teamwork results to staff through interactive visual communication. Changes can be added to the disk each month, and employees can run their disks at home or in the hospital. The next chapter will provide a more theoretical discussion of hospital and physician behavior.

REFERENCES

Ahmadi, M. (1989). "Traditional versus Nontraditional Work Schedules." *Industrial Management* 31:2 (March–April), 20–23.

Aiken, L. (1990). "Charting the Future of Hospital Nursing." *Image: The Journal of Nursing Scholarship* 22:2 (February), 72–77.

Aiken, L., and Mullinix, C. (1987). "The Nurse Shortage—Myth or Reality." *New England Journal of Medicine* 317:10 (October 18), 641–651.

Anderson, G. (1991). "The Number and Cost of Excess Hospital Beds." AHSI Consulting Report, Johns Hopkins University.

Arndt, M., and Bigelow, B. (1992). "Vertical Integration in Hospitals." *Medical Care Review* 49:1 (Spring), 93–115.

Arthur Young and Policy Analysis Inc. (1987). *Study of the Financing of Graduate Medical Education*. 2 vols. Report DHHS 100–87–0155. Washington, D.C.: DHHS (January).

Bennett, M., and Hylton, J. (1990). "Modular Nursing: Partners in Professional Practice." *Nursing Management* 21:3 (March), 20–24.

Booth, L. (1991). "Influence of Production Technology on Risk and the Cost of Capital." *Journal of Financial and Quantitative Analysis* 26:1 (March), 109–127.

Caldwell, C., McEachern, J., and Davis, V. (1990) "Measurement Tools Eliminate Guesswork." *Healthcare Forum Journal* 11:4 (July/August), 23–28.

Chambers, R.G. (1988). *Applied Production Analysis*. Cambridge: Cambridge University Press.

Charns, A., Cooper, W., and Thrall, R. (1981). "Evaluating Program and Managerial Efficiency: Application of DEA Analysis." *Management Science* 27:6 (June), 668–697.

Cleverley, W. (1990). "ROI: Its Role in Voluntary Hospital Planning." *Hospital and Health Services Administration* 35:1 (Spring), 71–82.

Congressional Budget Office. (1991). *Rising Health Care Costs: Causes, Implications, and Strategies*. Washington, D.C.: CBO, U.S. Congress.

Deming, W. (1986). *Out of the Crisis*. Cambridge, Mass.: Massachusetts Institute of Technology Press, Center for Advanced Engineering.

Eastaugh, S. (1991) Testimony in Multicare Medical Center vs State of Washington, U.S. District Court, March-April, C88–421Z.

————. (1990). "Hospital Nursing Technical Efficiency: Nurse Extenders and Enhanced Productivity." *Hospital and Health Services Administration* 35:4 (Winter), 561–573.

————. (1987). *Financing Health Care*. Dover, Mass.: Auburn House, 657–683.

————. (1985). "Improving Hospital Productivity under PPS: Managing Cost Reductions without Harming Service Quality or Access." *Hospitals and Health Services Administration* 30:4 (July/August), 97–111.

————. (1982). "Effectiveness of Community-based Hospital Planning: Some Recent Evidence." *Applied Economics* 14:5 (October), 475–490.

Eastaugh, S., and Eastaugh, J. (1991). "Economic Malpractice: Inappropriate Use of Cost Analysis." *Annals of Emergency Medicine* 20:8 (August) 944–945.

————. (1990). "Putting the Squeeze on Emergency Medicine: The Many Pressures on Today's E.D." *Hospital Topics* 68:4 (Fall), 21–26.

Eastaugh, S., and Regan-Donovan, M. (1990). "Nurse Extenders Offer a Way to Trim Staff Expenses." *Healthcare Financial Management* 44:4 (April), 58–62.

Feldstein, P. (1989). *Health Care Economics*. 3d ed, New York: Wiley Medical.

Finkler, S. (1979). "On the Shape of the Long Run Average Cost Curve. *Health Services Research* 14:4 (Winter), 281–289.

Friedman, B., and Pauly, M. (1981). "Cost Functions for a Service Firm with Variable Quality and Stochastic Demand: The Case of Hospitals." *Review of Economics and Statistics* 63:4 (November), 620–624.

Friedman, B., and Shortell, S. (1988). "Financial Performance of Selected Investor-owned and Not-for-Profit Systems." *Health Services Research* 23:2 (June), 188–211.

Fuchs, V. (1986). *The Health Economy*. Cambridge, Mass.: Harvard University Press.

Glandon, G., and Counte, M. (1992). "Measurement of Hospital Financial Position." *Public Budgeting and Financial Management* 4:1 (Spring), 57–82.

Grannemann, T., Brown, T., and Pauly, M. (1986). "Estimating Hospital Costs: A Multiple-Output Analysis." *Journal of Health Economics* 5:2 (June), 107–127.

Greene, J. (1990). "Do Mergers Work?" *Modern Healthcare* 20:11 (March 19), 24–36.

Grosskopf, S., and Valdmanis, V. (1987). "The Measurement of Productive Efficiency" *Journal of Health Economics* 6:1 (July) 89–97.

Guthrie, M. (1990). "Mergers in Health Care." *Journal of Healthcare Marketing* 10:1 (March), 47–52.

Health Care Investment Analysts (HCIA). (1991). *Changing Profitability: Investor-owned versus Public and Nonprofits*. Baltimore: HCIA.

Hellinger, F. (1975). "Specification of a Hospital Production Function." *Applied Economics* 7:2 (March), 149–160.

Hsia, C. (1991). "Estimating a Firm's Cost of Capital." *Journal of Business Finance & Accounting* 18:2 (January) 281–287.

Huang, Y., and McLaughlin, C. (1989). "Relative Efficiency in Rural Primary Health Care: Application of Data Envelopment Analysis." *Health Services Research* 24:2 (June), 143–157.

Johnston, J. (1989). *Econometric Methods*. 4th ed. London: McGraw-Hill.

Kalirajan, K., and Shand, R. (1989). "A Generalized Measure of Technical Efficiency." *Applied Economics* 21:1 (January), 25–34.

Keating, B. (1984). "Cost Shifting: An Empirical Examination of Hospital Bureaucracy." *Applied Economics* 16:3 (July), 279–289.

Kellermann, A., and Ackerman, T. (1988). "Interhospital Patient Transfer: The Case for Informed Consent." *New England Journal of Medicine* 319:8, 643–647.

Klein, L. (1989). "Experimental Nursing Tech Program Strengthens Staff." *Federation of American Health Systems Review* 22:4 (July–August), 27–30.

Lee, R. (1990). "The Economics of Group Practice: A Reassessment" in *Advances in Health Economics and Health Services Research*, ed. Scheffler, R., Greenwich: JAI. 111–129

Lenehan, G. (1988). "The AMA's Registered Care Technologist Proposal: Old Wine in New Bottles." *Journal of Emergency Nursing* 14:5 (May), 268–271.

Levit, K., and Cowan, C. (1992). "Business, Households, and Governments Health Care Costs," *Health Care Financing Review* 13:2 (Winter), 83–93.

Luke, R. (1991). "Spatial Competition and Cooperation in Local Hospital Markets." *Medical Care Review* 48:2 (Summer), 207–237.

Manthey, M. (1989). "Practice Partnerships: The Newest Concept in Care Delivery." *Journal of Nursing Administration* 19:2 (February), 33–35.

———. (1988). "Primary Practice Partners: A Nurse Extender System." *Nursing Management* 19:6 (June), 58–59.

———. (1970). "A Dialogue on Primary Nursing." *Nursing Forum* 9:4 (April), 356–379.

McCarthy, S. (1989). "The Future of Nursing Practice and Implications for Nurse Education." *Journal of Professional Nursing* 5:3 (March), 121–168.

McClain, J., and Eastaugh, S. (1983). "How to Forecast to Contain Your Variable Costs." *Hospital Topics* 61:6 (November/December), 4–9.

Medicus System Corporation. (1989). *Inpatient Nursing Productivity and Quality System (NPAQ)*. Evanston, Ill.: Medicus (and *Nursing Management* 20 (May 1989), 30–33).

Mitchell, S. (1991). "Medicare's Capital PPS." *Health Systems Review* 24:2 (March/April), 57–58.

Pauly, M. (1990). "Financing Health Care." *Quarterly Review of Economics and Business* 30:4 (Winter), 63–80.

———. (1988). "Market Power, Monopsony, and Health Insurance," *Journal of Health Economics* 7:2 (October) 111–128.

Pauly, M., and Wilson, P. (1986). "Hospital Output Forecasts and the Cost of Empty Hospital Beds." *Health Services Research* 21:3 (August), 403–428.

Powers, P., Dickey, C., and Ford, A. (1990). "Evaluating an RN/Co-Worker Model." *Journal of Nursing Administration* 20:3 (March), 11–15.

Robinson, J., and Luft, H. (1988). "Competition, Regulation, and Hospital Costs." *Journal of the American Medical Association* 260:18 (November 11), 2676–2681.

———. (1987). "Competition and the Cost of Hospital Care." *Journal of the American Medical Association* 257:23 (June 11), 3241–3245.

Salmon, J. (1991). *The Corporate Transformation of Health Care*. Part 2, *Perspectives and Implications*. Amityville, N.Y.: Baywood.

Schaafsma, J. (1986). "Average Hospital Size and the Total Operating Expenditures for Beds Distributed Over H Hospitals." *Applied Economics* 18:1 (April), 279–290.

Schwartz, W., and Mendelson, D. (1991). "Hospital Cost Containment in the 1980s. *New England Journal of Medicine* 324:15 (April 11), 1037–1042.

Secretary's Commission on Nursing. (1988). *Final Report to DHHS*. Vol. 2. Washington, D.C.: DHHS (December).

Sherman, D. (1988). *The Effect of State Certificate of Need Laws on Hospital Costs.* Washington, D.C.: Federal Trade Commission.

Shorr, A. (1991). *The Optimizer: Productivity Evaluation Methodology for Scheduling Staff with Linear Programming.* Tarzana, Calif.: Shorr Associates.

Shukla, R. (1983a). "Technical and Structural Support Systems and Nurse Utilization." *Inquiry* 20:4 (Winter), 381–389.

———. (1983b). "All RN Model of Nursing Care Delivery: A Cost-Benefit Evaluation." *Inquiry* 20:2 (Summer), 173–184.

Shultz, M. (1991). "Strategic Capital Planning: Systems Look Toward the Future." *Trustee* 44:10 (October), 10–12.

Siegel, J. (1989). "Interhospital Patient Transfer." *New England Journal of Medicine* 320:3 (January 19), 258–259.

Steinwachs, D. (1992). "Redesign of Delivery Systems to Enhance Productivity." In S. Shortell, ed., *Improving Health Policy and Management.* Chicago: ACHE.

Thorpe, K. (1988). "Why Are Urban Hospital Costs So High? The Relative Importance of Patient Source of Admission, Teaching, Competition, and Case Mix." *Health Services Research* 22:6 (February), 821–836.

Valdmanis, V. (1990). "Ownership and Technical Efficiency of Hospitals." *Medical Care* 28:6 (June), 552–561.

Vogel, R., and Frant, H. (1992). "On the Allocation of Revenues from User Fees." *Public Budgeting and Financial Management* 4:1 (Spring), 171–194.

Walton, M. (1990). *Deming Management at Work.* New York: G.P. Putnam.

Wedig, G. (1992). "Net Present Value Rules and Hospital Investment Decisions." *Public Budgeting and Financial Management* 4:1 (Spring), 33–55.

Young, W., and Maciose, D. (1992). "Product Line Analysis using PMCs versus DRGs." *Public Budgeting and Financial Management* 4:1 (Spring), 83–106.

II ECONOMIC MODELS AND PHYSICIAN BEHAVIOR

3 Economic Models of Physician and Hospital Behavior

The system is always driven by the factor in short supply. We now have a short supply of patients, not doctors.

—Walter McClure

The first step in the analysis of the medical-care market is a comparison between the actual market and the competitive model.

—Kenneth Arrow

The literature on physician and hospital behavior has been characterized by two approaches: utility-maximization models (Feldstein 1970; Eastaugh 1981) or profit-maximization models (Sloan 1976; Baumol 1988). Supporters of the first approach view classical maxims concerning simple profit maximization as totally unrealistic. Supporters of the profit-maximization approach view utility maximizers as unnecessarily fuzzy and complex. The situation is complicated because the hospital is an organizational anomaly. The principal input controlling the organization is a group of individuals—the physicians—who neither own nor work as employees of the firm. Rather than work with the unique aspects of the doctor-hospital interaction, most conservative economists have opted for standard competitive analysis of a two-element utility function (profit and slack or leisure) as the best first approximation to physician and hospital behavior (Pauly and Redisch 1973). Advocates of the profit-maximization model maintain that if a multifaceted model and a simple model work almost equally well, one should prefer the simpler version. Models with "excessive" realism are viewed as a mixed blessing, because they complicate empirical implementation. In some cases the simple and complex formulations perform equally well, but their explanatory power is too low to place any confidence in the models. Morrisey and Jensen (1990) provided an example of a hybrid hospital utility-maximization/profit-maximization model of the hospital's demand for physicians. They concluded that physicians should be concerned about reduced access to hospitals as the supply of hospital beds declines in the 1990s.

All economic models posit some degree of profit maximization in the physician's utility function, where profit is defined as net earnings above practice overhead costs and above an imputed basic wage for the profession. The specification of an imputed wage allows for formal consideration of the clinician's trade-off of leisure for income. The physician utility function (U) includes some of the following elements: profit, leisure time, professional status, internal ethics, complexity of case mix, study time to keep up-to-date, number of support staff under the physician's supervision, and so on. Sometimes the utility function is stated in negative terms; for example, the disutility of working more or the disutility to the physician of coercing doctor-induced patient visits. In stark contrast to more traditional markets, the percentage of patient visits that is supplier initiated is very high (39 percent; Wilensky and Rossiter 1980). We can infer little about the medical necessity of these patient visits. Both groups of theorists, profit maximizers and utility maximizers, agree that physician behavior is too complicated to explain merely by profit motives, but the first group is adamant in asserting that as in any other business, profit (net income plus perks) is the most important element.

Another element of the physician's utility function is the desire to treat an interesting complex of cases. Feldstein (1970) was the first to incorporate the need for interesting cases into a model. The inclusion of such provider-taste variables in a model is often ridiculed by conservative economists in spite of demonstrable physician mobility in pursuit of interesting cases. Many physicians are able to change their subspecialty, mode of practice, or locus of practice (HMO, hospital-based, private office) every few years to ensure an interesting patient case mix.

EARLY EVIDENCE OF SUPPLIER-INDUCED DEMAND

The conventional wisdom among many health economists studying pre–1972 data was that excess consumer demand grants physicians an unusually high degree of discretionary power to affect both the quantity and price of their services. Contrary to traditional competitive economic analysis, higher physician density per capita has been shown to correlate with higher (Dyckman 1978; Institute of Medicine 1976; Newhouse and Phelps 1974) or unchanged (Holahan et al. 1978) physician fees. One should introduce the caveat that correlation does not prove causality; for example, the direction of causality might be reversed. Physician density increases where fees are currently higher and more easily inflated in the future. However, there were three main hypotheses for explaining the mechanism by which physicians might maintain income levels in response to increased physician density and presumably somewhat more active competition among physicians.

Feldstein (1971) suggested that when physician density increases, physicians simply reduce the percentage of patient need that goes untreated in this market of permanent excess demand. Unpublished studies by the Canadian government supported this theory and suggested that one could increase physician density to five times the national average and still have excess demand. Feldstein and others ignored the issue of whether this excess demand is medically necessary. Health marketing practitioners are attempting to grasp the prickly nettle of how physicians affect consumer taste and induce the consumption of unnecessary medical services. In this respect, the growing discipline of marketing goes beyond the purview of traditional microeconomics; for example, one does not assume that preferences and taste are determined independently of the economic system. A second hypothesis advanced by a number of economists (Evans 1974; Fuchs and Kramer 1973) is that much of this new demand is physician generated rather than permanently existing.

Both of these aforementioned hypotheses postulate a unique ability of physicians to affect consumer demand. If physicians are unable to maintain a target level of demand, they can still maintain a target income by increasing fees in response to declining demand for their services. This third hypothesis has been reported by Newhouse (1970). These three hypotheses are not mutually exclusive. Physicians can maintain a target income by inflating prices, treating more elective conditions, or some combination of the two. As we shall see in a later section, one group of physicians (general practitioners) has been found to be less capable of maintaining a target income because the market for their particular services is relatively competitive. Therefore, they must act as price takers.

The question of the appropriate health manpower ratios per capita has been a subject for lively debate among public policy makers since 1960. The federal government has played a large role in providing the funds to expand medical school output. If an increased per capita supply of a given type of physician appears to cause both slightly higher prices and higher utilization, then Congress might consider more substantial controls on medical school capacity and residency training programs.

The benefits of a doctor oversupply (such as aggressive price competition) had not been flowing to the consumers because physicians would band together in tight trade-union groups and payers were naive enough to pay a provider-set price. The situation was largely reversed in the mid–1980s, and payers are "calling the tune," to paraphrase Fuchs (1986). One study suggested that physicians began to disperse to relatively underserved locations in response to competitive pressures as early as 1979 (Newhouse et al., 1982a). After a steep rise in physician supply in the 1970s, the annual number of physicians receiving licenses increased at a much slower rate in the 1980s (Moore and Priebe 1991). The slower rate of growth in physician supply per capita and changes in the epidemiology and treatment of disease (e.g., more AIDS cases, less inpatient surgery) render obsolete most predictions about physician supply (such as Graduate Medical Education National Advisory Committee [GMENAC] 1980). Physician manpower and reimbursement issues will be presented in chapter 4.

Supplier induced demand (SID) offers the obvious possibility of a conflict of interest: the physician provides extra service to generate income. The evidence is usually indirect by nature. For example, Broward County, Florida, has 19 doctor-owned Magnetic Resonance Imaging (MRI) machines and 41 MRI procedures per 1,000 population. Baltimore County, Maryland, has one doctor-owned MRI and two medical schools, but only 12 MRI procedures per 1,000 in 1991. Are the physicians at Johns Hopkins and University of Maryland underserving their patients, or is it more likely that the Florida physicians are generating unnecessary patient volume to cost-justify (break-even) or profit from their MRI business ventures? Is the urban number for utilization per 1,000 citizens too low in Baltimore or too high in Florida? Classical economic theory would predict that competition would keep the price of an MRI scan down in Florida. However, the charge in Broward County is nearly double the Baltimore price, and all the extra utilization is performed on nonpoor insured patients. Under the new 1992 regulations, in order to avoid prosecution under the anti-kickback law, a physician who has invested in an outside MRI facility or lab must meet the following six tests: (1) dividends must be related to the amount of capital contributed (not to the number of patients referred); (2) ownership does not impose a requirement on the physician to refer patients; (3) the equity and price of shares in the outside facility must be the same for referring physicians and all other investors; (4) the facility must not give loans to the physician; (5) no more than 40 percent of the revenue received by the outside facility can come from those who have investments in it, and (6) no more than 40 percent of the investors can be physicians.

SUPPLIER-INDUCED DEMAND, DENSITY, AND TARGET INCOMES

At the extreme, supplier inducement is characterized as a sinister form of demand creation in which clinicians provide large amounts of unnecessary or marginally helpful care for their own monetary gain. On the other hand, other analysts have argued that supplier inducement is an argument for strict government regulation of medical school class size (and bed capacity) because each additional doctor brought with him or her $400,000 of additional expense in the health budget. Supplier inducement was often simplistically explained by statements like "To know if you need to see a doctor you have to see a doctor, so demand does not exist, but patient needs do exist." However, subsequent empirical studies have demonstrated that demand is not largely supply determined, and both demand and supply are simultaneously driven by economic variables (Newhouse et al.1982b).

Supporters of the supplier-induced-demand (SID) theory have argued that doctors can create enough physician-initiated new services to counteract a rise in the markets' physician density and to maintain a target income without lowering fees. One physician was so bold as to state: "The doctor glut is not a problem, it's the undersupply of patients." Neurologists and plastic surgeons seem fully persuaded that they possess enough leeway to tell patients what they should "demand" (Mencken 1983; Reinhardt 1985). Advocates of the SID theory disregard the 6 percent annual decline in visits per physician during the period 1983–86 because it does not fit with their theory and argue that manipulative physicians will still make a target income by searching for frill markets catering to consumer fantasies. This may be true for noninsured services, catering to Yuppie boutique medicine, but insurers and employers will not reimburse for these services.

The SID theory for hospital-bed utilization has not received much support. The original Milton Roemer's law stated that a "bed built is a bed filled." While this may have been true in 1959, evidence by Ferguson and Crawford (1989) rejected the SID hypothesis. A more recent study by Rohrer (1990) suggested that Roemer's law is a statistical artifact of poor research design, because population data were not derived from actual population experience. Rohrer used patient-origin data in rural Iowa and found that bed supply per capita was not related to higher utilization rates. Instead, the number of unique hospital services was associated with higher utilization rates. In this context, one could postulate a Rohrer's law: An area with a greater variety of hospital services available will have somewhat higher hospital usage rates. This suggests that a hospital market with more specialization and less wide variety of service product-line availability will have lower hospitalization rates.

The major effect of increased physician density might be a shift in referral patterns among physicians and other providers. By comparing aggregated physician utilization data in 15 Michigan market areas, Stano (1985) concluded that the availability effect was due to the larger number of providers seen by patients in physician-dense markets. Physicians are more likely to refer, and patients are more likely to shop, in physician-dense areas. While aggregate data conformed to the SID hypothesis (e.g., a 1 percent increase in surgeon density increased per capita surgical use in the short run 0.14 percent in 1980), data from individual practices did not conform to the SID hypothesis. Data from the individual medical or surgical practices did not indicate that physicians treated their patients more intensely as physician density increased (Stano 1985). Moreover, the aggregate short-run inducement in per capita utilization reported by Stano may be dissipated in the long run by market forces, as is the case in the dental and lawyer markets (Satterthwaite 1979).

One could argue that the physician supply expansion is a major force in the development of managed-care systems, HMOs, PPOs, and the entire medical community's increased susceptibility to cost-containment initiatives. If consumers are increasingly in the driver's seat in the selection of a health plan, and physicians are no longer perceived as being in short supply, the health sector will become even more market driven. Any economic system is driven by the element in short supply—currently, patients. Increases in physician density may increase physician-initiated hospital visits or doctor visits, but as McCombs (1984) suggested, we shall begin to experience a physician-initiated attempt to restrict dollar flows to nonphysicians (e.g., anesthesiologists and Certified Registered Nurse Anesthetists [CRNAs]). McCombs accurately predicted a decline in hospital days per episode and a reduction in referrals to alternative providers (physician extenders, freestanding nurse practitioners) in market regions with increased physician density. Physicians are like any other professional group; they dislike competition and do not favor "professional helpers" developed in times of a doctor shortage when their volume of visits per week is on the decline.

The evidence for supplier inducement is weak in a poorly insured market segment such as primary ambulatory care. McCarthy (1985) examined the primary-care physician services market in over 100 cities in the 1975 AMA data base. The sample was restricted to urban areas since competitive forces, if they are to be found, should most likely exist in large urban areas. His results using 1975 data are consistent with monopolistic competition. Given the plentiful entry of physicians into primary care since 1975, the current marketplace should be even more competitive. Demand creation seems a trivial by-product of rising physician density in both the McCarthy (1985) and Sweeney (1982) studies. What little demand creation does exist might only be on paper.

Physicians can unbundle billings into several separately reimbursable activities. Physicians are intelligent professionals who may be tempted to minimize the decline in their incomes in a period of declining patient demand. Aggressive claims review and peer review actions will reduce the prevalence of such unbundling. One of the by-products of increased overseeing of physicians' activities is the increased production of information. Whether employers, insurers, and individuals utilize this information to value shop is the subject of chapter 9.

Fuchs (1986) studied the surgeon manpower supply equilibrium and the problem of provider-induced demand. If surgeons do partially shift demand upward by 3 to 3.5 percent to compensate for a 10 percent expansion in surgeons per capita and also increase price to minimize the potential reduction in income to a few percentage points, the current high number of surgical residency programs may be a major problem in cost containment. In the short term we could not reduce the supply of surgeon man-hours, because the postgraduate training pipeline prevents surgical subspecialists from reaching their maximum productive level for 7 to 10 years. Surgeons have suggested from time to time that surgery should be done only by specialists, but they have not supported a policy that would discourage medical students from entering the field; rather, they minimize the effects of competition by finding new patients and new conditions on which to operate (Wennberg 1986). According to Reinhardt (1989), econometric estimation can not divine what proportion of observed utilization was simply accepted by sick patients (or anxious relatives) and what proportion the patients would have demanded of their own free will had they been as well informed as their physicians. Pauly (1988) agreed that we will never solve the creation/information-imperfection question. As a practical matter the Physician Payment Reform Commission (PPRC 1991) has advised Congress to increase utilization and peer review efforts.

SERVICE-RATE VARIABILITY

A number of studies have evaluated small-area variations (SAVs) in per capita use rates of health services, surgery, and medical expenditures. Many of the early studies were done by Wennberg. Wennberg (1985) provided a classic case of the wide variability of clinical practice patterns with his small-area population-based methodology. Admission rates were analyzed based on epidemiologic techniques to track patients by location and not simply by hospital, such that transfers outside the service area were "charged back" to the patient's home area. Wide tenfold variations in surgical rates per capita were uncovered, with little apparent reason for such variability. Some of the more recent data on variability in surgical admission rates may be explained by differential use of ambulatory surgery. Of the 13 operations having wide inpatient operative variability in the Wennberg studies, 11 have been identified as prime candidates for ambulatory surgery (Lagoe and Milliren 1986). However, the volume of ambulatory surgery is sufficiently low and the variation in operative rates is sufficiently wide to ask the medical community to address this issue. Physicians in Iowa and Maine have successfully adjusted their hospitalization habits in reaction to such information of atypically high rates (Wennberg 1986). In contrast, the Massachusetts medical society has been rather unresponsive following two replications of the Wennberg approach (Barnes et al. 1985).

Excessive rates of elective hospitalization often occur in the last year of life. For example, Maine urologists were stunned to discover that 47 percent of their prostatectomy patients discharged to nursing homes were dead within a year after the procedure. The Maine urologists suddenly started doing fewer prostatectomies the next year (10 percent fewer in 1984, 15 percent fewer thereafter). One Maine urologist summarized the educational process: "Why do the surgery if this does nothing for the quantity of life of this subgroup of surgical-eligibles, especially when the act of surgery harms the quality of life?" On the more technical level, this example suggests that physicians can become more sensitive to the population-based destiny of certain patient groups. Obviously, the cost-saving potential if the operative rate for certain conditions is brought down 15, 25, or 35 percent is substantial, and therein lies the attraction of small-area analysis, in comparison to DRG price controls, as a cost-reduction strategy.

The Wennberg methodology raises a number of technical questions. For example, if one pools a number of years of data for each of the small areas, will the variability in operative rates be as significant? As Caper (1986) and Wennberg and Gittelsohn (1982) reported, the patterns of high-usage levels for a condition are generally stable over time, even after more than two years of data are pooled. Analysis of four years of data in Iowa and five to nine years' worth of data in Maine, Rhode Island, and Vermont indicates stable wide operative variations across demographically similar populations.

The variability in practice-style patterns, the "medical signatures," may be more significant outside of surgery. The admission rates for medical conditions, including chest pain, atherosclerosis, and congestive heart failure, are highly variable (California Health Facilities Commission [CHFC] 1985; Wennberg, McPherson, and Caper 1984). The necessity of inpatient care is less clearly defined for these conditions, and physicians differ widely from area to area as to when hospitalization is appropriate. In contrast, certain surgical procedures have low variability in operative rates: appendectomy, cholecystectomy, hernia repair, lens extraction, and mastectomy.

Chassin et al. (1986) reported on geographic differences in Medicare usage of medical and surgical services for 13 regions. This Rand Corporation study team reported that use rates were not consistently high in one region, but rates for procedures utilized to diagnose and treat a specific condition did vary together. Unfortunately for those who advocate reeducation or sanctions as a policy solution, the Rand results could not be explained by the actions of a small number of physicians. One does not know whether physicians in high-usage areas perform too many procedures or whether those in low-use areas perform too few. One former AMA president suggested that those who believe that economics alone should become the holy grail have a bias in favor of suggesting that the low rate is the correct rate (Boyle 1985). Wennberg (1986) suggested that some evidence exists in support of the low rate being closer to the "correct" rate, and that lowering the rates does no measurable harm.

A number of SAV studies have been done since Wennberg's early work. Holahan, Berenson, and Kachavos (1990) studied select Medicare procedures and concluded that a 10 percent increase in specialists per capita would increase dermatologists' workload for two popular conditions by 6.3 to 6.7 percent, would increase carotid endarterectomies (done by thoracic surgeons and general surgeons) by 6.7 percent, would increase arthrocentesis by 5.6 percent, and would increase colonoscopy by gastroenterologists by 3.3 percent. One should question the validity of SAV studies, although their utility to assist peer review programs in targeting areas of potential excess utilization is obvious. SAV advocates often have an implicit presumption at the ecological level that observations at the aggregate (county) level also imply similar relationships at the individual level of one doctor and one patient (McLaughlin et al. 1989; Howell and McLaughlin 1988). Folland and Stano (1989) tried to minimize this problem by studying five years of data for 15 service areas and doing microcase studies. SAV analysis is a good method to identify areas for study, but the best research for drawing valid and reliable conclusions comes from microlevel studies (Roos 1989; Gillespie et al. 1989; Folland and Stano 1990). In this regard Diehr et al. (1990) presented improved standards for presenting SAV results and statistics. Some conditions exhibit a lower variability in operative rate—e.g., prostatectomy—but perhaps should be utilized less frequently for certain population segments (such as nursing home institutionalized patients with low life expectancy). We will return to the question of provider-induced demand in chapters 11 and 12, but first let us survey the economic literature concerning physician behavior.

Figure 3.1
Physician Labor Supply Curve: Upward-sloping Normality (SF) or Backward-bending Response (SB)

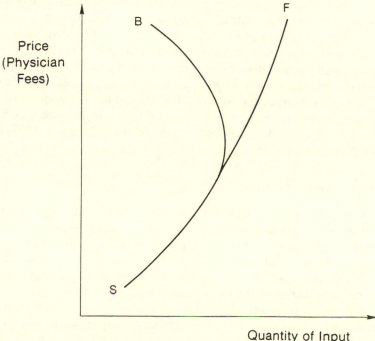

PHYSICIANS' SUPPLY CURVES

Whether a physician works more or less as a result of an increase or decrease in physician wages is an important subject for public policy. Depending on the physicians' labor supply curve, physicians could decide to work harder and substitute more patient care for leisure (the substitution effect). Alternatively, physicians could decide that their income is sufficiently high to afford increased leisure time in preference to a higher workload. They would consequently work less (the income effect). An important point to remember is that even if the supply curve for a given individual physician is backward-bending (*SB* in figure 3.1), the physicians' aggregate labor supply curve may instead be uniformly upward-sloping (*SF* in figure 3.1), as is usually the case in most labor markets.

The research results on this issue are mixed. Feldstein (1970) found strong support for the backward-bending supply curves. Sloan (1976) and Hu and Yang (1988) indicated no support for the position that physicians lie near the backward-bending portion of the labor supply curve and reported very low elasticities of supply. Vahovich (1977) reported empirical results intermediate between those of Sloan and Feldstein; he found slightly backward-bending supply curves and low elasticities of supply. In summary, physicians will not change their workload significantly in response to price controls or expanded health insurance coverage.

Brown and Lapan (1979) also corroborated the backward-bending labor supply hypothesis. Although they utilized aggregate time-series data, they operated under the hypothesis that physicians are price-taking utility maximizers rather than price setters. Their findings supported the view that physicians are on the backward-bending portion of the labor supply curve. A second interesting finding of this study was that nonphysician inputs (physician extenders, aides, and so on) substitute for declines in physician labor, so that the supply curve of physician-office services is always positively sloped (curve *SF* in figure 3.1). These findings utilizing aggregate data corroborate the results of Reinhardt (1975) using data for individual physician practices.

PHYSICIAN SUPPLY ESTIMATES

In 1980 the Graduate Medical Education National Advisory Committee (GMENAC 1980) estimated that by the year 2000 the nation would have 643,000 physicians, or 29 percent more than the perceived requirement according to the panel of distinguished physicians. Whether this estimate of a glut (oversupply) of 145,000 physicians will occur in the year 2000 depends on two factors: demand and supply. The demand curve for physician services should be recalculated in response to the unexpected rapid growth in HMOs and managed-care alternative delivery systems. For example, one proprietary study of a midwestern state suggested that if these prepaid systems control 80 percent of the market by 2000, 45 percent of the physicians (and 68 percent of the hospital beds) will be unnecessary. However, the market is dynamic, and conditions will change on the supply side. For example, the state medical school could admit 50 percent fewer students (following the Michigan example); physicians could work 15 to 25 percent shorter workweeks; foreign medical graduates could be substantially reduced (relative to GMENAC projections); and physicians could increasingly enter the field of administration. Therefore, hundreds of clinicians may receive training in administration, but few will resort to driving taxicabs or selling real estate because of a glut in the supply of physicians.

The original chairman of the GMENAC study later amended his manpower projections (Tarlov 1986). The projection of 643,000 physicians for the year 2000 can be downgraded by 17,000 to account for the lower number of first-year entrants to medical schools and transferees with advanced standing (from foreign schools to American schools; Crowley, Etzel, and Petersen 1985 reported 255 transfers in 1984). No definitive estimates were provided as to whether the estimate of 498,000 required physicians for 2000 should be downgraded by 20 to 40 percent. The estimate is highly dependent on the growth rate of prepaid systems, and to a lesser extent on the anticipated decline in the physician workweek. Steinwachs et al. (1986) utilized the GMENAC model to recalculate the requirements for certain physicians in HMOs. Extrapolating from productivity figures at three HMOs to 1990, they projected that HMOs will require only half the number of family physicians and internists and two-thirds the number of pediatricians in the GMENAC (1980) national estimates.

Competition between health plans might further improve the productivity figures over time, thus further reducing the required number of physicians. Declining consumer demand for clinical physician time bears a clear reciprocal relationship to increased availability of "free time" (for some combination of leisure, education, management activities, charity services, or research). Three trends seem apparent: In the future more physicians will be salaried, working less than 50 hours per week (even if not salaried), and involved in administration.

From 1966 to 1991 the estimated supply of physicians increased 122 percent, but the American population only increased 29 percent. The ratio of active physicians per 100,000 population increased from 169 in 1975 to 195 in 1980, 214 in 1985, and a projected 233 in 1991. Regulators favor the counsel of George Bernard Shaw in the preface to *The Doctor's Dilemma*: "Make up your mind how many doctors the community needs to keep it well, and do not register more or less than this number." However, the excess-supply problem is confined largely to specialists. Both the GMENAC (1980) study and Schroeder (1984) indicated that the European experience suggested that the most pressing health manpower problem is an oversupply of specialists. Whether this oversupply is a problem depends on one's point of view. For HMO or PPO managers negotiating fee discounts, this physician oversupply provides the bargaining leverage to save money and differentially select the most cooperative specialists. Specialists left out of managed-care systems in the 1990s are headed for two possible fates: serious financial trouble or membership in a union. As the formation of the AMA was a socioeconomic event to combat the cults in the nineteenth century, so specialty unions may form in the 1990s to combat the managed-care systems and "strike for quality care" (which helps defend their declining incomes). Ginzberg (1990) has argued for a number of years that physician incomes were bound to slide 40 percent relative to incomes of other Americans: "There is no reason for physicians to continue to earn 5.5 times as much as a skilled worker; a spread of 3.5 times is easier to justify."

PHYSICIANS' PRIVATE PRICING DECISIONS

Physician behavior has been presumed to vary on three very basic dimensions: (1) whether physicians act as price setters or price takers, (2) whether prices are sufficient to clear the market of excess demand, and (3) whether demand can be shifted or induced. Six types of physician pricing models have been developed by economists. The first three models we shall survey assume that the physician is a price setter; that is, third-party payers' reimbursement controls are not too constraining, and lack of competition allows the professional considerable freedom to set fees. According to the longest-standing physician pricing model, monopoly equilibrium (markets clear so that supply is brought into equilibrium with demand, and demand does not shift), physicians set prices as a discriminating monopolist (Kessel 1958; Newhouse 1970). Price discrimination involves charging what the individual patient can bear, not as an altruistic method of charging the poor less, but rather as a method of reaping monopoly profits by capturing all the area under the demand curve. (A demand curve is the schedule of quantity sold at various prices if a supplier offers one price to the entire marketplace. However, if a supplier could offer a spectrum of prices to the buyers so that each pays close to his or her maximum price, that would capture much more of the area under the demand curve; that is, the profits per unit of service would clearly be increased.) The growth in insurance coverage has all but eliminated the physician's ability to price discriminate, except in the case of out-of-pocket subspecialty fees paid by the rich for "star" physicians to perform transplants or heart surgery. A number of court cases made it impossible for organized medicine to maintain the discriminating pricing policies of the 1950s (Havighurst 1987).

The second model of physician pricing, monopolist demand creation, also assumes that the market clears, but demand is shifted as a result of price-setting decisions. This model assumes that the physician has the most power imaginable: Like a simple monopolist he can set fees irrespective of what the other physicians are doing, and he can manipulate consumer wants and inflate demands if necessary. Evans (1974) supported this difficult-to-test theory with empirical evidence on supplier-induced demand in Canada. The author also defended the omnipotent pricing powers of physicians in an earlier work (Evans 1973), which postulated that in markets with imperfect information on quality, the consumer is often led to believe that higher price means higher quality. Solid evidence of consumers searching for higher-priced providers would be a revolutionary attack against economic normality in medical markets. This pricing model has been rejected by Pauly (1980), Fuchs (1986), and Feldman and Sloan (1988).

A third physician pricing model involves simple monopolists' behavior in a market of chronic excess demand. This model is like model 2 in that physicians set prices irrespective of the market, but demand is not shifted and the market does not clear (excess demand is left unserved). This model is not manageable analytically; one can estimate neither a demand curve nor a supply curve. This model lacks advocates because it is largely untestable. It does have fleeting support from a number of different economists. Sloan (1976) advocated the idea of physicians acting as simple monopolists, and Feldstein (1970) in rejecting static and dynamic competitive models suggested that physician services are in a state of permanent excess demand, subject to various modes of nonprice rationing. Feldstein indicated that physicians benefit from a marketplace with permanent excess demand in which the profession can pick and choose among the most interesting case "material." In summary, none of these three models of physicians as price setters is firmly established as empirical fact, but the first and third models do have some support.

The last three models we shall survey are competitive models. Physicians are assumed to be such a small fraction of the marketplace that they must act as price takers. With the exception of the market for general practitioners and family practitioners, who comprise approximately 40 percent of all physicians, these competitive models are usually rejected by the econometric evidence of the authors. The fourth physician pricing model to consider is the classic competitive equilibrium model. Under conditions of competitive equilibrium, the market clears and demand is not shifted. This model has been tested on 20 years of time-series data by Feldstein (1970) and on cross-sectional data by Newhouse (1970), Fuchs and Kramer (1973), Newhouse and Phelps (1974), the Institute of Medicine (1976), and Dyckman (1978). Time-series data can be indicative of short-run behavior because practice resources are relatively fixed in the short or middle run of 5 to 15 years. Cross-sectional analysis provides more information concerning long-run behavior, assuming that the sample includes the range of various practice opportunities, in different stages of development. Analysis of a time series of cross-sections allows the researcher to construct a more complete set of structural equations for supply and demand relationships (Eastaugh 1981). All six of these studies rejected the competitive equilibrium hypothesis and reported positive coefficients for physicians per capita or surgeons per capita in their price equations. The positive association between price and physician supply ratios is inconsistent with competitive models. (The observed low price elasticities the studies surveyed in Table 3.1 are also not consistent with competition or simple profit-maximization theories. The price elasticity of demand for certain individual physicians will be substantially larger than the market price elasticities reported in the table.)

Many health professionals prior to the 1980s were quick to claim that competition had been eliminated in medical markets. Some of the aforementioned studies did not include the obvious caveat that physicians are not a homogenous group. The possibility exists that some subgroups of physicians or surgeons do exhibit competitive pricing behavior. Four studies supported this proposition. Steinwald and Sloan (1974) and Sloan (1976) reported mostly negative association between general practitioners' (GP) density and GP fees and a lower negative association between general surgeons' density and their fees. Holahan et al. (1978) also found the same relationships for GPs, but rejected any correlation in the case of general surgeons or internists. McLean (1980) derived structural equations for both the supply of and demand for GP services utilizing the American Medical Association's eighth periodic survey of physicians. McLean rejected the hypothesis that the market for GPs is perfectly competitive, but the high net price elasticity (-1.75) indicates a considerable degree of competition in the market. This price elasticity is larger than the price elasticity reported in any of the studies summarized in table 3.2. In summary, the competitive equilibrium model appears to have had validity in the case of general practitioners and possibly general surgeons as early as the 1970s.

The fifth physician pricing model can best be summarized as the oligopoly

Table 3.1
Summary of Nine Econometric Studies of Price Elasticity or Time Elasticity for Hospital and Physician Care

Data Source	Dependent Variable(s)	Elasticity with Respect to Price or Time
Phelps and Newhouse	Price elasticity for	
	(a) Physician home visits	-.35
	(b) Physician visits	-.14
	(c) Lab, X-ray, ancillary services	-.07
Davis and Russell	Outpatient visits	-1.00
Feldstein and Severson	Physician visits	-.19
Newhouse and Marquis	Physician visits	-1.00
Newhouse and Phelps	Physician visits	-.15 to -.20
Phelps	Physician visits (at 25% coinsurance)	-.20
Fuchs and Kramer	Physician expenditures	-.15 to -.35
Acton	Demand elasticity with respect to:	(Time Elasticity)
	(a) Travel time to M.D.'s office	-.25 to -.37
	(b) Waiting time for services	-.12
McGuirk and Porell	Travel time to hospital for obstetrics	-.45

target income hypothesis. The target income theory of pricing suggests markups in prices as input costs inflate or demand declines. The model presumes that the market clears, that demand will shift, and that demand can be manipulated by the physicians. The speed of adjustment depends on a number of factors, including information-collection costs. This model received some support from Feldstein (1970) and relatively less support from Vahovich (1977). Feldstein's study did not provide very strong statistical support for this theory, reporting mixed results in his demand and price adjustment equations. As Feldstein pointed out, reporting a low elasticity demand curve, finding a backward-bending supply curve, and inferring that price increases with excess demand seem very incompatible.

Sloan (1976) and Steinwald and Sloan (1974) soundly rejected the target income hypothesis. Green (1978) carried the argument one step further, reana-

Table 3.2
Money-Price Elasticities and Time-Cost Elasticities of Eight Econometric Studies of the Demand for Physician Services

Data Source	Dependent Variable(s)	Price Elasticity (computed at the mean)
Newhouse and Marquis	Hospital length of stay	-.05
Feldstein	Hospital days	
	(i) Short run	-.29
	(ii) Long run	-.13
Newhouse and Phelps	Hospital days	-.23
Davis and Russell	(a) Admissions	-.5
	(b) Hospital days	-.32 to -.46
Feldstein	(a) Admissions	-.43
	(b) Hospital days	-.26
Rosenthal	(a) Length of stay (depending on diagnosis)	0.0 to -.08
	(b) Patient days (depending on diagnosis)	-.01 to -.70
Rosett and Huang	Hospital and physician expenditures (at 20% coinsurance)	-.35
Manning	(a) Outpatient care	-.2 to -.29
	(b) All medical care	-.1 to -.14
	(c) Catastrophic coverage only of expenses above $1,000	-.2

lyzed the data from the Fuchs and Kramer (1973) study, and failed to reject the hypothesis that physicians cannot induce demand. Unfortunately, it is almost impossible to distinguish demand shifts resulting from changes in consumer tastes from shifts caused by physician manipulation of information to the consumer, or from shifts that are simply responses to changes in time price faced by the consumer. In summary, we can infer that "physician supply creating demand," or the so-called "availability effect," is not uniform or pervasive in either model 2 or model 5.

There is a sixth physician pricing model considered by Reinhardt (1975) and Pauly (1980), the possibility of competitive disequilibrium under price controls; that is, the market does not clear and demand is not shifted under private (insurance companies) or public (Economic Stabilization Program) price controls. Supply would consistently fall short of demand if the controls were too strict.

Figure 3.2
Taxonomy of Six Economic Models for Physician Behavior

1. Demand Shifts	2. Market Clearing Prices Achieved	3. Physicians Are Price-Setters	4. Physicians Are Price-Takers
NO	YES	**Model 1—** Monopoly Equilibrium	**Model 4—** Competitive Equilibrium
YES	YES	**Model 2—** Dynamic Demand Shifts	**Model 5—** Oligopolistic Target Income Levels
NO	NO	**Model 3—** Chronic Excess Demand Disequilibrium	**Model 6—** Exogeneous Price Ceilings

This is the traditional case of excess demand under price ceilings: Physicians acting as price takers only produce up to the point where marginal cost equals the price ceiling (typically less than what would be demanded of the physician at that "low" price; Ginsberg 1978). There is no empirical support for assuming that physicians presently pursue this sixth pricing model (Newhouse 1988).

In summary, there may be types of physicians for which all six of these economic models fail to work, while other significant groups of physicians behave in a manner that is reasonably consistent with a number of these models. As we shall observe in the next section, the Rand health insurance study provided strong support for the view that consumers are price sensitive and that physicians are increasingly price takers (consistent with models 4 and 6 in figure 3.2).

The early studies of price elasticity of demand were limited to small sample sizes, short time horizons, and most critically the total lack of randomization or selection of an appropriate control group (Newhouse 1988). Price elasticity refers to the responsiveness of the quantity of care demanded to changes in price, all other factors being held constant. For example, a -0.23 price elasticity with respect to hospital days translates into an expected 2.3 percent decline in hospital days resulting from a 10 percent increase in price. The price elasticity for minor or elective diagnoses is usually larger, but still inelastic (less than 1.0), whereas the price elasticity for life-threatening emergency care is very low; that is, price is of no consequence (table 3.1). Demand is also responsive to time cost, travel cost, and income (the Engel curve plots family income versus demand, yielding an income elasticity of demand). But patients are willing to sacrifice time and wages to seek a better-quality facility. Bronstein and Morrisey (1990) reported that a 5.0 percent increase in per capita income in the women's home county was associated with a 20 percent increase in actual travel distance for obstetrics services, other things being equal. The authors speculated that a rural hospital appears to be inferior goods in the economic sense: As incomes rise, rural citizens replace their small local hospital with better care in a neighboring city. A 1.0 percent increase in the per capita income in the county led to a 4.0 percent increase in the distance traveled for obstetrics services. Obstetrics is a special form of medical care, involving more time and opportunity to shop in comparison to acute-care emergency conditions. Other studies have looked at the opportunity cost of nonwork time (due to retirement) and the demand for physicians' services (Boaz and Muller 1989).

THE RAND HEALTH INSURANCE STUDY

The $60 million Rand health insurance experiment attempted to put some of the major research issues concerning the desirability and effectiveness of cost sharing to rest. Unlike the aforementioned retrospective studies, families in the Rand experiment were randomly assigned to different insurance plans. This randomization study, with long-run follow-up of the families, proved expensive but invaluable in overcoming the self-selection bias explicit in all previous studies of cost sharing. The experiment, which ran from November 1974 to January 1982, enrolled 7,706 people under age 62 at six study sites. Excluded from the experiment were rich families with incomes above the 97th percentile or persons too badly disabled and therefore eligible for Medicare. Families were assigned to one of 14 experimental insurance plans by a random-sampling technique that made the distribution of family characteristics as similar as possible (Manning et al. 1987). Each of the 14 plans was assigned to one of four basic categories (free care, 25 percent coinsurance, 50 percent coinsurance, or 95 percent coinsurance). There was a maximum loss provision of 5, 10, or 15 percent of family income, or $1,000 (in some sites during some years the maximum expenditure was limited to $750).

For both ambulatory care and hospital care, as the level of cost sharing increased, the family health expenditures declined (e.g., ambulatory-care annual expenses of $186 for free care, versus $149 under 25 percent coinsurance, $120 under 50 percent coinsurance, and $114 under 95 percent coinsurance, with a $1,000 maximum out-of-pocket cap). Contrary to the prevalent assumption in the 1970s, increased cost sharing for ambulatory care did not result in more use of inpatient services or increased overall costs. The probability of hospitalization actually declined with increased cost sharing (Manning et al. 1987). Ambulatory-care usage did not behave as a substitute or preventive service for inpatient care. The lower the cost sharing on ambulatory care, the greater the ambulatory utilization and the greater the likelihood of hospitalization. Once hospitalization began, cost sharing did not significantly affect hospital expenditures.

Insurance coverage did not affect the number of lab tests per ambulatory visit nor the duration of physician time during a visit (Danzon, Manning, and Marquis 1984). Other Rand study team reports indicated that cost sharing or insurance did not affect the cost of an ambulatory episode (Keeler and Rolph 1982). One should be careful about extrapolating these findings from a social experiment where Rand patients represented less than 1 percent of provider market share to a situation where providers might react to any activity affecting 15 to 50 percent of their patients (as in some two-company towns). In other words, Rand patients were a very small fraction of the business in any of the six sites.

Manning et al. (1987) also reported that expenditures by adults were more responsive to variation in cost sharing than expenditures for children. This suggests that families may not shop aggressively for price-competitive child care and perhaps suggests that a high proportion of child care represents truly "necessary services." However, adults covered by higher levels of cost sharing may often seek care less frequently or, if they have the information base on which to shop, may seek less costly sources of care (e.g., alternative providers). The rational consumers weigh the benefits of purchasing from their current suppliers against the costs and weigh the benefits of the search for lower prices or better value against the cost of this search (comparison shopping). There is little evidence to suggest aggressive shopping for lower-priced providers in the Rand data. Marquis (1985) found no evidence to suggest that consumers during the period 1974–81 shopped for lower-priced providers. As we shall see in chapter 6, employers will still promote cost sharing as a strategy to reduce the quantity, if not the direct price, of care. Perhaps the cost of search behavior will decline as more referral networks are set up for comparison shopping and more consumer handbooks are disseminated in the 1990s. Consumer shopping for a provider, on both a price and a quality basis, may become less costly and more fashionable in the near future (Eastaugh 1990). In chapters 5 and 6 we will discuss the long-run impact of cost sharing and HMO care on patients in the Rand study.

The Rand study team concluded that the poor are not more responsive to cost sharing if such payments are in proportion to family income. However, this income-related "ideal plan" may be the likely by-product of a political process that seems increasingly willing to compromise on the equity side to achieve overall cost savings in Medicaid or Medicare programs. If the probable changes in cost-sharing requirements are unrelated to family income, they will disproportionately reduce the buying power and provider contact (visits) among the sick poor. In the Rand study (Manning et al. 1987) the poor were more likely to exceed the maximum dollar expenditure of $1,000, as is consistent with the view that the economically disadvantaged are also the medically disadvantaged with a backlog of untreated health conditions (Brook et al. 1983). The administrative costs of a finely tuned, income-related cost-sharing program are substantial in the public sector. Government officials have trouble informing providers of beneficiary-program eligibility, for example, if Medicaid will pay a given individual's bill. However, the private sector has a proven track record of running an income-related cost-sharing program for more affluent employed populations. We shall discuss one such program in chapter 6.

GENERALIZABILITY OF THE RAND STUDY

One limitation in the Rand study was that subjects in the experiment faced no risk in joining the experiment. Any family assigned to a plan that offered less coverage than its current (preexperiment) insurance was reimbursed an amount equal to its maximal possible loss. This money was paid in installments every four weeks, and the family was not required to spend it on health care. Consequently, the effects of the coinsurance may have been underestimated. The participants who were covered by a high rate of coinsurance could not actually lose money in the experiment. The original Rand sample may have been additionally biased by participant refusals and attrition (net 35 percent).

The Rand analysis focused on the effects of cost sharing on consumer behavior, but what of the potential effects of cost sharing on provider behavior if a large fraction of their patient population is affected? Fahs (1992) studied physician treatment patterns before and after cost sharing was implemented on the United Mine Workers (UMW). She analyzed treatment patterns for three ambulatory conditions (diabetes mellitus, urinary-tract infection, and tonsillitis/pharyngitis/streptococcal infections) for 1,089 patient episodes. She divided components of an episode into patient-initiated and physician-initiated categories. After 30 years of free care the 800,000 members of the UMW agreed to imposition of cost sharing as of July 1977. The cost-sharing package included a $250 inpatient deductible, a 40 percent coinsurance on physician and most other outpatient services, and an annual maximum liability of $500. Immediately following the imposition of cost sharing, demand for physician visits decreased substantially. Scheffler (1984) found that UMW families and retirees were 36 percent less likely to have one or more physician visits in the second half of 1977.

Fahs's (1992) unique contribution to reanalyzing this unique natural experiment is that she indicated weak support for a target income hypothesis. The UMW physicians working in a stable group practice, the Russelton Medical Group, serving the UMW and steel workers, attempted to inflate the number of physician-initiated visits to compensate for declining patient revenues caused by the cost-sharing effects on 60 percent of their patients. The control group, the nonminers insurance plan, remained constant over the entire study period (1976–79). Fahs used a fixed-effects model that controlled for each managing physician over the episode, regressing patient-initiated and physician-initiated visits, and a number of independent variables (diagnosis, disease stage, age, sex, prior visits, and insurance). While total fees per episode, both ambulatory and inpatient fees, decreased by 10 percent for the UMW, the physicians found 17 percent more business (fees) in the control group that did not increase its cost-sharing requirements. Neoclassical competitive market analysis would not predict such an increase in the total fees per episode for other patients in the group practice. However, one could argue that one decade later, the 1987 solution to this finding might be twofold: to implement more stringent utilization review within the Russelton Medical Group and to offer alternative health plans (HMOs and PPOs) so that costs cannot be shifted onto nonminers by providers. All consumer groups, not the providers or the employers, can then decide which health plan offers a more appealing product.

The 17 percent cost shift of fees onto the control group in the Fahs (1992) study was barely significant at the 0.05 level. Patient-initiated visits were unchanged for the control group, but physician-initiated fees increased 11 percent in the nonminer group, and follow-up recall time improved (for the physicians) 24 percent. This provides weak evidence for the supplier-induced-demand (SID) hypothesis based on 1977 data. The SID effect manifests itself in increased physician-initiated recall visits. No published evidence involving more recent data exists to support either the target income or the SID hypotheses. Physicians are increasingly price takers, subject to utilization review and competition in the 1990s. Wickizer et al. (1991) reports that inpatient utilization review stimulates a measurable substitution effect: stimulating more outpatient care. In a study of 43 utilization review programs outpatient expenditures were 20 percent higher after adoption of utilization review, but their regression equations suggest a quite modest shift in utilization location ($9 per insured person per year).

Alternatives for Physicians

As a service becomes increasingly covered by insurance, the professionals become a subject for public study. According to the Congressional Budget Office (CBO 1991), consumers paid out-of-pocket 83 percent of total spending for physician services in 1950 and 60.4 percent in 1965, but this share dropped to 18.7 percent in 1990. This reduction since 1965 was related to increases in the proportion paid by government (28 percent in 1990, up from 1.0 percent in 1965) and the rise in the proportion paid by private insurance (48.4 percent in 1990, up from 32.9 percent in 1965).

Physician payment methods are increasingly a concern for public policy makers. Projections are that in 1992 Medicare's Part B physician services will exceed $50 billion (CBO 1991). Other alternative payment systems have been criticized. For example, DRG payments for doctors have been criticized on the grounds that the system would unfairly redistribute payments from physicians with genuinely more complex and costly practices to physicians with less complex and costly practices (Eastaugh 1990). In contrast to hospitals that serve large numbers of patients within a DRG category, individual doctors admit few cases per DRG and thus have few opportunities to offset high-cost cases with low-cost cases. The real potential for physician DRGs might reside in assisting medical staff, HMOs, PPOs, and hospital managers in monitoring physician practice styles.

In selecting a "fair price" for physician services (in chapter 4), four basic options are to be considered: (1) paying a variable rate for the same service depending on the professional, his or her credentials, and location, (2) paying a uniform rate per service, (3) paying a uniform rate per episode (e.g., DRGs), or (4) paying a per capita rate. The direction of public decision makers seems to be toward the last three options. Ultimately, capitation may become the most prevalent payment method because the physicians could not manipulate this system by increasing the quantity and complexity of services provided. If the private and public sectors continue to tighten physician payment rates, physicians will not be any more or less likely to treat public patients. However, the price Medicaid administrators pay in tightening physician rates excessively is that clinicians may discriminate against public patients (Holahan 1984).

THE FUTURE COLLAPSE OF THE SPECIALISTS' DREAM HOUSE

It is all too apparent that the fee-setting structure reimburses specialists and procedures more generously than cognitive physician-care outputs. This bias will be partially corrected in the new Medicare 1992 fee schedule outlined in chapter 4. The best early study of this bias in the incentive structure was provided by Hsiao and Stason (1979). The authors estimated that after adjusting for case complexity the doctors were paid four to five times as much per hour for surgery as for office visits. Moreover, procedures that have become automated or routine over time are highly profitable under Medicare (or other noncapitated payment schemes) because the relative-value (RV) scales have not been adjusted downward as the procedure has become less costly to perform. To promote efficiency, we should either recalibrate the RV scales (Hsiao 1989) or jettison the fee-for-service method of payment and move toward capitation systems (McClure 1984; Congressional Budget Office 1991). We shall discuss the capitated systems in depth in chapters 5 and 14. Medical journals contain a number of impassioned critiques of Medicare and private-sector managed care. The economic forces seem to favor continued downward pressure on physician fees (Pawlson 1991). American physicians who believe that they can take their case to the public should consider the failure to garner public support in recent Canadian physician strikes. The typical Canadian citizen reaction was contained in the following quote: "My physician is making a very adequate living without extra-billing, so let's cut their fees and continue to channel them into remote geographic areas. Cut the incomes of those who do not serve remote areas." In the United States the real rate of return from education in a primary-care specialty averages 13 percent, which is still a better return on training than getting a nonmedical

Table 3.3
Real Rates of Return from Medical Education

Specialty	Rate of Return to Training
Pediatrics	9%
General practice/family practice	11%
Psychiatry	13%
Internal medicine	14%
Obstetrics-gynecology	16%
Pathology	17%
Surgery	19%
Radiology	20%
Anesthesiology	22%
Total, all physicians	16%

Source: Sloan and Hay (1986).

doctorate (table 3.3). However, the real rate of return for specialists in the last four lines of the table is 20 percent (Sloan and Hay 1986).

Paying the doctor under statutory programs (e.g., Medicare, table 3.4) is inherently different from paying the hospital. From a historic perspective, hospitals are used to low profit margins, and the hospital rate of Medicare cost inflation per capita has slowed since the 1983 initiation of the DRG prospective payment system. However, physicians have grown familiar with high profit margins since the passage of Medicare and Medicaid reduced their cash-flow problems with the very poor and the aged. From the demand side, substantial problems still exist; for example, only 40 percent of the poor are eligible for Medicaid (Eastaugh 1991). From the physician provider's side, the doctors resent congressional passage of a resource-based relative-value scale (using the Hsiao model) to pay doctors for Medicare services in 1992. Physicians did not respond positively to the Medicare fee freeze, even if the cut in the inflation rate was impressive in 1984–85 (table 3.4, column 1). A cost saving for the Medicare program is correctly viewed as lost income by the physician community. Why did Congress target hospitals before physician expenditures in the cost-control discussions of 1982–83 and 1986? Hospitals involve a larger pool of dollars (with a deficit-reduction potential), and organized medicine is a more powerful special interest group in competition with the hospital sector. One could argue that the payment RVs should reflect the supply of physicians in the catchment area, but if one really wanted to reflect supply ratios in the payment system, one could pay on the basis of competitive bids. We shall discuss a quality-

Table 3.4
Annual Rates of Growth in Reimbursement under Medicare, 1975–1992

	Physician Services		Hospital Insurance	
	per *Enrollee*	*Total* *(billions)*	*per* *Enrollee*	*Total* *(billions)*
1975	$159	$ 3.8	$470	$11.3
1982	474	14.0	1,293 –	38.1
1985	651	19.5	1,572	47.6
1989	1,042	34.9	1,902	61.8
1991 est.	1,446	51.5	2,398	85.4
Average annual increase in constant dollars (using GNP deflator)				
1975-1982	8.05%	-	6.64%	-
1983	12.12%	-	4.64%	-
1984-1985	4.74%	-	4.22%	-
1986-1990	8.02%	-	4.13%	-

Sources: Congressional Budget Office 1991, and author's estimate for 1992.
Note: Enrollees increased from 25.0 million (1975) to 35.4 million.

enhancing system of competitive bidding based on price and quality in chapters 9 and 14.

REFERENCES

Acton, J. (1975). "Nonmonetary Factors in the Demand for Medical Services: Some Empirical Evidence." *Journal of Political Economy* 83:3 (May), 595–614.

Anderson, G. (1991). "Cost of Excess Beds." Report to ProPAC (April). Prospective Payment Assessment Commission, Washington, D.C.

Arrow, K. (1963). "Uncertainty and the Welfare Economics of Medical Care." *American Economic Review* 53:4 (December), 941–973.

Barnes, B., O'Brien, E., Comstock, C., D'Arpa, D., and Donahue, C. (1985). "Report on Variation in Rates of Utilization of Surgical Services in the Commonwealth of Massachusetts." *Journal of the American Medical Association* 254:3 (July 19), 371–376.

Baumol, W. (1988). "Price Controls for Medical Services and the Medical Needs of the Nation's Elderly." Paper commissioned by the American Medical Association, March 11.

Blomquist, A. (1992). "The Doctor as a Double Agent: Information, Insurance, and Medical Care." *Journal Of Health Economics* 10:4 (March), 411–422.

Boaz, R., and Muller, C. (1989). "Does Having More Time after Retirement Change the Demand for Physician Services?" *Medical Care* 27:1 (January) 1–15.

Boyle, J. (1985). "Regional Variations in the Use of Medical Services and the Accountability of the Profession.'' *Journal of the American Medical Association* 254:3 (July 19), 407–409.

Bronstein, J., and Morrisey, M. (1990). ''Determinants of Rural Travel Distance for Obstetrics Care.'' *Medical Care* 28:9 (September), 853–863.

Brook, R., Ware, J., Rogers, W., and Newhouse, J. (1983). ''Does Free Care Improve Adults' Health?—Results of a Controlled Trial.'' *New England Journal of Medicine* 309:23 (December 8), 1426–1434.

Brown, D., and Lapan, H. (1979). ''The Supply of Physicians' Services.'' *Economic Inquiry* 17:2 (April), 269–279.

Burstein, P., and Cromwell, J. (1985). ''Relative Incomes and Rates of Return for U.S. Physician Services.'' *Journal of Health Economics* 4:1 (March), 63–78.

California Health Facilities Commission (CHFC). (1985). ''Variations in Hospitalization Rates in California.'' California Health Facilities Commission Report IV–85–9. Sacramento, Calif.: CHFC.

Caper, P. (1986). ''How Medical Practice Affects Cost Containment.'' *Healthcare Executive* 1:2 (January/February) 29–31.

Chassin, M., Brook, R., Park, R., Keesey, J., Funk, A., Kosecoff, J., Kahn, K., Merrick, N., and Solomon, O. (1986). ''Variations in the Use of Medical and Surgical Services by the Medicare Population.'' *New England Journal of Medicine* 314:5 (January 30), 285–290.

Chilingerian, J., and Sherman, D. (1990). ''Managing Physician Efficiency and Effectiveness in Providing Hospital Services.'' *Health Services Management Research* 3:1 (March), 3–14.

Congressional Budget Office. (1991). *Trends in Health Expenditures by Medicare and the Nation*. Washington, D.C.: CBO.

———. (1986). *Physician Reimbursement under Medicare: Options for Change*. CBO Study Report (April), U.S. Congress, Washington, D.C.

Crowley, A., Etzel, S., and Petersen, E. (1985). ''Undergraduate Medical Education.'' *Journal of the American Medical Association* 254:15 (October 18), 1565–1572.

Danzon, P., Manning, W., and Marquis, M. (1984). ''Factors Affecting Laboratory Test Use and Prices.'' *Health Care Financing Review* 5:4 (Summer), 23–32.

Davis, K., and Russell, L. (1972). ''The Substitution of Hospital Outpatient Care for Inpatient Care.'' *Review of Economics and Statistics* 54:2 (May), 109–120.

Diehr, P., Cain, K., Connell, F., and Volinn, E. (1990). ''What Is Too Much Variation? The Null Hypothesis in Small-Area Analysis.'' *Health Services Research* 24:6 (February), 741–771.

Dyckman, Z. (1978). *A Study of Physician Fees*. Staff Report (March), Council on Wage and Price Stability, Executive Office of the President, Washington, D.C.

Eastaugh, S. (1991). ''Defining Medicaid Hospital Payment Levels.'' Affidavit in re Oregon Medicaid case 88–255-DA, Salem, Oregon.

———. (1990). ''Financing the Correct Rate of Growth of Medical Technology.'' *Quarterly Review of Economics and Business* 30:4 (Winter), 54–60.

———. (1981). *Medical Economics and Health Finance*. Boston: Auburn House.

Eben, M., and Pliskin, J. (1992). ''Incorporating Patient Travel Times in Decisions About Size and Location of Dialysis Facilities.'' *Medical Decision Making* 12:1 (January-March), 44–51.

Evans, R. (1974). ''Supplier-induced Demand: Some Empirical Evidence and Implications." In J. Perlman (ed.), *The Economics of Health and Medical Care*, 162–173. New York: John Wiley.

———. (1973). *Price Formation in the Market for Physician Services in Canada, 1957–1969*. Ottawa: Queen's Printer.

Fahs, M. (1992). "Physician Response to Cost Sharing." *Health Services Research* 27:1 (April), 20–28.

Feldman, R., and Sloan, F. (1988). "Competition among Physicians, Revisited." *Journal of Health Politics, Policy, and Law* 13:2 (Summer), 239–261.

Feldman, S., and Roblin, D. (1992). "Standards for Peer Evaluation: Hospital QA." *American Journal of Public Health* 82:4 (April) 525–528.

Feldstein, M. (1977). "Quality Change and the Demand for Hospital Care." *Econometrica* 45:7 (October), 1681–1689.

———. (1971). "Hospital Inflation: A Study in Nonprofit Price Dynamics." *American Economic Review* 61:5 (December), 853–872.

———. (1970). "The Rising Price of Physicians' Services." *Review of Economics and Statistics* 52:2 (May), 121–133.

Feldstein, P., and Severson, R. (1964). "The Demand for Medical Care." In *Report of the Commission on the Cost of Medical Care*, 56–76. Chicago: American Medical Association.

Ferguson, B., and Crawford, A. (1989). "Supplier-induced Demand: A Disequilibrium Test." *Applied Economics* 21:5 (May), 597–609.

Folland, S., and Stano, M. (1990). "Small Area Variations: A Critical Review of Propositions, Methods, and Evidence." *Medical Care Review* 47:4 (Winter), 419–465.

———. (1989). "Sources of Small Area Variations in the Use of Medical Care." *Journal of Health Economics* 8:1 (March), 85–107.

Friedman, B., and Pauly, M. (1981). "Cost Functions for a Service Firm with Variable Quality and Stochastic Demand." *Review of Economics and Statistics* 63:11 (November), 610–624.

Fuchs, V. (1986). *The Health Economy*. Cambridge, Mass.: Harvard University Press.

Fuchs, V., and Kramer, J. (1973). "Determinants of Expenditures for Physicians' Services in the United States, 1948–1968." Paper Series, National Bureau of Economic Research.

Gillespie, K., Romeis, J., Virgo, K., Fletcher, J., and Elixhauser, A. (1989). "Practice Pattern Variation between Two Medical Schools." *Medical Care* 27:5 (May), 537–542.

Ginsberg, P. (1978). "Impact of the Economic Stabilization Program on Hospitals: An Analysis with Aggregate Data." In M. Zubkoff et al. (eds.), *Hospital Cost Containment: Selected Notes for Future Policy*, 293–323. New York: Prodist.

Ginzberg, E. (1990). *The Medical Triangle: Physicians, Politicians, and the Public*. Cambridge, Mass.: Harvard University Press.

Glasser, W. (1989). "The Politics of Physician Payment." *Health Affairs* 8:4 (Winter), 87–96.

Graduate Medical Education National Advisory Committee (GMENAC). (1980). *Graduate Medical Education National Advisory Committee Report to the Secretary of DHHS*. 7 vols. Washington, D.C.: Public Health Service (September), Health Resources Administration.

Green, J. (1978). "Physician-induced Demand for Medical Care." *Journal of Human Resources* 13 (Supplement), 21–34.

Havighurst, C. (1987). "The Changing Locus of Decision Making in the Health Care Sector." In L. Brown (ed.), *Health Policy in Transition: A Decade of Health Politics, Policy, and Law*, 129–168. Durham, N.C.: Duke University Press.

Health Insurance Association of America (HIAA). (1991). *Source Book of Health Insurance Data*. Washington, D.C.: HIAA.

Hillner, B., Smith, T., and Desch, C. (1992). "Efficacy and Cost of Bone Marrow Transplant." *JAMA* 267:15 (April 15), 2055–2061.

Holahan, J. (1984). "Paying for Physician Services in State Medicaid Programs." *Health Care Financing Review* 5:3 (Spring), 99–110.

Holahan, J., Berenson, R., and Kachavos, P. (1990). "Area Variation in Selected Medicare Procedures." *Health Affairs* 9:4 (Winter), 166–175.

Holahan, J., Hadley, J., Scanlon, W., and Lee, R. (1978). *Physician Pricing in California*. Urban Institute working paper, report 998–10.

Howell, D., and McLaughlin, C. (1989). "Regional Variation in Health Care Expenditures." *Medical Care* 27:8 (August), 772–788.

Hsiao, W. (1989). "Potential Effects of an RBRVS-based Payment System on Health Care Costs and Hospitals." *Frontiers of Health Services Management* 6:1 (Fall), 40–43.

Hsiao, W., and Stason, W. (1979). "Toward Developing a Relative Value Scale for Medical and Surgical Services." *Health Care Financing Review* 1:2 (Fall), 23–38.

Hu, T., and Yang, B. (1988). "Demand for and Supply of Physician Services in the U.S.: A Disequilibrium Analysis." *Applied Economics* 20:8 (August), 995–1006.

Hughes, J. (1991). "How Well Has Canada Contained the Cost of Doctoring?" *Journal of the American Medical Association* 265:18 (May 8), 2347–2351.

Institute of Medicine (1976). *Medicare-Medicaid Reimbursement Policies*. Part 3, vol. 3. Washington, D.C.: National Academy of Sciences.

Keeler, E., and Rolph, J. (1982). *The Demand for Episodes of Medical Treatment*. Rand Report R–2829-HMS. Santa Monica, Calif.: Rand Corporation.

Kenny, G. (1991). "Understanding the Effects of PPS on Medicare Home Health Use." *Inquiry* 28:2 (Spring), 129–139.

Kessel, R. (1958). "Price Discrimination in Medicine." *Journal of Law and Economics* 1:1 (October), 20–53.

Lagoe, R., and Milliren, J. (1986). "A Community-based Analysis of Ambulatory Surgery Utilization." *American Journal of Public Health* 76:2 (February), 150–153.

Mann, S., and Sicherman, N. (1991). "Agency Cost of Free Cash Flow: Acquisition Activity and Equity Issues." *Journal of Business* 64:2 (April), 213–227.

Manning, W., Newhouse, J., Duan, N., Keeler, E., Leibowitz, A., and Marquis, M. (1987). "Health Insurance and the Demand for Medical Care: Evidence from a Randomized Experiment." *American Economic Review* 77:3 (June), 251–277.

Marquis, M. (1985). "Cost Sharing and Provider Choice." *Journal of Health Economics* 4:2 (June), 137–157.

McCarthy, T. (1985). "The Competitive Nature of the Primary Care Physician Services Market." *Journal of Health Economics* 4:2 (June), 93–117.

McClure, W. (1984). "On the Research Status of Risk-adjusted Capitation Rates." *Inquiry* 21:3 (Fall), 205–213.

McCombs, J. (1984). "Physician Treatment Decisions in a Multiple Equation Model." *Journal of Health Economics* 3:2 (June), 155–171.

McGuire, T., and Pauly, M. (1992). "Physician Response to Fee Changes with Multiple Payers." *Journal of Health Economics* 10:4 (March), 385–409.

McGuirk, M., and Porell, F. (1984). "Spatial Patterns of Hospital Utilization: The Impact of Distance and Time." *Inquiry* 21:1 (Spring), 84–89.

McLaughlin, C., Normalle, D., Wolfe, R., McMahon, L., and Griffith, J. (1989). "Small-Area Variation in Hospital Discharge Rates: Do Socioeconomic Variables Matter?" *Medical Care* 27:5 (May), 507–521.

McLean, R. (1980). "The Structure of the Market for Physicians' Services." *Health Services Research* 15:3 (Fall), 271–280.

Menken, M. (1983). "Consequences of an Oversupply of Medical Specialists: The Case of Neurology." *New England Journal of Medicine* 308:22 (May 12), 1224–1226.

Mick, S. (1990). *Innovations in Health Care Delivery: Insights for Organization Theory*, San Francisco: Jossey-Bass.

Moore, F., and Priebe, C. (1991). "Board-certified Physicians in the United States, 1971–1986." *New England Journal of Medicine* 324:8 (February 21), 536–543.

Morrisey, M., and Jensen, G. (1990). "Hospital Demand for Physicians." *Quarterly Review of Economics and Business* 30:1 (Spring), 16–25.

Newhouse, J. (1988). "Has the Erosion of the Medical Marketplace Ended?" *Journal of Health Politics, Policy, and Law* 13:2 (Summer), 263–278.

———. (1970). "A Model of Physician Pricing." *Southern Economic Journal* 37:2 (October), 174–183.

Newhouse, J., and Marquis, M. (1978). "The Norms Hypothesis and the Demand for Medical Care." *Journal of Human Resources* 13 (Supplement), 159–182.

Newhouse, J., and Phelps, C. (1976). "New Estimates of Price and Income Elasticities of Medical Care Services." In R. Rosett (ed.), *The Role of Health Insurance in the Health Services Sector*, 261–312. New York: Watson Academic.

———. (1974). "Price and Income Elasticities for Medical Care Services." In M. Perlman (ed.), *The Economics of Health and Medical Care*, 139–161. New York: John Wiley.

Newhouse, J., Williams, A., Bennett, B., and Schwartz, W. (1982a). "Where Have All the Doctors Gone?" *Journal of the American Medical Association* 247:17 (May 7), 2392–2396.

———. (1982b). "Does the Geographical Distribution of Physicians Reflect Market Failure?" *Bell Journal of Economics* 13:2 (Autumn), 493–505.

Pauly, M. (1988). "Market Power, Monopsony, and Health Insurance Markets." *Journal of Health Economics* 7:1 (July), 111–128.

———. (1980). *Doctors and Their Workshops: Economic Models of Physician Behavior*. Chicago: University of Chicago Press.

Pauly, M., and Redisch, M. (1973). "The Not-for-Profit Hospital as a Physicians' Co-operative." *American Economic Review* 63:1 (March), 87–99.

Pauly, M., and Wilson, P. (1986). "Hospital Output Forecasts and the Cost of Empty Hospital Beds." *Health Services Research* 21:3 (August), 403–428.

Pawlson, G. (1991). "Medicare as a System." In J. Moreno (ed.), *Paying the Doctor*, 157–169. Westport, Conn.: Auburn House.

Peden, E., and Lee, M. (1992) "Output and Inflation Components of Medical Care." *Health Care Financing Review* 13:2 (Winter), 75–82.

Phelps, C. (1975). "The Effects of Insurance on the Demand for Medical Care." In R. Anderson et al. (eds.), *Equity in Health Services: Empirical Analyses in Social Policy*. Cambridge, Mass.: Ballinger.

Phelps, C., and Newhouse, J. (1972). "The Effect of Coinsurance: A Multivariance Analysis." *Social Security Bulletin* 35:6 (June), 20–29.

Physician Payment Reform Commission (PPRC). (1991). *Annual Report to Congress*. Washington, D.C.: PPRC.

Reinhardt, U. (1989). "Economists in Health Care: Saviors, or Elephants in a Porcelain Shop?" *American Economic Review* 79:2 (May), 337–342.

———. (1985). "The Theory of Physician-induced Demand: Reflections after a Decade." *Journal of Health Economics* 4:2 (June), 187–193.

———. (1975). *Physician Productivity and the Demand for Health Manpower*. Cambridge, Mass.: Ballinger.

Rosenstein, A. (1991). "Health Economics and Resource Management: A Model for Hospital Efficiency." *Hospital and Health Services Administration* 36:3 (Fall), 313–330.

Rohrer, J. (1990). "Supply-induced Demand for Hospital Care." *Health Services Management Research* 3:1 (March), 41–48.

Roos, N. (1989). "Predicting Hospitalization Rates by the Elderly: The Importance of Patient, Physician, and Hospital." *Medical Care* 27:10 (Oct), 905–917.

Rosenthal, G. (1970). "Price Elasticity of Demand for Short-Term General Hospital Services." In H. Klarman (ed.), *Empirical Studies in Health Economics*, 104–124. Baltimore: Johns Hopkins University Press.

Rosett, R., and Huang, L. (1973). "The Effect of Health Insurance on the Demand for Medical Care." *Journal of Political Economy* 81:2 (March–April), 281–305.

Satterthwaite, M. (1979). "Consumer Information, Equilibrium Industry Price, and the Number of Sellers." *Bell Journal of Economics* 10:2 (Autumn), 483–502.

Scheffler, R. (1984). "The United Mine Workers' Health Plan: An Analysis of the Cost-sharing Program." *Medical Care* 22:3 (March), 247–254.

Schroeder, S. (1984). "Western European Responses to Physician Oversupply." *Journal of the American Medical Association* 252:3 (July 20), 373–384.

Sloan, F. (1976). "Physician Fee Inflation: Evidence from the Late 1960s." In R. Rosett (ed.), *The Role of Health Insurance in the Health Services Sector*, 321–354. New York: Watson Academic.

Sloan, F., and Hay, J. (1986). "Medicare Pricing Mechanisms for Physicians' Services." *Medical Care Review* 43:1 (Spring), 33–45.

Soumerai, S., Ross, D., and Avorn, J. (1991). "Effect of Medicaid Drug-payment Limits on Admission to Hospitals and Nursing Homes." *New England Journal of Medicine* 325:15 (October 10), 1072–1077.

Stano, M. (1985). "An Analysis of the Evidence on Competition in the Physician Services Market." *Journal of Health Economics* 4:3 (September), 197–211.

Steinwachs, D., Weiner, J., Shapiro, S., Batalden, P., Coltin, K., and Wasserman, F. (1986). "A Comparison of the Requirements for Primary Care Physicians in HMOs with Projections Made by the GMENAC." *New England Journal of Medicine* 314:4 (January 23), 217–222.

Steinwald, B., and Sloan, F. (1974). "Determinants of Physicians' Fees." *Journal of Business* 47:3 (October), 493–511.

Sweeney, G. (1982). "The Market for Physicians' Services: Theoretical Implications and an Empirical Test of the Target Income Hypothesis." *Southern Economic Journal* 48:1 (January), 594–614.

Tarlov, A. (1986). "HMO Enrollment Growth and Physicians: The Third Compartment." *Health Affairs* 5:1 (Spring), 23–35.

Thorpe, K. (1992). "Health Care Cost Containment." In S. Shortell (ed.), *Improving Health Policy and Management.* Chicago: ACHE.

Vahovich, S. (1977). "Physicians' Supply Decisions by Specialty: TSLS Model." *Industrial Relations* 16:1 (February), 51–60.

Welch, W. (1991). "Defining Geographic Areas to Adjust Payments to Physicians, Hospitals and HMOs." *Inquiry* 28:2 (Spring), 151–160.

Wennberg, J. (1988). "Improving the Medical Decision-making Process." *Health Affairs* 7:2 (Summer), 99–106.

———. (1986). "Which Rate Is Right?" *New England Journal of Medicine* 314:5 (January 30), 310–311.

———. (1977). "Changes in Tonsillectomy Rates Associated with Feedback and Review." *Pediatrics* 59:7 (July), 821–826.

Wennberg, J., and Gittelsohn, A. (1982). "Variations in Medical Care among Small Areas." *Scientific American* 246:4 (April), 120–135.

Wennberg, J., McPherson, K., and Caper, P. (1984). "Will Payment Based upon DRGs Control Hospital Costs?" *New England Journal of Medicine* 311:6 (August 9), 295–300.

Wennberg, J., and Servi-Share of Iowa. (1985). "A Comparative Study of Iowa Hospital Utilization, 1980–81." Des Moines: Servi-Share of Iowa.

Wickizer, T., Wheeler, J., and Feldstein, P. (1991). "Have Hospital Inpatient Cost Containment Programs Contributed to the Growth in Outpatient Expenditures?" *Medical Care* 29:5 (May), 442–451.

Wilensky, G. (1990). "Technology as Culprit and Benefactor." *Quarterly Review of Economics and Business* 30:4 (Winter), 45–49.

Wilensky, G., and Rossiter, L. (1980). *The Magnitude and Determinants of Physician-Initiated Visits in the United States.* Proceedings of the World Congress on Health Economics, September 8–11, Leiden University, the Netherlands.

Zuckerman, S., Welch, W., and Pope, G. (1990). "Index for Physician Fees." *Journal of Health Economics* 9:1 (June), 39–69.

4 Physician Payment Options for the 1990s

Concerning the coming surplus of 60,000 physicians, I use "surplus" with caution because I do not believe the United States will ever see a surplus such as exists in some Western European countries, where trained physicians have taken jobs as taxicab drivers and have applied for welfare.

—Alvin Tarlov, M.D., Chairman of the 1980
Graduate Medical Education National Advisory Committee

In analyzing physicians a useful mnemonic is TUMS: tantalized by technology, uncomfortable with uncertainty, motivated by money, scared by suit.

—Richard Riegelman, M.D.

Since the publication of the Tarlov GMENAC study in 1980, the concept of a doctor glut (oversupply) has become part of the conventional wisdom. In the context of the 1990s the term "glut" might be a misnomer, like the term "doctor shortage" in the 1960s. In Rashi Fein's classic book *The Doctor Shortage* (1967) Fein pointed to the two real problems: maldistributions of physician supply by geographic location and specialty choice (too many specialists). As a number of economists from the Rand Corporation have pointed out, these maldistribution problems have diminished as the supply of physicians per capita has increased. However, perception of a "glut" of doctors is still the conventional wisdom among policy makers regardless of the data.

A number of so-called procompetition measures were initiated in the 1980s to stimulate cost-decreasing behavior. In reaction to regulations and payer-driven fee negotiations, the physician community has been more willing to accept utilization review programs and discount pricing because of the so-called doctor glut (Schloss 1988). Consequently, the perceived doctor glut has served as a primary catalyst for change in payment policies even if the projected oversupply of 60,000 physicians in 10 to 20 years never becomes a reality. The GMENAC (1980) study overestimated supply, as fewer doctors are being trained and clinicians are working shorter hours each month doing patient care. A study by Schwartz, Sloan, and Mendelson (1988) suggested that a slight shortage of physicians might exist by the year 2000 if the capitated health plans (HMOs, PPOs, and other managed-care plans) do not achieve a 28 percent market share of the American population. Such predictions of a shortage of 30,000 physicians due to AIDS and inefficient fee-for-service medical-staffing ratios are highly suspect, as Schwartz, Sloan, and Mendelson concede. Demand-expanding and demand-constraining forces flow like a tide over a medical community hardly conscious of economic forces. Technological change could increase patient demand beyond all projections, whereas corporate and federal attempts to ration services could decrease the demand for physician services. Whether society has an under- or oversupply of doctors depends on two factors: demand (highly unpredictable) and supply (stable in the 1990s compared to the rapid growth in the period 1965–82; Moore and Priebe 1991).

RECENT TRENDS IN PHYSICIAN SUPPLY

In 1978 medical schools received over 45,000 applications. By 1988 the number of applications for 16,400 medical school slots had declined to under 24,000, and many of the applicants were multiple reapplicants. The demand for medical education had declined by 50 percent in one decade. The reasons that fewer students are applying to medical school are complex. Physicians are fighting to maintain their authority and their incomes. Third-party payers wish to constrain prices and volume levels. Payers implement peer review programs to affect the style of medical care and have some sentinel effect in determining unnecessary or inappropriate medical care (Shroder and Weisbrod 1990; Eisenberg 1989). It is ironic that countries where doctors have economic freedom (e.g., where they are not salaried employees of a public system) practice medicine with less clinical freedom (Reinhardt 1987). Cost containment has replaced the cost-is-no-concern view of medical practice in America.

The data from the American Medical Association and the Health Resources and Services Administration of the Department of Health and Human Services (HRSA, DHHS) in table 4.1 review recent trends in physician supply. One can observe in line 2 the steady climb in the supply of physicians per capita. A geographic maldistribution of physicians still exists beyond what can be expected from trends in urban group practice and the need to create citadels for medical education in urban centers. New York State is still 44 percent above the national average of physicians per capita, and Mississippi is 37 percent below average physician supply. Some of the growth in the physician supply ratio is necessary due to the aging of the population, but some of the additional physicians specialize in quality-of-life subspecialty care (e.g., plastic surgery; Eastaugh 1991). A very slight tendency toward more primary-care physicians has been observed. In the

Table 4.1
Supply of Allopathic M.D.s and M.D. Characteristics, 1963–2000

	1963	1970	1980	1985	1990[b]	2000[b]
Number of active M.D.s[a]	258,958	314,217	440,357	512,849	568,000	664,000
M.D.s per 100,000 population[c]	135	151	189	211	227	248
M.D.s per 100,000 population:						
General and family practice		27.8	26.0	27.6	28.7	26
Internal medicine		20.1	30.9	37.2	42.4	49
Other medical specialty		17.0	23.5	28.5	34.3	38
Surgical specialties		41.3	47.9	52.8	58.6	69
Anesthesiology		5.2	6.9	9.1	11.0	13
Psychiatry[d]		11.2	13.4	14.9	16.0	19
Radiology		6.4	8.8	10.4	10.2	10
Other specialties		21.6	31.1	30.1	26.2	24
Major locus of activity as a percentage of active M.D.s:						
Office-based		57.6%	58.2%	59.7%	58.9%	57%
Hospital-based		25.8	22.3	21.5	20.2	19
Teaching/research/admin.		9.7	8.2	8.7	9.3	12
Other activities		6.8	11.2	10.1	11.5	12
Percentage of foreign medical graduates 9FMGs)	13%	20%	23%	22%	21%	18%
FMGs as a percentage of residents	28%	33%	25%	16%	13%	11%

[a]These figures do not include osteopathic doctors (D.O.s): 12,000 in 1970; 17,100 in 1980; 22,000 in 1985; 28,000 in 1990; 40,000 in 2000.
[b]1990 and 2000 estimates by Eastaugh (1991).
[c]Inactive M.D.s vary from 19,000 to 39,000 depending on the AMA survey year for *Physician Characteristics and Distribution.*
[d]Psychiatry includes child psychiatry.

1980s the supply of primary-care physicians grew faster than that of all non-primary-care physicians (30 percent compared to 23 percent). The primary locus for physician activity seems to change at a glacial pace toward more administration and research activity and less office-based fee-for-service self-employment. Those who think that office-based practitioners will decline at a faster pace in the future should reflect on the 1910 Flexner Report. Those who predicted the demise of the private practitioner following publication of the 1910 report were grossly inaccurate (Starr 1982).

One last trend that is apparent in table 4.1 is the decline in foreign medical graduates (FMGs) since the mid–1980s. Congress took action to restrict the flow of immigrant physicians during the 1980s. Public hospitals and small marginal teaching hospitals are still highly dependent on a FMG work force to deliver patient care (Ginzberg 1990). One educational response to the perceived doctor glut in the 1980s was to lengthen the period of graduate medical education. For example, plastic-surgery residents spent 50 percent more time in graduate training in 1989 than they did in 1981. The elder senior medical staff may lengthen the apprenticeship to enhance quality of care and also may keep their competition in the educational pipeline for as long as possible. On a national average, 38 percent of the physicians who will be in practice in 1999 were in training in 1990. Some of the younger doctors in training wish that their elders would listen to Hippocrates and reflect that "life is so short and the craft so long to learn." Lucky Hippocrates never faced a $50,000 debt service from his medical education.

A career in medicine is being viewed as increasingly regulated and less profitable than in prior decades. According to the AMA survey of socioeconomic characteristics of medical practice, physician incomes after inflation increased a total of only 5.4 percent from 1979 to 1988. However, the cost of a medical education markedly outpaced inflation. Average tuitions at medical schools outpaced inflation by 194 percent over the decade. Those without substantial wealth have to incur a substantial debt before graduation day. Nearly one in every four graduates was more than $50,000 in debt by graduation. Because of the rise in bureaucratic paperwork and the increasing competition within the profession, some doctors are steering young people away from a career in medicine.

Clearly, nonfinancial factors such as loss of autonomy or prestige contribute to the downward trend in applications to medical schools. Medicine is not a poverty profession. As an index of physicians' economic status within a society, one can consider the ratio of physicians' net income to gross domestic product per capita within a nation. In 1988 by that yardstick the West German physician (BASYS 1989) outpaced the general public in Germany by a ratio of 7.2 to 1, closely followed by American and Japanese physicians in their countries (6.6 to 1). However, these pretax medical-practice figures understate the economic advantage among Japanese physicians. The Japanese physicians have such high status that by law they pay no income taxes. In contrast, the physicians in most of Western Europe outpace the general public by 3.9 to 4.2. Because of the high tax rates in these countries with national health insurance, it is futile to negotiate higher salaries, so the clinicians negotiate about working hours and working conditions (Iglehart 1991).

While American physicians fear the idea of government-negotiated salaries, the cost-escalation problem is driving Congress to consider broad systemic reforms in the payment of physicians. In 1989 physicians' income represented 23 percent of personal health expenditures and 2.24 percent of the gross national product. Unconstrained, physician expenses will rise to $1,400 per capita by the year 2000. This chapter cannot survey all physician manpower issues, but many analysts believe that there is a maldistribution of types of physician (too many surgeons and subspecialists and not enough primary-care or internal-medicine specialists). However, some economic analysis suggests that even in the year 2000 some large cities will have a deficit of most types of subspecialists (Schwartz et al. 1989). Before surveying the payment options, one should survey the incentives implicit in the three basic methods of paying the doctor.

PRINCIPAL METHODS FOR PAYING THE DOCTOR

The three basic methods for compensating clinicians are salary, capitation, and fee-for-service. Each method has relative strengths and weaknesses. (For a more extended discussion of these methods, see Berenson 1991.) The primary advantages of a salaried system are cost control and a controlled workweek (many young doctors like the life-style advantage of working a salaried shift and going home). If a doctor is salaried (paid per unit of time), the organizational risk involves poor productivity and the potential underprovision of care. The salaried individual can try to come late, leave early, and do a minimum amount of work per hour. Because of this obvious moral hazard to underprovide service, salaried contracts increasingly come with an incentive compensation provision to pay more for enhanced productivity. Clever salaried contracts try to promote the carrot (additional pay for additional work above the average) rather than to emphasize the stick (sanctions if one fails to meet a quota for workload per month).

The second method for paying physicians involves capitation. Pure capitation pays the doctor a fixed payment per person joining his or her panel of potential patients. The incentives are to keep the patients happy and healthy (happy so they do not disenroll and healthy so they do not overutilize expensive health care resources). Capitation offers no incentive to overprovide expensive care, and it offers the long-run incentive to provide preventive care (thus saving money in future years). In our mobile American society this last incentive is probably overstated because subscribers change jobs and health plans often. Thus the capitated system providing the preventive care accrues only a small fraction of the financial benefits. Capitated managed-care systems make the doctor a gatekeeper with the dual responsibility to do no harm to the patient while acting as an explicit guardian of the health plan's financial welfare. Capitated systems run the risk of undercare, so quality must be closely monitored. Capitated systems also run the risk of overreferral, in that gatekeepers may minimize their workload by shunting too many patients to specialists elsewhere in the health plan (this can be controlled through the process of utilization review and reinforced through financial incentives by providing less holdout pay at year's end). A number of managed-care systems have demonstrated that physicians can practice excellent and cost-effective medicine under a capitated contract. Unnecessary admissions and routine tests (e.g., chest roentgenograms) can be reduced without detriment to the patient. Consequently, capitated payment was the most rapidly growing method of paying physicians in the 1980s. A study by Pauly et al. (1990) suggested that HMO for-profit ownership does enhance the power (or the need) of management to offer effective rewards for parsimonious use of resources.

The predominant, but declining, method for paying the doctor is fee-for-service (AMA 1991). Under fee-for-service payment per unit of work the clinician's income is directly related to work ethic and business acumen. However, just as capitation runs the potential risk of conflict of interest for financial reasons, fee-for-service offers the conflict of interest to steer patients to tests or facilities in which the doctor reaps financial returns (e.g., the doctor owns the equipment that does the test or receives kickback incentive pay for referrals). For example, it looks greedy to the public if the clinician is a business partner with the laboratory and the radiology imaging center. Congress is increasingly wary of the argument that the physician is unconcerned with cash flow and only owns such facilities to ensure the quality of patient care. Fee-for-service doctors get paid more if they provide more services, but they also get paid more (1) if they are paid as owners of the equipment that does the test or procedure and paid again to interpret the results, and (2) if they are paid for upcoding (upgrading) the coded work done to receive higher payment rates. The fee-for-service system has been very inflationary because all the incentives stimulate overprovision of inappropriate or unnecessary care. In contrast, salaried or capitated physicians have no incentive to own health care facilities or upcode the patient record in current procedural terminology (CPT) coding. For example, a total hysterectomy (58150) might be coded as exploration of the abdomen (49000), removal of ovaries and tubes (58720), appendectomy (44955), and lysis of adhesions (58740). According to the CPT manual, this coding is incorrect, because all of these procedures are bundled together as total hysterectomy (58150), and the moral hazard exists to select the code that maximizes payment.

WANTED: A BETTER DISTRIBUTION OF PHYSICIANS

To the general public, physicians are like cops: The aggregate supply appears to be adequate, but there is never one around when you need one. The growing supply of physicians is important because they add to the medical cost-inflation problem. Grumbach and Lee (1991) reported that depending on whether expenditures per physician grow at the historical 1980s rate or at the projected rate of the consumer price index, the rising supply of doctors could add between $40 or $21 billion (in 1986 dollars), respectively, to national health expenditures in the year 2000. Physician supply is an interesting manpower issue because physicians have some control over the volume of patient demand and, as Christensen (1990) pointed out, can partially offset the impact of fee freezes (price controls) by expanding volume. Christensen studied 1,000 internists and general practitioners in Colorado and reported a volume offset of approximately 50 percent. Mitchell, Wedig, and Cromwell (1989) studied the 1984–86 Medicare fee freeze and reported that expenses per capita increased 30 percent while fees were frozen. Volume increased most rapidly for radiological procedures and diagnostic surgery. In addition to the quantity and adaptability of the physician community, the composition of doctors by specialty distribution is a major issue for public policy because specialists are more expensive than generalists (Baumgardner and Marder 1991).

Capitation systems are growing in popularity because governments and insurance companies want to negotiate with bundles of services, fewer sellers, and risk-contracting care organizations (e.g., a few hundred plans willing to take an annual per person check as payment in full). Both in terms of cost control and administrative simplicity, capitated plans are superior to dealing separately with 500,000 physicians and each and every ancillary service provider and their unbundled pile of bills. However, organized medicine fears declining professional autonomy and loss of the prerogative to exceed the employers' norms for standard care if clinicians are only salaried or capitated employees of some faceless corporation. An emerging change in physician attitudes may result over the 1990s as guidelines and models are developed for plans that have excellent quality as well as excellent cost-efficiency. Billions of dollars could be saved each year if physicians practiced in the same style as those at Stanford, the Mayo Clinic, or Case Western Reserve (Caper 1988). Such facilities are what Jack Ott (1991) referred to as competitive medical organizations (CMOs), acting as islands for 5 to 20 percent of the physicians in an area, enhancing quality, taking responsibility for patient needs, and making prudent decisions concerning discretionary care.

Naive policy makers question the concept of discretionary care, saying that the world is black or white, that care is either unnecessary or necessary and there is no middle category. One could expand Ott's concept of the CMO one step further and suggest that such organizations represent pathway guidelines for better medical practice at a reasonable cost in the community. Pathway guidelines serve as yardsticks for cost-effective clinical decision making and as a standard to demonstrate that good medicine and good economics can coexist. Too much attention has been focused on a second type of guideline: boundary guidelines for payers to define the range of medical practice beyond which a clinician incurs the wrath of the payers. If the practitioner exceeds the boundary, the computer suggests an administrative sanction, and after a number of due-process hearings a monetary penalty may result. This second type of guideline gives the topic a bad reputation and has led to the phrase ''cookbook medicine.'' Physicians are not ignorant or venal, but many clinicians need help with the positive, proactive type of pathway guideline. If physicians wish to preserve their autonomy, they should actively participate in the development of pathway guidelines. Case management can remain a caring art and not a cold cookbook formula if beacons are established to assist experienced practitioners in developing pathway guidelines. The guidelines are suggestions, and the microcomputer is more of an educational tool than an enemy to be consorted with as a part of standard federal operating procedure (Derzon 1988). In summary, boundary guidelines clamp down on ''bad'' physicians, whereas pathway guidelines assist the profession.

The federal government recognizes 12 classes of visits: new and established patient office visits, initial and subsequent hospital visits, initial and follow-up consultations, initial and subsequent nursing facility visits, initial and subsequent rest home visits, and new and established patient home visits. This allows payment per level of service to vary, reflecting differences in effort (work per unit time) and practice costs for different types of visits and for visits in different sites. The following terminological definitions are used:

New patient (ambulatory settings): A visit with a patient who is new to the physician's practice or who has not been seen within the past three years. The transfer of care from one physician to another constitutes a new patient visit.

Established patient (ambulatory settings): A visit with a patient who has been seen by the physician's practice within the past three years. Concurrent care constitutes an established patient visit.

Initial care (inpatient settings): The initial visit by the admitting physician in which the medical record is established for an admission. The transfer of care from one physician to another constitutes initial care.

Subsequent care (inpatient settings): Follow-up visits in an institution during an inpatient stay. Concurrent care constitutes subsequent care.

Initial consultation (all settings): A visit in which a physician, at the request of another health care provider, renders an initial opinion regarding a specific problem. The consultant must document the need for the consultation, his or her opinion, and any services that have been ordered or performed. In addition, the consultant must document that this information has been communicated to the health care provider who requested the consultation.

For medical conditions within each category of visits, what constitutes appropriate care and an optimal pathway can be established in three basic ways: the implicit ad hoc method, the risk-benefit method, and the cost-benefit method. Decision trees in academic settings focus on the cost-benefit method (an action is appropriate if the marginal benefit exceeds the marginal cost, with the intangible benefits shadow priced). The risk-benefit approach suffers because this method only includes traditional medical risks and excludes monetary costs. The implicit approach used in hospital utilization review is hard to export to other settings and has questionable validity, given that we know little of what the reviewer had in mind during the ad hoc process of making judgments (Wennberg 1988; Chassin et al. 1987; Eastaugh 1991).

CONTROLLING THE VOLUME OF SERVICES

The great equation in medical economics involves the control of expenditures (E), which are equal to price (P) times quantity (Q). All payers desire to control their expenditures by trimming P and constraining Q (the volume of services). The health care system is a very adaptable balloon, where squeezing down on only one factor (e.g., P) can cause a bulge in another area (increased volume). Medicare Part B services, which pay for physician services, averaged an 18.7 percent annual increase from 1975 to 1984 until Congress imposed a price freeze in 1984. During the first year of the freeze the growth rate declined to 8.3 percent per year, but it rebounded to 16.2 percent in 1985 and 14.3 percent in 1986. The price freeze was co-opted by an obvious expansion in volume. Congress lifted the freeze as part of the October 1986 Consolidated Omnibus Reconciliation Act (Mitchell, Wedig, and Cromwell 1989). However, in the 30 months following the lifting of the fee freeze, the Part B expenditures per capita increased at 17 percent per annum, while prices only rose at 2.4 percent on average. Price controls without volume controls yield little in the way of cost control. Service volume per capita is clearly out of control. Physicians can expand volume by a stepped-up quantity of procedures, operations, and provider-initiated follow-up visits. Moreover, with 7,200 codes available to label physician services, including six subjective codes for the basic office visit, code creep (upcoding) becomes prevalent. The fine detail of the codes allows the smart physician to unbundle the patient experience or upcode individual items (e.g., the minimal visit is upcoded as brief, and the extended visit is upcoded as a comprehensive office visit). Hospitals played the same game in the 1980s with DRG creeping of patient classifications to the better-paying higher-code groups.

Some of the added volume and intensity might represent real health benefits to patients, but some of the increase has been clearly labeled unnecessary and inappropriate by the federal Health Care Financing Administration (HCFA; Roper 1988). The number one physician reimbursement issue seems to involve controlling the growth in per capita service volume. The most effective single solution is capitation. Capitation decentralizes decisions about which patient receives what and how much while heightening the need for quality assurance and minimizing the chance of underprovision of care. Capitation will not be the voluntary choice of all Americans, as evidenced by the fact that capitated Medicare only covers 1.4 million Americans. Since 1988 HCFA has pilot tested in six HMOs an improved average adjusted per capita cost (AAPCC) formula by adding a health-status adjustment factor based on demographic data to place individuals in diagnostic cost groups (DCGs; Ash and Ellis 1989). A ratebook has been established in which enrollees will be classified in a particular cost-weight category based on age, sex, welfare status, and the highest number of eight possible DCGs associated with a hospitalization in the previous 15 months (DCG 0 = no hospitalization or a discretionary one- to two-day hospitalization). Ash and Ellis's (1989) DCGs may eliminate any incentive that exists for discouraging sick enrollees from joining a capitated plan. Capitation cures the incentive to game the payment system through increased volume of unnecessary services and will leave the plan with the discretion to divide the annual payments among the various physicians and facilities.

The number two physician reimbursement issue involves selecting a fair work-load scale for equitable payment among physician specialties. Hsiao (1989) worked for five years to develop a resource-based relative-value scale (RBRVS) as an alternative to the current charge-based system. Resource inputs by physicians include (1) total work input performed by the physician for each service, (2) practice costs (including office overhead and malpractice premiums), and (3) the cost of specialty training (e.g., the opportunity costs for spending 13 years going to medical school and training to become a cardiac surgeon). The Hsiao study, with the help of the AMA and a number of specialty societies, presented fairly valid and reliable estimates of physicians' work according to four dimensions: time, psychological stress, mental effort and judgment, and technical skill plus physical effort.

The Hsiao et al. (1988) study has been subject to one minor and one major criticism. The minor point revolves around the heavy emphasis on time measurement. Other professionals (e.g., lawyers) do not have their charges related so fully to their work time expended. This minor point is easily dismissed: (1) in the name of scientific accuracy, resource based relative value units (RBRVUs) are better than perpetuating tradition, (2) time orientation may stimulate physicians to enhance productivity, and (3) other professions make less use of government funds or insurance dollars (e.g., if we had government paying half the legal fees, then RBRVUs would be necessary for that profession). On a more important point, the RBRVS study methodology could be improved if a refined estimate for health-status improvement to the patient could become a major measure of workload. Hsiao could only equate physician activity with workload. If activity were replaced by health-status improvement as the purists' measure for effective workload, the providers who offer better care could be paid better. In the business world this mechanism would be labeled pay for performance. Obviously, not all activity proves to be beneficial, given that the real output in an ideal study would be health-status improvement. If we had a refined health-status measure, the clinicians who produce higher-quality patient outcomes could get paid more for their effort and skill (Shortell 1990).

The basic research question the Hsiao study answers is how much to pay for cognitive services relative to procedures. The payment system is biased toward paying for procedures done to the patient, rather than for talking to or thinking about the patient. The specialist who spends 60 minutes doing an invasive

Table 4.2
Physicians' Charges and Workloads under a Resource-based Relative-Value Scale

Service Workload	Charge (1987)	Work Units	Charge per Work Unit
Follow-up visit of family physician to nursing home patient, with extended service	$37	159	$0.23
Diagnostic proctosigmoidoscopy examination of colon	53	118	0.45
Simple repair of superficial wound, 2.5 to 7.5 cm	66	75	0.88
Delivery of child (vaginal)	481	407	1.18
Repair of inguinal hernia (in the groin)	732	476	1.54
Triple coronary artery bypass	4,663	2,871	1.62
Insertion of permanent pacemaker (ventricular)	1,440	620	2.32

procedure on a patient who has heart failure receives $700, but the doctor who spends 60 minutes doing a history and physical on the same patient arrives at the diagnosis and is only paid $70. Under the Hsiao scheme, physicians would be paid more equitably per unit of work (there would not be a tenfold variation in the last column of table 4.2). If the gains and losses among physicians had been redistributed in a zero-sum fashion between the various specialties, $140,000 of income would have been carved out of the average thoracic surgeon's $350,000 in 1988. Most surgeons would lose money, but urologists and otolaryngologists would lose only a fraction. Primary-care fees would rise by more than 60 percent, which might (1) cause physicians to spend more time talking with their patients and (2) reenergize the declining supply of filled residency positions in internal medicine (many medicine programs have gone begging for residents since 1986).

In the period 1988–90 Hsiao developed vignettes describing a typical patient for the service to be provided for a representative sample of services for each physician specialty. Each vignette was intended to represent the average service for its corresponding current procedural terminology (CPT) code. Data from both the Hsiao study and the Visit Survey suggest that physicians responding to vignettes may have overestimated the share of time they spend in pre/post activities in actual practice. According to the Physician Payment Reform Commission (PPRC 1991), the Visit Survey demonstrated that physicians spend most of the encounter performing the history, physical examination, and counseling. By contrast, most pre/post time is spent in activities that would be expected to be less intense, such as scheduling, reviewing records, and contacting other providers. Hsiao and the PPRC will continue working on the Medicare adjuster, and they will need to determine whether intraservice work is different when certain surgical global services are performed on elderly and all-age populations. PPRC will also need to obtain information about age-related differences in intraservice work and pre/post work for nonoperative technical procedures (such as endoscopy or angioplasty).

THE HSIAO RELATIVE-VALUE APPROACH

The Hsiao resource-based relative-value units will be the basis for the new Medicare fee schedule in 1992. In the short run, primary-care doctors may be energized by the higher fee schedules. However, critics argue that in the long run government fee schedules may eventually lose all receptivity to market signals from consumers (Pauly 1988; Glasser 1990). Under a worst-case scenario competition among physicians may decrease, and they may channel their energies to political negotiation with government for higher pay (which is what British physicians have done since the 1950s, and what South Korean doctors have done since the passage of national health insurance in 1989). Physicians may spend more time in unionization activities to negotiate with the government, managed-care systems, and insurance companies (Eastaugh 1991). Other payers should be expected to copy the Medicare approach as the list of RVUs expands (Becker et al. 1990). These payers need only change the conversion factor ($32 for Medicare in FY 1993).

Ginsburg, LeRoy, and Hammons (1990) and Lasker et al. (1990) have projected the impact of the new RBRVUs. Recent projections by the AMA suggest that Medicare payments to family practitioners may rise only half as much (28 percent) in 1992, and thoracic surgeons may anticipate a dip in Medicare prices of only half as much (23 percent). Some analysts have worried that Medicare may attract fewer physicians in the long run (Kay 1990; Pauly 1990). The PPRC (1991) supported the concept of prospective payment for ambulatory procedures (surgery, medical services, and tests) done in outpatient settings, including physicians' offices. Prospective payment by DRG for most physicians' services may not be far behind in the late 1990s. The HCFA is already studying a system of 400 ambulatory patient groups (APGs) based on the outpatient principal diagnosis, treatment (CPT codes), age, sex, and status as a new or established patient.

To collapse the current 7,000 CPT codes and 1,900 lab codes into 400 APG groups will not be easy. Physicians also face a number of new legal and paperwork limits on medical practice.

Congressman Pete Stark's (Democrat of California) Ethics in Patient Referrals Act 1992 is one attempt to constrain physician income-generating options. Such proposed bills are reactions to studies suggesting a conflict of interest in the physician-patient relationship. Hillman (1990) reported that diagnostic imaging involving self-referring physicians (having the equipment) resulted in 4.5 times as many films and average charges 4.4 to 7.5 times as expensive as episodes involving imaging done by referrals. A self-referral pattern has the obvious moral hazard of conflict of interest. The problem may exist beyond films and lab tests done in private offices. Referral patterns, friendships, and complex factors bind providers into a network of mutual obligations and courtesies. Even the Joint Commission on Accreditation of Healthcare Organizations (JCAHO 1991) is looking into the possibility that the quality of care could be regrettably compromised by informal arrangements and conflict-of-interest relationships.

Perceived equity implicit in the new payment system will affect physician reaction to the Hsiao approach. Zuckerman, Welch, and Pope (1990) have developed an improved geographic index of physician practice costs using relative prices for four practice inputs: physician time, employee wages, office rents, and malpractice insurance. In this Laspeyres index each input price is weighted by the share of physicians' gross revenues spent on that input. The index is useful in explaining geographic variation in physician fees.

Hsiao (1989) and the PPRC (1991) utilized the human-capital concept that resources devoted to increasing an individual's skills or knowledge, such as education, can be thought of as investment in future income. Income is not limited to monetary compensation, but includes the psychic benefits from any undertaking. For example, most people derive monetary income from their jobs and psychic income from leisure activities. Most theoretical discussions of human capital include all forms of income as the result of the stock of human capital that individuals are endowed with at birth and any subsequent investment in human capital (medical school education, varying lengths of time in residency, and fellowship programs). An individual's pool of skills and knowledge is the input he or she can use to create a product, whether a good or service or leisure activity, that will generate monetary or psychic income. Economic studies with regard to human capital have led to many estimates of the implicit return in earnings from investments in different levels of education. The weakness of these analyses is that they cannot include the psychic income that people derive from their work and leisure activities. Conservative physicians will continue to protest any "comparable-worth" attempts to set fair payment levels, given different levels of education. To determine fair payments, it is necessary to determine what rate of return nonphysician practitioners should realize on their investment in education. One measure that could be used is the rate of return to education realized by all professionals, including nonphysician providers (chapter 10).

A number of medical reporters gave rather imperfect examples of the Hsiao study; for example, ''The specialist who spends 25 minutes inserting a tube into a patient with a stomach ulcer receives $350, but the cognitive doctor who spends 60 minutes talking to the patient arrives at the same diagnosis at a price of only $70.'' This example is imperfect, because the gastroscopy procedure is a better diagnostic tool for gastrointestinal bleeding than history with physical; one needs to know the area and the specific pathology of the stomach ulcer. Table 4.3 offers a simple example of how Medicare fees will be set in 1992. Table 4.4 provides an example of the variation in expenses for different physician specialties.

Surgeons and other specialty groups most affected by the Hsiao study suggest that redistribution of physician fees could worsen the volume of services (e.g., more discretionary operations might be performed and might not be detected by peer review or second-opinion surgery programs). In a pessimistic worst-case scenario the RBRVS would not stimulate many more primary-care doctors to accept assignment under Medicare and the government check as payment, but a massive number of surgeons already on assignment with Medicare (because surgical fees are difficult to collect) would either drop assignment (and charge more) or drop out of the Medicare program. This scare scenario seems unlikely because surgeons are in need of the cash flow. From 1979 to 1991 the number of surgeons increased from 8,514 to above 13,000, but the average number of operations per surgeon declined 28 percent, thus proving that supply and demand are alive and well in the surgical marketplace. Surgeons need Medicare business too much to drop out of the Medicare program. Moreover, the HCFA never hoped that a RBRVS scheme would induce a flood of demand for primary care by the elderly, given the tight budgets.

The importance of the Hsiao study is not simply in its proposal of a cost-control mechanism to keep the FY 1992 Medicare budget from exceeding $124 billion. The RBRVS will give all payers the device to implement a type of aggressive price competition unknown to physicians. Each insurance company could go to the medical community and ask for a single number, on a sealed bid, for their minimum contract price relative-value multiplier. Insurance companies will then have a simple device and one confidential number on a piece of paper to force physicians to bid down their prices (and incomes) each year.

ALTERNATIVES TO ''OVERHAUL GRADUALLY''

The phrase ''overhaul gradually'' is a classic oxymoron, two words that do not go together. Yet we know that the physician community will resist major changes in payment policies, even as we know that the policy must be dramatic to curtail a 16 percent inflation rate in Medicare Part B expenditures (PPRC 1991). A number of alternatives, not all mutually exclusive, have been suggested. One could simply reform the existing system to prevent upcoding by reducing the number of available billing codes. This idea worked in the Canadian context with Quebec physicians, but may not prove as effective with American doctors who see their incomes protected by code creeping into better-paying classification

Table 4.3
Medicare Fees for an Intermediate-Length Office Visit with a New Patient in Three Locations, 1992

	Work		Overhead		Malpractice		Conversion Factor	Payment
	RVU[a]	GCI[b]	RVU	GCI	RVU	GCI		
Ithaca, N.Y.		1.009		1.031		1.140		$38.95
New York, N.Y.	20.6 x	1.059	+ 15.4 x	1.255	+ 2.0 x	1.865	x $1 =	$44.88
Paris, Texas		0.961		0.825		0.447		$33.41

Note: Starting in 1992, Medicare fees will be set by Meshing Seven Components, including geography, variation in overhead, malpractice, and work.
[a]RVU = Relative value units (Hsiao et al., 1988).
[b]GCI = Geographic cost index.

Table 4.4
Variation in Expenses as a Percentage of Practice Revenue for Six Types of Physicians

	Practice Costs as Percentage of Revenue	Salaries and Fringes	Administration	Malpractice
Family practice	52	42	3	12
Gen'l surgery	45	38	3	29
Internal medicine	48	43	3	10
Ophthalmology	48	41	3	8
Orthopedics	51	45	3	20
Urology	44	41	5	17

Source: PPRC (1991).

categories (Fuchs and Hahn 1990). The second reform idea, fee schedules, involves implementing the Hsiao RBRVS concept such that a uniform price list pays the same rate for similar services (in marked contrast to uniform customary rates that have wide variability). A third reform idea, payment for packages of services, sets a prospective rate that puts doctors at financial risk for the use and cost of those services (Mitchell 1985; Culler and Ehrenfried 1986). For example, the DRG prices could be expanded to include physician fees (e.g., if the care is done more efficiently, the physician receives a higher residual share of the check, and the payer provides extra outlier payments for severely ill patients). Ambulatory care could be reimbursed through an analogous DRG mechanism of ambulatory visit groups (AVGs; Lion et al. 1989). The problem with the third reform idea is that it may fall prey to the law of small numbers. Consider the use of DRGs to pay hospitals. Hospitals are partly protected from undue financial risk by the effect of large numbers if each DRG has over 75 or 100 cases. But individual physicians may have only 1 to 2 patients in each category and may experience a poverty wage if their patient mix is more severely ill than the average. AVG payments would unfairly redistribute payments from those clinicians with genuinely more complex and costly cases for a given AVG to their peers who have less complex cases.

The fourth reform idea, capitation, is currently the most popular initiative. Whether the nation moves to capitation or tougher fee schedules, specialists left out in the cold are headed for two possible fates: serious financial trouble and/ or membership in a union. As the payers get tougher with doctors, they must respond with a countervailing force that acts as a bargaining unit (Ginzberg 1990).

JOIN TOGETHER OR SUFFER ALONE

As the formation of the AMA was an event to combat the cults in the nineteenth century, aggressive specialty unions may form in the future to defend specialists' declining incomes and strike for better-quality patient care. Unionization, once a dirty word in the medical world, is spreading. The California-based Union of American Physicians and Dentists has 29 state chapters. Politically conservative physicians may have to face two economic truths: (1) Unions are not always bad, and (2) clinicians in overdoctored locations can properly go broke. Going broke is a major cost-containment agenda for those who pay for medical services. Payers report with joy that economic failure of excess doctors and hospitals will eject the pathology from the system and drive costs down. Physicians require better productivity and a voice to negotiate on their behalf (Koska 1991). If the profession does not act together as a group and continues to pursue only individual business interests, medicine will be no more protected or respected than a used-car dealership. Likewise, those who disrespect business skills, productivity, marketing to the public, and patients' shifting tastes will also face an early retirement.

HCFA administrator Gail R. Wilensky has characterized the RBRVS payment system initiated for Medicare in 1992 as the dawn of government-administered pricing in medicine. If our goal is to contain the growth in expenditures, a product of price times volume, a simple system of price controls can be ineffective because of expansion in volume. Global-based budgets (GBB) that constrain expenditures, with so-called behavioral offsets (for volume expansion), have proved successful in countries like Germany, Sweden and South Korea. Annual social arbitration over spending caps could set incomes for all sectors of the health economy: physicians, hospitals, home health care, and long-term care. If the volume growth outpaces the global budget by 4.5 percent, prices are subsequently deflated by 4.5 percent. In the decentralized German system, fee negotiations between hospitals and sickness funds require final approval from state governments, but the overall management of policy is typified by compromise and consensus building. Federal and state governments, sickness funds, labor unions, hospitals and physician groups (geographic-based councils known as the Arztekammern, with an average membership of 7,000 doctors) annually agree on fees and expenses in each sector of the health economy. If physician fees exceed their target in one time period, they are subsequently reduced in future periods to penalize providers for cost overruns due to unplanned volume shifts. In the jargon of accounting, this political process is described as variance analysis under a limited budget (the global pie of dollars for local health care). If the budget variance is unfavorable (overbudget) the fees are deflated in proportion to the "unnecessary part of the increase in volume."

All nations with GBB spend one-third less of GNP on health care. Moreover, creation of a GBB might be the catalyst that breaks the gridlock against national health insurance for 31 million uninsured Americans. Implementation of GBB will not cause the United States to spend 4.0 percent of Gross National Product (GNP) less on health care; but it could free up the resources necessary to make national health insurance more affordable. GBB could also reduce or eliminate the need for explicit rationing (e.g., the Oregon Medicaid program).

Will the Hsiao (1992) methodology lead to a better (more equitable) distribution of incomes and services? Germany has tried a broad approach with a major revision of physician fees in 1987. The impact was minimal in that: (1) no substantial substitution effect occurred between technical procedures and patient-centered communication, and (2) income rankings of the top specialties did not change by more than two points (Brenner and Rublee 1991). However, average income at the lowest end of the physician scale, gynecology and pediatrics, did increase substantially. The German context for global budgetting and rate setting is discussed further in chapter 14.

It is difficult to forecast the impact of the new Medicare physician fee schedule (Lee and Ginsburg 1991). By law the new fee schedule was to be implemented in a ''budget-neutral way.'' Therefore, all four federal estimates agree that physicians were scheduled to receive $191 billion over the five budget years FY1992–96. However, the AMA and other physician groups lobbied against the expense-neutral interpretation of the law, and suggested that physicians receive $211 billion over the five years. HCFA argued in 1991 that the prices be down-adjusted 6.4 percent (or $7.5 billion over 1992–96) to exactly compensate for the predicted 6.4 percent upsurge in volume ($7.5 billion) so that no more than $191 billion is spent on Medicare physician fees 1992–96. The initial spring 1991 HCFA estimate of 16.3 upsurge in volume over the period 1992–96 was rejected for political reasons to appease physician groups.

Is a 16.3 percent upsurge in volume over five years possible? Not only is it possible, but it is half the historic rate of physician volume inflation. The AMA's spokesman on the Physician Payment Review Commission (PPRC), Thomas Reardon, reports that historically volumes have gone up 7.0 percent a year and not 3.1 or 1.1 percent (Iglehart, 1991). The average number of services provided per Medicare beneficiary has increased from 12 in 1978 to 28 in 1991. The Medicare fees are also asymmetric in transition: increased fees for undervalued services will be more rapid than the decreases in fees for surgeons. For example, in 1992 family practice and general practice physicians will see their Medicare fees enhanced by 14 percent, while thoracic surgeons will have their fees deflated by only 5.6 percent. However, by 1996 thoracic surgeons will experience a nearly 30 percent five-year deflation in Medicare fees, while family and general practice fees will be inflated by a five-year total of 15.5 percent. The net impact on physician income is harder to predict. Two policy questions remain. Is HCFA correct that physicians who lose income will only offset half their losses with a volume shift (above 1.1 percent), and the physicians who gain income (price hikes) will not also increase their volume? If every physician lets their volume go up 4.5 percent per year, the profession will earn a windfall profit of $23.9 billion (over and above $191 billion) over the five years 1992–96. Physicians are smart people, and like any profession they can adapt to the new game in order to make more money (unless the PROs are successful in curtailing unnecessary service volume). Shifts in physician income may be insufficient to convince many (or any) young doctors to work in a rural area or choose a primary care specialty. The Medicare fee schedule differentials between specialties must be more substantial to affect new physicians unless we go to an all-payer global budgeting system for setting prices and expense targets for all patients and providers.

REFERENCES

AAMC, Association of American Medical Colleges. (1992). *Supplying Physicians for Future Needs: Report of the Task Force on Physician Supply*, Washington, D.C.: AAMC.

American Hospital Association. (1991). *The Emerging Roles of Physicians*. Chicago: AHA.

American Medical Association. (1991). *Physician Characteristics and Distribution in the United States*. Chicago: AMA.

Ash, A., and Ellis, R. (1989). "Diagnostic Cost Groups DCG Methodology." Presented at the American Public Association meeting in Chicago.

BASYS. (1989). "Wirkungen von Verguetungsystemen auf die Einkommen der Aerzte, die Preise, und auf die Struktur aerzlicher Leistungen im Internationalen Ergleich." Augsburg, Bavaria, Germany: BASYS GmbH, mimeo.

Baumgardner, J., and Marder, W. (1991). "Specialization among Obstetrics Gynecologists: Another Dimension of Physician Supply." *Medical Care* 29:3 (March), 272–281.

Becker, E., Dunn, D., Braun, P., and Hsiao, W. (1990). "Refinement and Expansion of the Harvard Resource-based Relative Value Scale." *American Journal of Public Health* 80:7 (July), 799–803.

Berenson, B., and Holahan, J. (1992). "Medicare Physician Expenditures." *JAMA* 267:5 (February 5), 687–691.

Berenson, R. (1991). "Payment Approaches and the Cost of Care." In J. Moreno (ed.), *Paying the Doctor*, 63–74. Westport, Conn.: Auburn House.

Brenner, G., and Rublee, D. (1991). "The 1987 Revision of Physician Fees in Germany." *Health Affairs* 10:3 (Fall), 147–156.

Caper, P. (1988). "Solving the Medical Care Dilemma." *New England Journal of Medicine* 318:23 (June 11), 1535–1536.

Chassin, M., Kosecoff, J., Park, R., and Brook, R. (1987). "Does Inappropriate Use Explain Geographic Variations in the Use of Health Care Services? A Study of Three Procedures." *Journal of the American Medical Association* 258:26 (December 27), 2533–2537.

Christensen, S. (1990). "Estimate of Behavioral Responses." In Congressional Budget Office, *Physician Payment Reform under Medicare*, Appendix B. Washington, D.C.: Congressional Budget Office.

Cohen, A., Cantor, J., Barker, D., and Hughes, R. (1990). "Young Physicians and the Medical Profession." *Health Affairs* 9:4 (Winter), 138–147.

Crane, M. (1991). "Annual Fee Survey." *Medical Economics* 68:19 (October 7), 124–142.

Culler, S., and Ehrenfried, D. (1986). "On the Feasibility and Usefulness of Physician DRGs." *Inquiry* 23:1 (Spring), 40–55.

Derzon, R. (1988). "The Odd Couple in Distress: Hospitals and Physicians Face the 1990s." *Frontiers of Health Services Management* 4:3 (Spring), 4–18.

Eastaugh, S. (1991). "Financial Methods for Paying the Doctor: Issues and Options." In J. Moreno (ed.), *Paying the Doctor*, 49–62. Westport, Conn.: Auburn House.

———. (1990). "Financing the Correct Rate of Growth of Medical Technology." *Quarterly Review of Economics and Business* 30:4 (Winter), 54–60.

Eddy, D. (1991). "What Care Is 'Essential'? What Services Are 'Basic'? *Journal of the American Medical Association* 265:6 (February 13), 782–788.

Fahey, D. (1992). "Projected Responses to RBRVS: Induced Demand versus Contingency Theory." *Medical Care Review* 49:1 (Spring), 67–91.

Fein, R. (1967). *The Doctor Shortage*. Washington, D.C.: Brookings Institution.

Frech, H. (1991). *Regulating Doctors' Fees: Competition, Benefits and Controls under Medicare*, Washington, D.C.: American Enterprise Institute Press.

Fuchs, V., and Hahn, J. (1990). "How Does Canada Do It? A Comparison of Expenditures for Physician Services in the U.S. and Canada." *New England Journal of Medicine* 323:13 (September 27), 884–890.

Ginsburg, P., LeRoy, L., and Hammons, G. (1990). "Medicare Physician Payment Reform." *Health Affairs* 9:1 (Spring), 178–188.

Ginzberg, E. (1990). *The Medical Triangle: Physicians, Politicians, and the Public.* Cambridge, Mass.: Harvard University Press.

Glasser, W. (1990). "Designing Fee Schedules by Formula, Politics, and Negotiation." *American Journal of Public Health* 80:7 (July), 804–809.

Glenn, J. (1989). "Hospitals and the Ecology of Primary Care." *Hospital and Health Services Administration* 34:3 (Fall), 371–384.

Graduate Medical Education National Advisory Committee (GMENAC). (1980). *Graduate Medical Education National Advisory Committee Report to the Secretary of DHHS*. Washington, D.C.: PHS:HRA.

Grumbach, K., and Lee, P. (1991). "How Many Physicians Can We Afford?" *Journal of the American Medical Association* 265:18 (May 8), 2369–2372.

Herger, T. (1990). "Two-Part Pricing and the Mark-ups Charged by Primary Care Physicians for New and Established Patient Visits." *Journal of Health Economics* 8:4 (February) 399–414.

Hillman, A. (1990). "Frequency and Costs of Diagnostic Imaging in Office Practice: A Comparison of Self-referring and Radiologist-referring Physicians." *New England Journal of Medicine* 323:23 (December 6), 1604–1608.

Hsiao, W. (1989). "Potential Effects of an RBRVS-based Payment System on Health Care Costs and Hospitals." *Frontiers of Health Services Management* 6:1 (Fall), 40–43.

Hsiao, W., Braun, P., and Becker, E. (1992). *Managing Reimbursement in the 1990s: Physician's Reference to Resource-based RVS*. New York: McGraw-Hill.

Hsiao, W., Braun, P., Yntema, D., and Becker, E. (1988). "Estimating Physicians'

Work for a Resource-based Relative-Value Scale.'' *New England Journal of Medicine* 319:13 (September 29), 834–841.

Hughes, R., Barker, D., and Reynolds, R. (1991). ''Are We Mortgaging the Medical Profession?'' *New England Journal of Medicine* 325:6 (August 8), 404–408.

Iglehart, J. (1991). ''The Struggle over Physician-payment Reform.'' *New England Journal of Medicine* 325:11 (September 12), 823–828.

———. (1990). ''The New Law on Medicare's Payments to Physicians.'' *New England Journal of Medicine* 322:17 (April 26), 1247–1252.

Joint Commission on Accreditation of Healthcare Organizations (JCAHO). (1991). *Report of the Joint Commissions Survey*. Chicago: Joint Commission on Accreditation of Healthcare Organizations.

Kay, T. (1990). ''Volume and Intensity of Medicare Physicians' Services.'' *Health Care Financing Review* 11:4 (Summer), 133–146.

Koska, M. (1991). ''RBRVS and Hospitals: The Physician Payment Revolution.'' *Hospitals* 65:4 (February 20), 24–30.

Kowalczyk, G., and Harden, S. (1992). ''Physician Customary Charges and Medicare Payment,'' *Health Care Financing Review* 13:2 (Winter), 57–73.

Lee, P., and Ginsburg, P. (1991). ''The Trials of Medicare Physician Pay Reform.'' *Journal of the American Medical Association* 266:11 (September 18), 1562–1565.

Lion, J., Henderson, M., Malbon, A., and Noble, J. (1989). ''Ambulatory Visit Groups AVGs: A Prospective System for Outpatient Care.'' In N. Goldfield and S. Goldsmith (eds.) *Financial Management of Ambulatory Care*, 3–18. Rockville, Md.: Aspen.

McCurren, J. (1991). ''Capitated Primary Physicians in Medicare HMOs.'' *Health Care Management Review* 16:2 (Spring), 49–53.

Mitchell, J. (1985). ''Physician DRGs.'' *New England Journal of Medicine* 313:11 (September 12), 670–675.

Mitchell, J., Wedig, G., and Cromwell, J. (1989). ''The Medicare Physician Fee Freeze: What Really Happened?'' *Health Affairs* 8:1 (Spring), 21–33.

Moore, F., and Priebe, C. (1991). ''Board-certified Physicians in the United States, 1971–1986.'' *New England Journal of Medicine* 324:8 (February 21), 536–543.

Newhouse, J. (1988). ''Has the Erosion of the Medical Marketplace Ended?'' *Journal of Health Politics, Policy, and Law* 13:2 (Summer), 263–278.

Orsund-Gassiot, C., and Lindsey, S. (1991). *Handbook of Medical Staff Management*. Rockville, Md.: Aspen.

Ott, J. (1991). ''Competitive Medical Organizations: A View of the Future.'' In J. Moreno (ed.), *Paying the Doctor*, 83–92. Westport, Conn.: Auburn House.

Parks, C., Cashman, S., Winickoff, R., and Bicknell, W. (1991). ''Quality of Acute Episodic Care in Investor-owned Ambulatory Health Centers.'' *Medical Care* 29:1 (January), 72–86.

Pauly, M. (1990). ''Objectives for Changing Physician Payment.'' *Frontiers of Health Services Management* 6:1 (Fall), 44–47.

———. (1988). ''Market Power, Monopsony, and Health Insurance.'' *Journal of Health Economics* 7:2 (October), 111–128.

Pauly, M., Hillman, A., and Kerstein, J. (1990). ''Managing Physician Incentives in Managed Care: The Role of For-Profit Ownership.'' *Medical Care* 28:11 (November), 1013–1024.

Physician Payment Reform Commission (PPRC). (1991). *Annual Report to Congress.* Washington, D.C.: PPRC.

Pope, G. (1990). "Physician Inputs, Outputs, and Productivity." *Inquiry* 27:2 (Summer), 151–160.

Radecki, S., Ginsburg, P., and Lasker, R. (1992). "RBRVS: Objections." *JAMA* 267:13 (April 1), 1824–1825.

Reinhardt, U. (1987). "Resource Allocation in Health Care: The Allocation of Lifestyles to Providers." *Milbank Quarterly* 65:2 (Summer), 153–176.

Riegelman, R. (1991). "Taming Medical Technology." In J. Moreno (ed.), *Paying the Doctor*, 75–82. Westport, Conn.: Auburn House.

Rizzo, J., and Zeckhauser, R. (1991). "Advertising and Entry: Physician Services." *Journal of Political Economy* 89:3 (May), 436–54.

Roper, W. (1988). "Perspectives on Physician Payment Reform: The RBRVS in Context." *New England Journal of Medicine* 319:13 (September 29), 865–867.

Scheffler, R., Sullivan, S., Haochung, T. (1991). "Impact of Blue Cross and Blue Shield Plan Utilization Management Programs." *Inquiry* 28:3 (Fall), 263–275.

Schloss, E. (1988). "Beyond GMENAC—Another Physician Shortage from 2010–2030?" *New England Journal of Medicine* 318:14 (April 7), 920–922.

Schwartz, W., Sloan, F., and Mendelson, D. (1988). "Why There Will Be Little or No Physician Surplus between Now and the Year 2000." *New England Journal of Medicine* 318:14 (April 7), 892–896.

Schwartz, W., Williams, A., Newhouse, J., and Witsberger, C. (1989). "Are We Training Too Many Medical Subspecialists?" *Journal of the American Medical Association* 259:2 (January 8), 233–239.

Shortell, S. (1990). "Revisiting the Garden: Medicine and Management in the 1990s." *Frontiers of Health Services Management* 7:1 (Fall), 3–31.

Shroder, M., and Weisbrod, B. (1990). "Medical Malpractice, Technological Change, and Learning-by-doing." in *Advances in Health Economics and Health Services Research*, ed. Scheffler, R., Greenwich, Conn.: JAI Press, 185–199.

Starr, P. (1982). *The Social Transformation of Medicine.* New York: Basic Books.

Tarlov, A. (1990). "How Many Physicians Is Enough?" *Journal of the American Medical Association* 263:4 (January 26), 571–572.

Welch, W. (1991). "Giving Physicians Incentives to Contain Costs under Medicaid." *Health Care Financing Review* 12:2 (February), 103–111.

Wennberg, J. (1988). "Improving the Medical Decision-making Process." *Health Affairs* 7:2 (Summer), 99–106.

Zuckerman, S., Welch, W., and Pope, G. (1990). "Index for Physician Fees." *Journal of Health Economics* 9:1 (June), 39–69.

III COST SHARING, MANAGED CARE, AND COMPETITION HEALTH PLANS

5 Competition Health Plans: Managed Care and the Use of Case Managers

The ultimate purpose of pro-competitive proposals is to motivate doctors, hospitals, and other providers to compete with each other to offer health care in less costly ways. There is merit in this theory.

—Walter J. McNerney

Consumers want value for their money, and that means shopping on the basis of quality and effective price. Much of the credit for lower rates of cost containment rests with private initiatives, not just the federal prospective payment system.

—Willis Goldbeck

Demands are infinite, whereas the resources are finite, regardless of whether the care is funded through health insurance or from public funds. The marketplace system encourages demand and diversity, whereas the controlled system leads to uniformity, rationing, and possibly mediocrity.

—John Lister, M.D.

Most countries view the U.S. health care system as being very market oriented and competitive. Some of these nations look to the U.S. approach for alternatives to total government regulation. The preference in Canada and Western Europe is for some degree of private management of the national health service or national health insurance plan. In the United States, physicians and administrators who distrust regulatory approaches have advocated the injection of more competitive relationships between health care providers. However, not all physicians have a truly procompetitive bias. Many hospital managers and doctors who have had experience with competition and are now facing declining patient volume dream of returning to a less competitive era. Nobody likes competition in what he or she produces, but we all like competition in what we buy. Physicians searching

Table 5.1
Number of HMOs and Enrollment, Select Years, 1970–1991

Year	Number of Prepaid Plans (HMOs)	Enrollment (in millions)	Percentage of U.S. Population
1970	26	2.9	1.4
1973[a]	140	5.2	2.5
1975	178	5.7	2.6
1977	165	6.3	2.9
1979	215	8.2	3.6
1981	243	10.2	4.4
1982	265	10.8	4.7
1983	280	12.5	5.3
1984	306	15.1	6.4
1985	392	18.9	7.9
1986	585	23.3	9.4
1987	636	26.2[b]	10.4
1988	653	30.6	12.0
1989	607	32.6	12.7
1990	575	34.7	13.4
1991	555	37.7	14.4

Sources: Interstudy (1991) and the National HMO Census, Office of HMOs, U.S. Public Health Service.

[a]The HMO Act, Pub. L. 93-222, was passed in 1973.

[b]A small number of open-ended HMO enrollees have been included in the totals since 1987 (e.g., 858,000 in 1990).

for fiscal security are increasingly working with their local managed-care plans (American Hospital Association [AHA] 1990).

Over 34.7 million Americans, 13.4 percent of the population, were in HMOs in 1990 (table 5.1). HMOs have obvious incentives to curtail hospital utilization and specialist referrals (Clancy and Hillner 1989). The model of the incentive-based physician as a "gatekeeper" places the clinician under some financial risk. For example, secondary resource pools (funds) are set up, and if the primary physician needs to refer, the cost comes out of his or her pocket up to a certain point ($1,500, $2,000). After that point, reinsurance kicks in, but the gatekeeper is still liable for enough financial risk to discourage inappropriate referrals. Some specialists argue that this creates restricted access to some appropriate referrals. Advocates of gatekeeper HMOs argue that underutilization is not a major problem and that specialists desire a continued supply of inappropriate referrals to guarantee their target incomes. Short-run profit taking may not lead to long-run inefficient referral patterns, assuming ethical clinician behavior. At the end of the year, if there is any money left in the primary pool, the primary-care physician gets a share. However, physicians realize that failure to make appropriate referrals often results in failure to obtain early diagnoses, resulting in more costly (and more frequent) inpatient expenses (and withdrawals from their risk-pool fund; Wrightson 1990).

In staff-model HMOs the primary-care physicians are salaried. Capitated or salaried "gatekeepers" lack the direct financial incentive to improve earnings by restraining costs. They may still prove effective as gatekeepers for reasons of professional pride, preventive medicine, and long-run concern for balancing service and solvency in their HMO. However, in an understaffed staff HMO, the gatekeepers may refer too many inappropriate cases to the specialists, especially if they are very busy (or uncompensated for working any harder). Under no circumstances do HMOs offer an incentive to overhospitalize (Seaman 1990).

The basic rationale behind the competitive model is to keep the insurance companies, and hopefully providers, under constant pressure to find the means to provide care at lower costs (Atkinson and Eastaugh 1984). Third-party payers and HMOs will on occasion make management mistakes, create long patient queues, or provide unacceptable patient-care conditions, but the strength of competitive markets is that the good-quality, lower-cost operators will grow. Advocates of competition recognize consumer ignorance, insured consumers' indifference to costs, and strong physician influence on demands as three strong arguments for regulatory activity (Enthoven 1980; Hreachmack and Stannard 1990; Kirkman-Liff 1989).

The public policy question is not simply one of whether to allow competition or regulation, but rather, what the proper balance of regulation and competition is and how much price and nonprice competition should be encouraged. As we have observed in chapters 1–3, the strongest argument for regulatory limits on competition—significant economies of scale leading to excessive monopoly power—does not exist in the medical sector.

A number of barriers impede competition in the health field. While there is sufficient time to shop for maternity care, there is seldom enough time to shop in most hospital "purchase" situations. Conventional analysis says that there is seldom a real "purchase" choice to be made, since the consumer, acting with minimal knowledge of medicine, goes to the doctor and says "save me." The doctor acts as the patient's agent. One might counterargue that an economist who purchases a jacuzzi has less knowledge of the equipment than the typical high-school graduate has concerning medicine. Yet the economist, with the aid of *Consumer Reports*, can make an intelligent purchase decision. The ignorance problem does not preclude competitive markets in the case of high-technology consumer goods. However, this problem is compounded in the medical sector when "rival" providers and hospitals act in a collusive fashion—for example, when they restrict advertising or quality-disclosure activities.

TYPES OF HMOs

There are four basic types of HMOs: staff HMOs, medical-group HMOs, independent practice associations (IPAs), and networks. Staff-model HMOs hire physicians as salaried employees. IPAs are fee-for-service HMOs and tend to be smaller (Interstudy 1991). IPAs represent 63 percent of the HMO plans, but only 42 percent of the national HMO enrollment. There are a few large IPAs, including Physicians Health Plan of Minnesota, Blue Choice of New York, HMO of Pennsylvania, Bay State Health Care, and Humana Health Plan in Kentucky. Group-model HMOs tend to be larger, including the three largest HMOs, Kaiser Northern California, Kaiser Southern California, and HIP (Health Insurance Plan of Greater New York). Group-model HMOs are 11 percent of the plans and have 28 percent of the national HMO enrollment (Interstudy). Network HMOs are 15 percent of the HMO plans and have 17 percent of the enrollment. Large network-model HMOs include PacifiCare of California, Health Net in California, HMO Illinois, and the troubled Humana Medical Plan of Florida. Staff-model HMOs represent 11 percent of the plans and 13.3 percent of the enrollment.

Each of the four HMO types has for-profit and tax-exempt forms. IPAs and network HMOs tend to be for-profit, but nearly half the staff- and group-model HMOs are also for-profit. Nonprofit HMOs tend to be larger than average. Over 51 percent of HMO enrollees are members of the one-third of HMOs that are tax-exempt (nonprofit). The stock values of most for-profit HMO chains took a major nosedive in 1988 when Congress rewrote the 1973 HMO Act to allow a form of experience rating, thus permitting employers to pay less for HMO coverage than they do for indemnity insurance. For-profit HMOs had been earning record-high price-to-earnings ratios because of the high premiums HMO enrollees were paying relative to their expenses.

A BETTER TAXONOMY FOR TYPES OF HMOs

Welch, Hillman, and Pauly (1990) outlined a better taxonomy for classifying HMOs by payment incentives and organizational structure. The five payment-incentive types in the 1991 context are the following: (1) Prepaid group-practice HMOs (42 percent of HMOs) have salaried physicians seeing only HMO patients (95 percent of staff HMOs and 80 percent of group HMOs do this). (2) Salary IPAs (4.9 percent of HMOs) have clinicians on salary and sharing a HMO-wide risk pool (holdout pool in case expenses exceed revenues, with the residual going to the providers at year's end) (15 percent of group-model HMOs). (3) Capitation IPAs (19 percent of HMOs) pay a fixed fee per enrollee per clinician each quarter or year. The doctors also see non-HMO private patients (35 percent of IPAs and 50 percent of network HMOs). (4) Fee-for-service IPAs with subgroup risk pools (18 percent of HMOs) have the clinician (self) or peers as a risk-pool subgroup (holdout pool to be distributed at year's end). The doctors are paid fee-for-service and see non-HMO patients privately (30 percent of IPAs and 35 percent of network HMOs). (5) Foundation-type IPAs (16 percent of HMOs) pay all the physicians fee-for-service, and they all share one risk pool as a group (33 percent of IPAs and 2.2 percent of group-model HMOs).

The five organizational-structure categories in the 1991 context are the following: (1) Prepaid group-practice physicians (42 percent of HMOs) see only HMO patients (95 percent of staff HMOs and 80 percent of group HMOs do this). (2) Two-tiered IPAs with a single risk pool (13 percent of HMOs) have physicians contract directly with the IPA and place doctors in a single risk pool, but the doctors can privately see fee-for-service patients (one-third of IPAs). (3) Two-tiered IPAs with subgroup risk pools (20 percent of HMOs) have physicians contract with the IPA and subdivide the physicians into risk pools by location and type of doctor (specialty, referral, or primary-care). The doctors also see their own fee-for-service patients (40 percent of IPAs). (4) Three-tiered IPAs with subgroup risk pools (19 percent of HMOs) pay medical groups that in turn pay their physician membership—the groups have specialty, referral, and primary-care risk pools, and the doctors also see their own fee-for-service patients (15 percent of IPAs and 4.5 percent of staff HMOs). (5) Three-tiered IPAs with a single risk pool (8 percent of HMOs) pay medical groups that in turn pay their physician membership, and doctors also see fee-for-service patients (4.5 percent of IPAs and 13 percent of group model HMOs).

HMO physicians are concerned with the mechanism by which holdout risk pools are distributed. The physicians have full knowledge of the fee schedule or age-adjusted capitation rate of reimbursement from the HMO plan, but the risk pool can be handled a number of ways. Each clinician may have a referral fund to ensure that he or she does his or her work and does not shunt it off to other physicians (does not overrefer). Deficits in the referral fund might be covered with a 20 percent across-the-board holdout risk pool (a withhold), which means that the referral funds with a surplus are making up the loss. Each physician has a hospital fund, and the HMO absorbs 100 percent of all losses (because the HMO doctor cannot be held to blame for this "unexpected" event), but the HMO would pay 40 to 60 percent of any hospital-fund surplus to the physicians. Even HMOs without explicit risk pools or withholds offer some incentive to hold costs down. For example, a prepaid group-practice HMO like Harvard Community Health Plan may budget physician bonus pay at 5.5 percent of salaries, but depending on cost-control effectiveness, the bonus may vary from 0 to 10.5 percent of salaries. The decision to issue bonus pay is decentralized for a large three-tiered HMO like Health Insurance Plan (HIP) of Greater New York, which contracts with 8 physician groups and 49 hospitals.

CONSUMER TASTE FOR MANAGED CARE

Concerns over the quality of HMO service have been brought up by government (General Accounting Office [GAO] 1989) and the general public. But HMOs appear to be performing quality control adequately, according to Berwick,

Godfrey, and Roessner (1990) and Eisenberg and Kabcenell (1988). Consumers are also concerned with the time cost and restrictions of choice associated with HMO care.

From the patient perspective, the access to specialty referrals may pose a problem. Referrals are less of a problem for consumers in large staff- or group-model HMOs, where they can simply walk down the hall to the specialist's office. However, in an IPA-model HMO, the consumer often has to travel to a different office building. A second potential problem involves consumer expectations. Some consumers unrealistically expect a plastic surgeon for every small cut and a specialist for every minor complaint. This segment of the market would be wise to avoid enrolling in HMOs. Moreover, any HMO that caters to such whims must either go out of business or find subspecialists willing to work for $10 per hour.

Rural communities are less likely to be served by HMOs, presumably because of the lack of a critical mass (volume) of potential enrollees. This generality is not valid in all rural communities; for example, some rural areas have active business coalitions that have fueled the development of HMOs with sufficient initial start-up resources and promotional campaigns. A HMO offers certain rural areas the opportunity to retain resources and patients within the community. The percentage of rural communities served by HMOs has been on the increase: an estimated 15 percent of counties with fewer than 10,000 residents had HMOs in 1990 (up from only 4 percent in 1980); 25 percent of rural counties with 10,000–49,999 residents had HMOs in 1990 (up from 11 percent in 1980). Virtually 100 percent of urban communities had one or more HMOs available by 1985.

Do sick patients have a bias against HMO enrollment and instead prefer fee-for-service care? Feldman, Finch, and Dowd (1989) studied 6 HMOs and 17 employer groups and concluded that employees with poor health habits do not prefer fee-for-service plans compared to HMOs. They also speculated that HMOs have not gained long-term cost advantages by enrolling employees with favorable habits (nonsmokers, people who exercise, no heavy drinkers).

Although most HMOs charge copayments per visit in the range of $10 to $25 on the East Coast, more modest copayments can have a significant impact on utilization. Cherkin, Grothaus, and Wagner (1989) indicated that introduction of a $5 copayment per HMO office visit resulted in an 11 percent decrease in primary-care visits and a 3.3 percent decline in specialty-care visits. These copayments had much greater impact on enrollees who were high users (more than 10 visits per year) during the year before the introduction of cost-sharing expenses. Since no decline in health status has been detected, Davis et al. (1986) referred to such forgone patient visits as an example of the "worried well" avoiding unnecessary additional visits to save the copayment expense.

The style of medicine practiced in HMOs may reduce expenditures by 15 to 25 percent, principally through a 25 to 40 percent reduction in hospital admissions

(Luft 1981), but is this style of medicine quality neutral? In other words, for certain patient groups, does the quality of care seem to be worse (or better) in HMO settings than in fee-for-service care? One study by Ware et al. (1986) suggested that for one HMO the economical style of care may erode patient health status for the sick poor over a period of years. The Puget Sound HMO, a well-established plan, was studied as part of the Rand health insurance experiment from 1975 to 1983. The initially sick (at enrollment) low-income (bottom 20 percent of the population) participants appeared to fare better in the group randomized into fee-for-service settings than in the group in HMO care. However, the sick and nonsick high-income participants (top 40 percent of the income distribution) experienced a higher health-rating index in the group randomized into HMO care than in the group in traditional care. For the high-income enrollees, there are thus two reasons for joining an HMO: cost savings and gains in health status. The observed increases over time in bed days and serious symptoms were confined to the initially sick low-income HMO enrollees. The sick poor appeared worse off at the end of the study period than both the free-care and cost-sharing-care patients who were treated by traditional fee-for-service providers.

One lesson that could be drawn from the Rand study is that HMO care places more responsibility on the patient for compliance than the more aggressive and paternalistic fee-for-service system. Fee-for-service providers may cost more, but they have strong financial interests to coerce the additional follow-up care by telephone and mail. A follow-up study by Davis et al. (1986) suggested that poor people in the Puget Sound HMO were less likely to maintain continuity with the same physician than Medicaid patients in the fee-for-service sector. In addition to problems in communication or continuity of care, the poor may also have greater difficulty in arranging transport to the HMO's centralized locations. What is disturbing about these two studies is that the Puget Sound HMO has two decades of experience in treating the poor and providing outreach programs. In HMOs without such an established track record and social orientation, the initially sick poor may not fare as well as the Puget Sound enrollees.

There are a number of study limitations in the Rand data base. Ware et al. (1986) pointed out that one should not conclude that Medicaid patients are better off in fee-for-service settings than in HMO care. The Rand experiment had a supply-side effect on Seattle physicians in that the researchers paid fee-for-service providers charges that were 20 to 60 percent more generous than those of the Washington State Medicaid program. Consequently, physicians would be potentially more aggressive in following up a more profitable Rand Medicaid patient than an ordinary Medicaid patient. That initially sick poor enrollees in the Rand study would have fared better under the standard Medicaid program seems unlikely. Underlying many media reports lurks the presumption that the quality of patient outcomes is directly related to the quantity of care provided. No such link that "more is better" has ever been established.

DO HMOs SAVE MONEY?

There is disagreement whether HMOs are more cost-effective than other in-surance options (Feldman et al. 1990). The GAO (1989) and Wrightson (1990) stated that HMOs today are more cost-effective than pure 1982 indemnity plans. The problem in this comparison of apples and oranges is that pure indemnity plans no longer exist. By 1990 every private insurance plan engaged in personal benefits management: an organized effort to identify high-cost patients as early as possible, access lower-cost quality treatment options, and manage the average-cost patients more cost-effectively. Over 130 million Americans are covered by managed-care plans that perform utilization review with varying degrees of effectiveness (half of these employees are in PPOs). In the period 1988–91 managed-care indemnity plans experienced annual cost inflation of 17.9 percent, in contrast to 10.1 percent for staff-model HMOs and 14.4 percent for other HMOs. Therefore, the 4.9 million Americans in the 50 largest staff-model HMOs (like Harvard Community Health, Group Health of Puget Sound, Group Health of Minnesota, CIGNA, and FHP Inc.) are receiving a real social dividend: a less inflationary style of quality medical care. But for the 32.8 million Americans in other types of HMOs there is less circumstantial evidence to suggest that HMOs save money in comparison to the competition (other managed-care alternatives).

There is no evidence that quality of care is any different in HMOs from that in traditional fee-for-service medicine. In the Rand health insurance experiment enrollee health status was tracked for eight years for a randomized cohort of enrollees in Group Health of Puget Sound and a control group. The researchers (Sloss, Keeler, and Brook 1987) reported that the cost savings achieved by this staff-model HMO through 30 percent lower hospitalization rates were not re-flected in lower levels of health status after 1976. Another staff-model HMO, Harvard Community Health, has reported high levels of quality care resulting from the Deming method of quality control (Berwick, Godfrey, and Roessner 1990).

Business leaders are beginning to report a cost savings from certain HMOs. One unpublished study by A. Foster Higgins and Company in 1991 suggested that select HMOs save employers and employees $4.1 billion annually. Business leaders should also be equally concerned with the risk that HMOs might un-derprovide service. HMOs have a powerful incentive to avoid overusing services, but do some underutilize services? The federal professional review organizations (PROs) monitor HMO care to ensure that Medicare beneficiaries are protected, but most of the private-sector quality-of-care studies for all age cohorts of en-rollees have been performed in staff-model HMOs. More quality-of-care research must be performed on the other types of HMOs to assure the public that certain plans are not ''prepaid ghettos'' (a few such unethical HMOs have been sanc-tioned in Florida). Ethical exclusive provider organizations (EPOs) that lock in a limited set of providers are an increasingly popular hybrid product. The EPO has stricter utilization controls than a PPO but does not do as much review as a HMO (and therefore has a lower administrative expense; Madlin 1991).

PREPAID MEDICARE

Medicare HMO volume in the form of Medicare risk contracts has grown since 1979. In 1985, 119 HMO plans had enrolled 560,000 elderly beneficiaries. Langwell and Hadley (1990) reported that risk contracting has resulted in higher levels of satisfaction among Medicare beneficiaries. By 1991, 95 HMOs had enrolled 1.2 million Medicare beneficiaries. Congress and the health care industry are interested in two basic risk-contracting issues: price and equity. The risk-contracting program offered a slim 1.4 percent price rise in 1991, yet 11 new HMOs joined the risk-contracting program, and 13 dropped out (thus the number of HMOs in the program declined from 97 to 95 from 1990 to 1991). The second issue is more basic: How fair is the adjusted average per capita cost (AAPCC) methodology if it explains only 1.0 percent of the variation in cost per capita? Consequently, Congress specified in the November 5, 1990, budget bill that the HCFA come up with an improved AAPCC alternative by FY 1993 that explains at least 15 percent of the variation in cost and utilization among enrollees. Ash et al. (1989) reported that incorporating prior utilization by the individual into the model, defining nine distinct diagnostic cost groups (DCGs), helped to explain 4 to 9 percent of the variance in cost and utilization per capita. These results from a prior-use model were confirmed by Porell and Turner (1990), but the policy maker should still be left with a nagging question. Granted, using prior-year utilization data improves the statisical model, but how much of this prior utilization was unnecessary care, discretionary care, or required care? These issues will be addressed in subsequent chapters of this book when we consider technology assessment and cost-effective clinical decision making. An alternative payment formula yet to be developed has the potential to reduce favorable selection bias in Medicare HMOs, ensure payer equity, and reduce fiscal risk for both parties (Riley, Rabey, and Kasper 1989).

A more comprehensive alternative to DCGs is the payment amount for capitated systems (PACS) developed at Johns Hopkins University. PACS establishes a payment rate for the HMO based on two factors: the health status of the individual who actually enrolls in the HMO and the input costs faced by the HMO. Anderson et al. (1990a) tested their model on random samples of Medicare beneficiaries from Florida and Pennsylvania and concluded that while DCGs may be four times as good as AAPCC, the PACS model beats DCGs in most closely approximating costs per capita. PACS performs well because it explicitly differentiates between acute and chronic conditions and offers higher payment rates for beneficiaries who experienced multiple hospitalizations during the prior year. PACS employs a continuous model, rather than clustering individuals into nine discrete groups like DCGs. The fourth advantage of the PACS model is that its incorporation of the Medicare Part B deductible variable helps differentiate those healthy people who have little or no contact with the health care system. Neither PACS nor DCGs can accurately predict which individuals will have multiple hospitalizations in the future. Therefore, Anderson et al. (1990b) suggested a separate payment mechanism to pay for high-cost outliers.

According to the theory of consumer choice, under the assumption of perfect information, the elderly would pick the HMO that best meets their needs. Unfortunately, the elderly are a high-cost cohort of individuals operating with less than perfect information (on their providers and concerning their future health needs). However, the HMO option may be a great deal for patients with serious chronic illnesses. Medicare supplemental insurance plans are poorly coordinated, overpriced, and poorly designed (Berenson 1986). Therefore, it would be difficult for the sick elderly not to find a better deal in joining prepaid plans. However, the elderly with many preexisting conditions seem most concerned with staying with their existing sources of care and not shopping for a HMO unless their current physician is a member of a plan. Participating in Competitive Medical Plans (CMPs) or HMOs offers an ethical dilemma for the clinicians, because to do what is best for the elderly may minimize their long-run income.

If low disenrollment rates are any indication of the enrollees' acceptance of HMOs and CMPs, it is apparent that the elderly are satisfied with the services they receive. Advocates of prepaid Medicare are fond of pointing out this fact, in addition to citing an actuarial phenomenon known as "regression to the mean" (Lichtenstein et. al. 1991). If the plan experiences adverse selection (expensive cases), its cost experience tends to regress down to the mean (get lower over time). Lubitz, Beebe, and Riley (1985) reported that high-risk elderly experienced Medicare costs 4.7 times higher than the mean, but by the next year their experience had fallen to 1.8 times the mean of all beneficiaries. On the other hand, favorable selection of the low-risk elderly also results in a regression up to the mean (in the first year the low-risk group may spend 1.8 percent of the national average Medicare expenses, but within a year this figure will have risen to 55 percent). Moreover, if the HMO or CMP can only selectively market to a small fraction of its enrollees, and if their behavior tends to regress to the mean, the question of selection bias may be labeled "much ado about nothing" by the health plans (Wilensky and Rossiter 1986). However, if the prepaid business evolves into a highly competitive market, a difference of a few percentage points in cost behavior could mean the difference between plan growth, stagnation, or closure. Four rural plans have already announced that they will stop their Medicare contracts because the rural AAPCC rate was $110 lower than the local urban rate, and their enrollees were heavy users of the expensive urban hospitals.

The General Accounting Office (GAO 1989) is obviously concerned with offering too much of a profit in the market with a generous AAPCC formula. However, the GAO will have a difficult task determining whether the plans underpromote to the sick elderly, overpromote to the low-risk elderly, or work

Table 5.2
Comparison of Operating Expenses as a Percentage of Premium Revenues in Two Large National HMOs, 1991

		U.S. Health Care	United Health Care
1.	Inpatient hospital	26%	29%
2.	Physician services	38%	37%
3.	Ambulatory care	5%	6%
4.	Other medical	8%	6%
5.	SGA overhead	10%	8%
6.	Total operating expenses	87.1%	86.3%
7.	Number of plans	6	16
8.	Number of states	6	10[a]
9.	Year the company became a national firm	1983	1979
10.	Inpatient days per 1,000 enrollees	331	342
11.	Physician visits per 1,000 enrollees	3.6	3.5

[a]Has IPA management contracts for physician groups in 18 other states.

with their physicians to improve utilization review activities. Is any reduction in utilization the result of patient selection or provider education?

TRENDS: MARKET SHAKEOUT AND MORE FOR-PROFITS

Prior to 1981 the HMO industry was wedded to nonprofit ownership status. Since the elimination of federal grants in 1982, almost half of the HMOs have converted to for-profit status. If the two large HMO chains listed in table 5.2 are well-managed HMO chains, Maxicare is an example of overreaching, out-of-control costs, and poor planning. In 1986–87 Maxicare had administrative overhead and inpatient hospital payments that were 25 to 35 percent higher than the figures in table 5.2. Maxicare proved that a HMO could grow bigger and drive a business into the ground. In 1985 Maxicare had 686,000 enrollees in 9 states and made $20 million in profit, and the central office amassed $330 million in cash for further expansion. In 1986 Maxicare had 1.96 million enrollees in 19 states, and profits fell to under $4.8 million. In 1987 Maxicare had 2.3 million enrollees in 25 states and lost $71 million. Maxicare senior management still tried to retain the dream of approaching national employers with a national HMO network in 25 of the 30 largest cities in the nation. It is not a smart strategy to take on service-delivery burdens faster than the firm has learned how to contain the cost behavior of the providers. At the end of 1987 Maxicare's net worth was negative $29.3 million, Standard and Poor's credit rating declined to B −, and the firm was placed on the Credit Watch list. In 1988 the two senior managers in Maxicare resigned, 20 months after being profiled by *Fortune* magazine as "among the 50 most fascinating business people of the year." In March 1989 Maxicare filed for protection from creditors under chapter 11 of the Federal Bankruptcy Code. The good news is that the phoenix emerged from the ashes: Maxicare concentrated on operating in 7 states, emphasized cost control for its 405,000 enrollees, and reported its first quarterly profit in five years in the fall of 1990.

There has been a paucity of research concerning what an optimal scale is for HMOs. Gurnick (1991) did a survival analysis of HMOs in the 1980s and concluded that (1) an optimal size for communication and fiscal survival is 40,000 to 60,000 enrollees; (2) to survive, a HMO should achieve a critical mass of 25,000 enrollees in four to five years; and (3) if the HMO is too large, it should subdivide into smaller segments (Kaiser Oakland subdivides into decentralized segments of 50,000 enrollees, and thus produces better communication with the medical staff). Future research should consider long-run average cost curves and a more traditional economic analysis. Survivor analysis and market-share statistics (Gurnick 1991) only provide indirect evidence. But the HMO industry will not have the necessary uniform audited financial data until the mid–1990s.

If one assumes that the retailer controls the production channel, as in the case of a HMO, the plan can achieve maximum profits by hiring physician services at below-market prices. A second alternative is to assume that the physicians and hospitals or HMO plans pursue profit maximization while allowing a "necessary" profit margin to the other party. Such a compromise may result in an inefficient equilibrium at a price between P' and P'' producing a quantity of service ranging between Q' and Q'' in Figure 5.1. To maximize profits, physicians set marginal physician revenue equal to their marginal costs, implying a transaction with the hospital involving Q' units of care at price P'. To maximize hospital revenues in excess of costs, hospitals would prefer a transaction with the physicians involving fewer units of service (Q'') at a higher level of reimbursement (P'').

Prepaid group health plans are one of the few markets where health facility managers and physicians are on a relatively equivalent bargaining basis. The management of new HMOs must frequently report to the private risk bearers who supplied the venture capital. The HMO sponsors are always putting on the pressure and searching the market for better managers. The market for HMOs is less stable than the hospital industry, in that there is a higher chance of exit (going out of business). However, the opportunity for growth is very large. Consequently, the owner-sponsors of the HMO search for the best-quality managers to deal with the potential growth opportunities in the market for prepaid group health care (Dolinsky and Caputo 1991).

Figure 5.1
Potential Equilibrium in the Doctor-Hospital Producer-Retailer Production Channel for Hospital Services

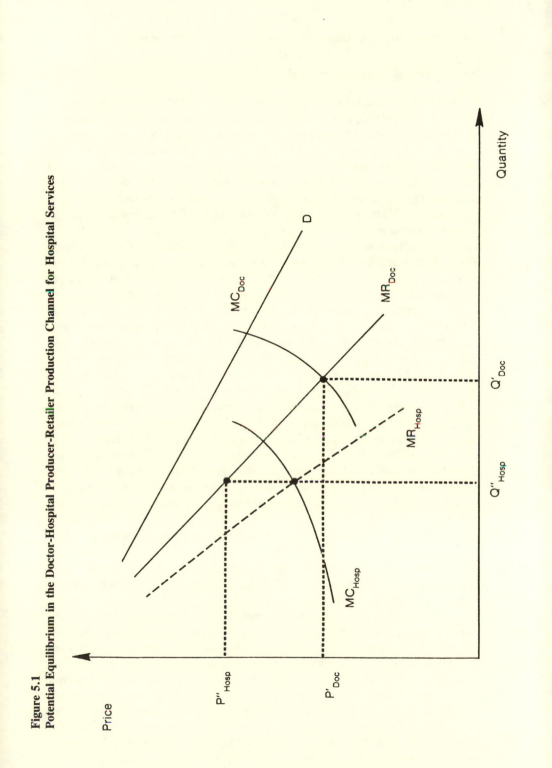

SOCIAL HMOs FOR THE ELDERLY

Protection from catastrophically high health care costs is becoming an increasingly recognized public problem. One alternative delivery system, the social HMO (SHMO), attempts to efficiently coordinate care for older people who are most likely to have multiple health problems requiring the attention of multiple providers. SHMOs are prepaid managed-care systems for long-term care and medical care geared toward elderly enrollees. The sponsoring organization takes responsibility for integrating a wide range of services for a membership. Under the 1983–89 SHMO Demonstration Project with HCFA, members of a representative sample of the elderly, both disabled and able-bodied, were paid on a prepaid capitation basis at four SHMOs (Kaiser Portland, Elderplan Brooklyn, Ebenezer Minneapolis, and Senior Care Action Plan Long Beach). The SHMO is at risk for service costs, taking responsibility for operating within a budget and generating a profit (or loss) depending on how effectively costs are managed.

If the SHMOs are successful, it is hoped that they will interest employers, insurance carriers, and government to encourage greater prefunding of long-term care (McCall, Knickman, and Bauer 1991). We shall discuss long-term-care insurance later in this chapter, but HMOs face a number of the same generic problems (e.g., adverse selection). There are three basic methods by which a SHMO can protect itself from attracting a disproportionate share of the sicker elderly enrollees. First, the SHMO could provide less than full chronic-care benefits and a lower premium (to attract the healthier elderly). Second, one could cheat the system by screening potential enrollees on the basis of health factors outside the HCFA adjusted average per capita cost (AAPCC) formula, but the demonstration prohibited such skimming behavior. Third, queuing, with a significant waiting period to join the SHMO, is one formal mechanism to minimize adverse selection, be fair to the payer, and collect a representative share of high-risk elderly.

Two of the SHMOs in the demonstration project did not achieve the projected financial break-even level of 4,000 enrollees by 1989. The SHMOs are enrolling Medicare-only beneficiaries and Medicare beneficiaries who receive Medicaid assistance and are designed to be budget neutral for both payer groups. Considering a study demonstrating how one long-standing HMO appears to have discounted quality for poor enrollees (Ware et al. 1986), government officials should continue to monitor quality of care. The innovative impulse behind SHMOs resides in the integration of services and funding sources, so that the elderly are not shuffled from one provider to another. The business community should be attracted to the idea of "living within a budget," and consumer groups should like the idea of reduced fragmentation of services. The HMO incentive structure encourages the substitution of earlier, less expensive, "low-tech" services prior to the need for expensive inpatient services. Reducing hospital use is essential to the SHMOs' ability to support expanded long-term-care benefits. In addition to promoting increased use of community-based alternatives, SHMOs should (1) decrease inappropriate nursing home admissions and (2) slow the Medicaid "spend-down" rate at which elderly beneficiaries expend personal resources. To advise Congress on what levels of cost sharing are most appropriate for the elderly, the SHMO demonstration sites offered different cost-sharing packages (Leutz et al. 1990).

Gerontologists and psychologists will be interested in the degree to which the SHMO case management system strengthens or erodes the informal principal-care-person and family support system for the enrollee. In theory, as the difficulty of caring for frail elders increases due to the stress of precipitating events, the informal support network should be less likely to break down. Such a prediction assumes that the extensive SHMO case management placement system works well. However, the system could break down if the case manager is perceived as an enemy who is forcing a too severely ill patient to be treated at home by overworked family and friends. SHMOs have a clear financial incentive to shift more burdens to the family, even though their efficient placement services should be faster and more effective at final institutional placement. There comes a point where the sicker home care patients are better served in an institution, yet SHMOs have a financial incentive to underadmit.

If the SHMOs are not providing good service or overextend the patience of unpaid family and friends, one would predict that disenrollment levels would be high. If the demonstration proves a success, perhaps in the late 1990s Congress will enact a SHMO entitlement for Medicare enrollees that will do for long-term care what Pub. L. 97–248 did for hospice care. If we enact a national SHMO program, shoddy "fast-buck" operators may have less interest in ethics, equity, and service than these four model SHMOs.

After a slow start the four SHMOs are beginning to improve operating performance. Three of the first SHMOs reported substantial losses in their first three years, primarily because of slow enrollment and resultant high marketing and administrative costs (Leutz et al. 1990). After assuming full risk, two of the three showed surpluses in the most recent fiscal year (1989). Management and service costs for expanded long-term care were similar across the four sites and are affordable within the framework of Medicaid and Medicare payment rates (Harrington and Newcomer 1991; Birnbaum et al. 1991).

Case managers can help channel patients to cost-effective providers within the context of SHMOs and also in the context of more flexible organizations. For example, one report on the National Channeling Demonstration Project (Kemper 1990) suggested that case managers are not yet cost-effective at substituting home health care services for nursing home care. The reason the case managers were not successful at limiting costs is that they had no financial incentive to do so. Kemper and Murtaugh (1991) suggested giving the case managers more autonomy and incentive to channel home care services to the patients that will in turn be most likely to substitute this care for inpatient nursing home care. In theory, case managers can also assist in the quality-assurance process and help negotiate prices below the prevailing market rates. Case managers will begin to justify their 6 to 10 percent administrative expense when they have the monetary incentive to trim costs, make home care a substitute for bed care, and not simply make home care an extra add-on service (without economic benefit).

We need to provide case managers with the tools to predict nursing home admissions and length of stay (Liu, Coughlin, and McBride 1991; Short, Cunningham, and Mueller 1991) and to assess the quality of care (Ferris and Wyszewianski 1990). Greater reliance on geriatric nurse practitioners has some potential to reduce cost per case (Buchanan et al. 1990).

SLOW GROWTH FOR LONG-TERM-CARE INSURANCE

The aging of the population clearly represents a major public policy challenge, and new public programs may have difficulty getting funded in an era of budget austerity. Therefore, increasing attention has turned to the development of private insurance funds for long-term care. The pioneer in the private long-term-care insurance business was Acsia Insurance Services. Acsia of California began issuing policies through Fireman's Fund Insurance in 1976. Fireman's will issue the policy to a person over age 79 if the spouse is under age 80 and insured for an equivalent or greater amount of indemnity (Phillips 1984).

Insurance to cover the costs of long-term care has failed to develop in the private sector for a number of reasons. While a total of 120 companies sell some form of long-term-care insurance for 2.7 million Americans, the market penetration in any given state was disappointingly small in 1991. Members of the group for which the premiums are the most reasonable, the middle-aged, have little incentive to purchase such insurance in our prevailing youth culture. They have numerous other pulls on their income, from the mortgage to their children's education. The insurance industry would have to structure premiums to reflect actual risk at a certain age, rather than the lifetime risk, in order to encourage greater participation by the population aged 45 to 69. Moreover, some public subsidy would be required to encourage significant market growth. The Heritage Institute has advocated an individual retirement medical account (IRMA) to encourage prefunding of long-term care. The investment return would be taxable and, although earmarked for health care, would be owned by consumers to do with as they choose.

Pricing of long-term-care insurance must be based on careful actuarial data. Kemper and Murtaugh (1991) reported that the probability that a person had used a nursing home increased sharply with age at death: 17 percent for those aged 65 to 74, 36 percent for those aged 75 to 84, and 60 percent for those aged 85 to 94. Of those turning 65 in 1990, 43 percent are projected to need a nursing home at some time before they die. A surprising 21 percent of this 43 percent requiring a nursing home will have total lifetime use of five years or more. The expense of a five-year nursing home stay, discounted to 1992 dollars, should exceed $140,000. If these trends continue, some 200,000 Americans turning 65 during 1992 will spend more than $140,000 on nursing home stays exceeding five years. Who will pay the bills? Government? Private long-term-care insurance? Studies like these may prompt the middle-aged population to purchase long-term-care insurance (Kane and Kane 1991).

A private 1991 Gallup Poll indicated that 22 percent of Americans said that they expect to need a nursing home at some point. Over 62 percent of adults said that they would be willing to purchase long-term-care insurance, and the mean respondent would be willing to pay $42 per month in premiums, with 14 percent willing to pay $61 or more. Greater reliance on long-term care might benefit the general economy if it would free up informal caregivers (spouse, family) to do other productive activities (Stone and Short 1990). However, documented cases of policyholders being denied benefit payments due to prior-hospitalization and prior-skilled-care clauses in the contract (Wilson and Weissert 1989) may limit the public interest in purchasing long-term-care insurance. Rice et al. (1991) emphasized the point that the premiums would be more affordable if they were purchased in the middle years, ages 40 to 64. However, many families have other consumption needs during that period (raising a family, education costs). Estimates of how much a federal subsidy program to purchase long-term-care insurance would cost annually range from $20 billion (Health Care Financing Agency [HCFA] 1991) to $4 billion (Stan Wallack 1991, private study for the Health Insurance Association of America [HIAA]). The current restrictive clauses in long-term-care policies have done little to reduce uncertainty and financial risk (National Association of Insurance Commissioners [NAIC] 1991). Setting the inflation-protection clause and the duration of policy coverage are problematic (Luft 1991).

McCall, Knickman, and Bauer (1991) have outlined a number of ways in which the Robert Wood Johnson Foundation is trying to promote long-term-care insurance for the elderly in eight states. In Oregon and California the minimum amount of insurance required in the program is two years or at least a $50,000 lifetime maximum benefit. Oregon is initiating state tax credits on the long-term-care premiums paid. New York State has expanded the minimum amount of insurance required to three years. Massachusetts has expanded its program to include 2,500 working-age citizens and 7,500 people aged 65 to 69. The Massachusetts program sets the minimum amount of insurance required to the amount purchased with a maximum of 5.0 percent of income (including annuitization of nonhousing assets). Five states offer a more liberal pilot program whereby policyholders are eligible for Medicaid after their private insurance is exhausted (Connecticut, California, Indiana, New Jersey, and Wisconsin). Massachusetts and New York do not link asset protection to the actual amount of private benefits paid out (Somers and Merrill 1991).

HOME HEALTH CARE

That the home health care sector is a creature of public policy is undeniable. In some nations home health care is centuries old (China), whereas in other nations the home health care center is having difficulty surviving because the physicians refuse to allow competition (Korea). In the American context, as payment rates remain flat, so has business remained flat at $6.2 billion annually in the home health sector (1988–91). The only growth segment in the home care business is the high-tech home infusion-therapy market (Wagner 1990). Infusion-therapy firms grew from 330 in 1988 to 890 in 1991 because of advances in drugs, drug-delivery technology, and insurance coverage. It is obvious to health insurance companies that it is more cost-effective to shift patients from expensive hospital settings to home infusion therapy (Shaughnessy and Kramer 1990). AIDS patients are more cost-effectively treated at home ($188 per day for home infusion antibiotics and $160 per day for nursing care, compared to over $1,000 per day for an inpatient hospitalization; National Underwriter [NU] 1991). It is less obvious to federal public policy makers that national coverage of home health care would be cost-effective (Williams et al. 1990; HCFA 1991; Kemper 1990). The economies of scale are inconsequential for home health firms (Kass 1987). If the entitlement to home health care creates a demand-pull inflation of questionable home health care seekers (people wanting custodial care for the first time because its price is reduced by insurance), it may not be good public policy. The Pepper Commission's call for "full social insurance" was largely ignored because the price tag, $13 to $16 billion annually for additional home health and custodial care, was judged too costly by Congress (Rockefeller 1990). There is a wide level of agreement that families would be relieved of the burden of providing unreimbursed home care for relatives if the government could afford to pay for it. There is a less salient level of agreement as to the "crushing impoverishment" that long-term care represents to the frail elderly without family and friends. Some policy makers misinterpret a study like that of Burwell, Adams, and Meiners (1990) by jumping to the conclusion that Medicaid spend-down in nursing homes (impoverishment before eligibility for Medicaid) is not a substantial problem. The study by Burwell, Adams, and Meiners (1990) indicated that during a single nursing home episode only 10 percent of patients who entered as private payers received Medicaid at discharge. There is a need for a longitudinal study of multiple episodes tracking individuals over a long period of time to assess the fiscal burden of the Medicaid spend-down provision on elderly patients and their relatives.

Home health care grew from 1.6 percent of Medicaid expenditures in 1975 to 3.2 percent in 1985 and 3.9 percent in 1989–91. Medicare has also paid for $1.6 to $1.9 billion of home health care per year since 1984 (1.6 million people served and 24 visits per person per year, on average; HCFA 1991). Policy makers are currently considering prospective payment for the 5,500 home health care firms. In this era of DRGs for hospitals and resource utilization groups (RUGs) for some nursing homes, it is inconsistent that home health care is still cost reimbursed. In the interest of containing home health care expenses, more payers will begin to replace cost reimbursement with prospective payment.

Some researchers refer to the subacute care that hospitals had traditionally

Table 5.3
Medicare Beneficiaries' Usage of Home Health Care and Skilled Nursing Facilities by Age, 1970–1990

| | Utilization per 1,000 Medicare Enrollees | | | |
| | Home Health Agency | | Skilled Nursing Facility | |
Patient Age	1970	1990	1970	1990
65-69	5	39	5	6
70-74	7	65	10	6
75-79	9	88	19	11
80-84	12	106	36	21
85 and over	12	115	54	36
Total	8	74	16	12

Source: Health Care Financing Administration, 1991.

provided but that is now provided on an ambulatory basis (in response to PPS or utilization review) as *transitional care*. Transitional care can be provided in a nursing facility, intermediate-care facility, at home (with the assistance of home health workers), and sometimes in hospital-based, subacute-care-bed sections. Some of the eliminated hospital days—168 million between 1983 and 1991—result in increased days of care in other transitional settings. Russell (1990) may have overstated the $17 billion in savings to the Medicare program. The savings from shorter stays and fewer admissions among public and private patients are partially offset by the costs incurred in transitional care. Medicare enrollees, other patients, and families are finding that some of the financial burden for this transitional care has shifted onto them. By definition, some cost shift has to occur because transitional care is less well insured (more consumer out-of-pocket cost sharing) than hospital care.

Much of the growth in transitional care has been in the home health care arena (table 5.3). The nature of home health service is changing. The 1986 survey of Area Agencies on Aging (AAA) reported a fivefold increase in case management services, a threefold increase in home skilled nursing care, and a twofold increase in personal care services and housekeeping following the first three years of PPS (1983–86). In contrast, the 1991 survey suggested a fourfold increase in high-tech home health care since 1987.

Data on the development of hospital-based subacute-care beds will become available from the American Hospital Association in 1992–93. HCFA officials fear that some hospitals may place financial concerns above the clinical concerns of the patients by moving some individuals prematurely so as to "game" the system and receive supplemental payments for rehabilitation or other transitional types of care. Unfortunately, it will be nearly impossible to judge how much of this is "gaming" versus a medically appropriate transfer or discharge to a lower-cost service setting. These lower-cost service settings not only represent an alternative source of revenue, they also help minimize losses that might have been incurred by a PPS patient sitting in an inpatient bed any longer than deemed necessary. However, when medically appropriate, transitional care is a good loss minimizer and revenue-generating strategy. If medically inappropriate, the transfer or early discharge may cause the PPS patient to relapse and be rehospitalized, much to the embarrassment (e.g., in PRO oversight) and financial loss of all concerned at the hospital.

Most ethical providers argue that transitional care is more properly and less expensively delivered in less resource-intensive settings. Officials at HCFA and in the HMO industry can observe (with some smugness) that this discovery of lower-cost alternative care settings was largely prompted by hospital prospective payment formulas and employer interest in prepaid care. The most critical policy question is whether this movement to transitional care will decrease total per capita costs. Three other key questions are (1) whether increasing severity-of-illness levels among transitional-care patients pose a threat to patient quality of care, (2) whether access to services is a problem for certain patient groups, and (3) whether theorized continuity-of-care benefits accrue if the patients receive all their transitional care from one institution. Future research may provide answers.

One major stimulus to the rapid growth in Medicare home health payments, in addition to the PPS hospital payment scheme, was Pub. L. 96–499 to liberalize home health benefits in 1980. This bill provided for the first time coverage for an unlimited number of home health visits and eliminated the three-day prior-hospitalization requirement as a condition for the receipt of home health services.

The policy debate concerning home care versus institutionalization has raged since precolonial Elizabethan poor laws. In the American context, pioneering hospitals developed home care "hospitals without walls" in the 1950s to compensate for the decline in the rate of physician house calls. Physicians in markets of oversupply have provided a modest rebirth of the home health care market, but home care is unlikely to become physician dominated. If anything, experts argue that physician involvement has been too minimal (Koren 1986). House calls as a percentage of the 1.1 billion physician visits with noninstitutionalized Americans increased from 0.6 percent in 1982 to 2.9 percent in 1991. Payment rates will limit the expansion in house calls. Rates set for a home visit by a physician will never be commensurate with those for other hospital or office visits.

HCFA is playing its part in curtailing the growth of a booming home health market (Department of Health and Human Services [DHHS] 1986). The rate increases fall substantially short of any inflation-adjustment levels, and the regulatory requirements are increasing (HCFA 1991). Still, many hospitals plan continued expansion into home health care, which led analysts at Kurt Salmon and Associates (1989) to predict a glut of home health care agencies in the future. Lower payment rates are the traditional payer response to any glut in supply.

Policy trends in home health care currently point in all different directions, like a pile of jackstraws. The marketplace is littered with the wreckage of well-intentioned home health agencies and meals-on-wheels programs disbanded. On the other hand, high-tech home care has been rapidly promoted by manufacturers. Insurers, HMOs, and PPOs are eager to pay for these high-tech services if they substitute for higher-cost hospital care. Antibiotics, chemotherapy, central intravenous lines, peripheral lines, cardiac pressor agents, and parenteral nutrition have become major product lines in home health care since 1983. For example, some 260,000 Americans have digestive problems each year and require total parenteral nutrition (TPN). If TPN can be done for $5,000 per month at home, it is substantially more cost-effective than paying $12,000 to $19,000 per month for inpatient TPN.

Some 6.6 million elderly require help in the tasks of daily living. Approximately 80 percent of this help comes in the form of unpaid assistance from friends and relatives. Home health care assists all concerned in maintaining the activities of daily living, so that the elderly are not forced into an institution. According to one survey, home health care patients are younger and less functionally disabled than nursing home patients (Kramer, Shaughnessy, and Pettigrew 1985). For years advocates of home health care had hoped that "low-tech" provision of services would prove cost-effective relative to inpatient care.

Hedrick and Inui (1986) surveyed 12 economic evaluations of home health services. Home health care had no impact on patient functioning, mortality, nursing home placements, and acute hospitalization (in three studies hospitalization actually increased with home care provision). The total cost of care was either not affected or actually increased by 15 percent. Poor organization and fragmentation of services could explain why home health care has yet to live up to its promise for cost-benefit. For example, Medicare-reimbursed home health care not only lacks homemaker/chore services, but also needs more stringent case management and referral services to prevent fragmentation. A new delivery style, managed care, allows the broker or case-managing agency to assess needs for care, develop a comprehensive care plan, refer the patient, and monitor the individual's situation so that the care plan can be readjusted if necessary.

Case management in home health care has typically been very poor. Medicare requires that a beneficiary be homebound and need skilled nursing, physical therapy, or speech therapy in accordance with a physician's treatment plan, but physician intervention is so minimal as to involve but a few minutes of time (Koren 1986). This is not to suggest that the case manager must be a physician, but cost-benefit is only achievable if the case manager takes the time to closely monitor the case. If the case manager does not get the appropriate services delivered on a consistent basis, very costly events will be forthcoming (hospitalization or nursing home placement). The challenge for home health care has been particularly strong since 1984. Because of the DRG payment system, home health care patients are sicker, and coordination of care is even more critical than before. Nurses or social workers, who may work for the organization to which they refer patients, have not been effective as case managers seeking to maximize either quality or cost-efficiency (Kemper 1990).

Our understanding of home health care agencies' shortcomings is equally matched by federal analysts' misunderstandings of the patient population. Very few patients who use home-based services would have become long stayers in nursing homes in any case (Weissert and Cready 1989). Long stayers tend to be older, more dependent, and poorer in social resources than those who use home care. Few patients who actually use home care have their institutional stay averted or shortened. Patients who use "high-touch, low-tech" home care are most often using it as an add-on (complement) to existing services, rather than as a substitute for institutional care. The sickest and most dependent cases may be less expensive to serve in a nursing home or a clinic than in the home, except in the case of a few high-tech home health conditions.

Public support for home health care might best focus on functionally dependent people rather than on the aged per se. Home health agencies might be able to market their services on a cost-benefit basis with better case management. However, "low-tech" home health care might still have to resort to intangible quality-of-life benefits for justification, like reduced feelings of isolation or improved cognitive functioning. Methods to shadow-price intangible benefits will be considered in chapter 13.

REFERENCES

Abou, F., Falle, V., and Matsuwaka, R. (1991). "Hospice Care Can Yield Savings to HMOs, Patients." *Healthcare Financial Management* 45:8 (August) 84–86.

Aluise, J., Konrad, T., and Buckner, B. (1989). "IPAs and Fee-for-Service Medical Groups." *Health Care Management Review* 14:1 (Winter), 55–63.

American Hospital Association. (1990). *Physicians in the Management of Risk in Managed Care Contracts.* Chicago: AHA.

Anderson, G., Steinberg, E., Powe, N., Antebi, S., Whittle, J., and Horn, S. (1990a). "Setting Payment Rates for Capitated Systems: A Comparison of Various Alternatives." *Inquiry* 27:3 (Fall), 225–233.

Anderson, G., Steinberg, E., Whittle, J., Powe, N., and Antebi, S. (1990b). "Development of Clinical and Economic Prognoses from Medicare Data Claims." *Journal of the American Medical Association* 263:7 (February 11), 967–972.

Ash, A., Porell, F., Gruenberg, L., Sawitz, E., and Beiser, A. (1989). "Adjusting Medicare Capitation Payments Using Prior Hospitalization Data." *Health Care Financing Review* 10:4 (Summer), 17–29.

Atkinson, G., and Eastaugh, S. (1984). "Guaranteed Inpatient Revenue: Friend or Foe to PPOs and Alternative Delivery." *Maryland HFMA Quarterly* 18:5 (May), 1–4.

Baloff, N., and Griffith, M. (1982). "Managing Start-up Utilization in Ambulatory Care." *Journal of Ambulatory Care Management* 5:2 (February), 1–12.

Beebe, J., Lubitz, J., and Eggers, P. (1985). "Using Prior Utilization Information to

Determine Payments for Medicare Enrollees in HMOs." *Health Care Financing Review* 6:3 (Spring), 31–49.

Berenson, R. (1986). "Capitation and Conflict of Interest." *Health Affairs* 5:1 (Spring), 141–146.

Berwick, D. (1991). "Blazing the Trail of Quality," *Frontiers of Health Services Management* 7:4 (Summer), 47–50.

Berwick, D., Godfrey, A., and Roessner, J. (1990). *Curing Health Care: New Strategies for Quality Improvement*. San Francisco: Jossey-Bass.

Birnbaum, H., Holland, S., and Lenhart, G. (1991). "Savings Estimate for a Medicare Insured Group." *Health Care Financing Review* 12:4 (Summer), 39–48.

Boland, P. (1990). "Joining Forces to Make Managed Health Care Work." *Healthcare Financial Management* 44:12 (December), 21–25.

Buchanan, J., Arnold, S., Bell, R., and Witsberger, C. (1990). *Financial Impact of Nursing Home-based Geriatric Nurse Practitioners*. Santa Monica, California: Rand Corporation.

Burwell, B., Adams, E., and Meiners, M. (1990). "Spend-down of Assets before Medicaid Eligibility among Elderly Nursing-Home Recipients." *Medical Care* 28:4 (April), 349–362.

Cherkin, D., Grothaus, L., and Wagner, E. (1989). "Effect of Office Visit Copayments on Utilization in a HMO." *Medical Care* 27:11 (November), 1036–1045.

Clancy, G., and Hillner, B. (1989). "Physicians as Gatekeepers: The Impact of Financial Incentives." *Archives of Internal Medicine* 149:4 (April), 917–920.

Cohodes, D. (1985). "HMOs: What Goes Up Must Come Down." *Inquiry* 22:4 (Winter), 333–334.

Davis, A., Ware, J., Brook, R., Peterson, J., and Newhouse, J. (1986). "Consumer Attitudes toward Prepaid and Fee-for-Service Medical Care: Results from a Controlled Trial." *Health Services Research* 21:2 (July), 429–452.

Davis, K. (1991). "Expanding Medicare and Employer Plans to Achieve Universal Health Insurance." *Journal of the American Medical Association* 265:19 (May 15), 2525–2529.

Department of Health and Human Services. (1986). "Limits on Home Health Agency Costs—Final Notice." *Federal Register* 51:104 (May 30), 19734–19741.

———. (1985). "Medicare Program: Payment to HMOs and CMPs —HCFA Final Rules and Comment Period." *Federal Register* 50:7 (January 10), 1314–1418.

Dolinsky, A., and Caputo, R. (1991). "Assessment of Employers' Experiences with HMOs." *Health Care Management Review* 16:1 (Winter), 25–31.

Eastaugh, S. (1992). "Healthy Management Alternatives for Better Productivity." *Harvard Business Review* 70:1 (January-February), 161–162.

———. (1986). "Differential Cost Analysis: Judging a PPO's Feasibility." *Healthcare Financial Management* 40:5 (May), 44–51.

Edelston, J., Valentine, S., and Ginoza, D. (1985). "PPO Contracting: A California Experience." *Hospitals* 59:19 (October 1), 81–83.

Eisenberg, J., and Kabcenell, A. (1988). "Organized Practice and the Quality of Medical Care." *Inquiry* 25:1 (Spring), 78–89.

Enthoven, A. (1980). *Health Plan*. Reading, Mass.: Addison-Wesley.

Enthoven, A., and Kronick, R. (1991). "Universal Health Insurance Through Incentives Reform." *Journal of the American Medical Association* 265:19 (May 15), 2532–2537.

Feldman, R., Chan, H., Kralewski, J., Dowd, B., and Shapiro, J. (1990). "Effects of HMOs on the Creation of Competitive Markets for Hospital Services." *Journal of Health Economics* 9:2 (September), 207–220.

Feldman, R., Finch, M., and Dowd, B. (1989). "The Role of Health Practices in HMO Selection Bias." *Inquiry* 26:3 (Fall), 381–387.

Ferris, A., and Wyszewianski, L. (1990). "Quality of Ambulatory Care for the Elderly: Formulating Evaluation Criteria." *Health Care Financing Review* 12:1 (Fall), 31–38.

Gabel, J., and Ermann, D. (1985). "Preferred Provider Organizations: Performance, Problems, and Promise." *Health Affairs* 4:1 (Spring), 24–40.

General Accounting Office. (1989). *Medicare: Physician Incentive Payments by Prepaid Health Plans Could Lower Quality of Care*. GAO Report HRD–89–29 (January). Washington, D.C.: U.S. Government Printing Office.

Ginsburg, P., and Hackbarth, G. (1986). "Alternative Delivery Systems and Medicare." *Health Affairs* 5:1 (Spring), 6–22.

Goldberg, L., and Greenberg, W. (1979). "The Competitive Response of Blue Cross and Blue Shield to the HMOs in Northern California and Hawaii." *Medical Care* 17:10 (October), 1019–1028.

Goldfield, N., and Goldsmith, S. (1989). *Financial Management of Ambulatory Care*. Rockville, Md.: Aspen.

Green, P., and Schaffer, C. (1991). "Importance Weight Effects on Self Explicated Preference Models: Some Empirical Findings." *Advances in Consumer Research* 18 (Spring), 476–482.

Grossman, W. (1990). "Risk Contracting." *Topics in Health Care Financing* 16:4 (Summer), 24–30.

Group Health Association of America. (1991). *HMO Industry Profile*. Washington, D.C.: GHAA, annual book.

Gurnick, D. (1991). "HMO Survival: Determination of Optimal Size. "Unpublished AUPHA paper, Medical College of Virginia, Richmond.

Harrington, C., and Newcomer, R. (1991). "Social HMOs Service Use and Cost." *Health Care Financing Review* 12:3 (Spring), 37–52.

Harvard Community Health Plan. (1991). *Annual Report, Harvard Community Health Plan*. Boston.

Health Care Financing Administration (HCFA). (1991). "Trends in the Utilization of Medicare Home Health Agency Services." Washington, D.C.: DHHS.

Health Insurance Plan of Greater New York. (1991). *HIP Annual Report*. New York: HIP.

Hedrick, S., and Inui, T. (1986). "The Effectiveness and Cost of Home Care: An Information Synthesis." *Health Services Research* 20:6 (part II, February), 851–880.

Hillman, A., Pauly, M., and Kerstein, J. (1989). "How Do Financial Incentives Affect Physicians' Clinical Decisions and the Financial Performance of HMOs?" *New England Journal of Medicine* 321:2 (July 13), 86–92.

Hillman, A., Welch, W., and Pauly, M. (1992). "Contractual Arrangements Between HMOs and Primary Care Physicians: Three-tiered HMOs and Risk Pools." *Medical Care* 30:2 (February), 136–148.

Hornbrook, M., and Berki, S. (1985). "Practice Mode and Payment Method." *Medical Care* 23:5 (May), 484–511.

Hreachmack, P., and Stannard, R. (1990). "The Managed Care Environment." *Employee Assistance* 11:6 (July), 12–14.

Iezzoni, L., Schwartz, M., and Restuccia, J. (1991). "Role of Severity Information in Health Policy Debates: A Survey of State and Regional Concerns." *Inquiry* 28:2 (Spring), 117–128.

Interstudy. (1991). *The Interstudy Edge.* Vols. 1–2. Excelsior, Minn.: Interstudy.

Johns, L. (1989). "Selective Contracting in California: An Update." *Inquiry* 26:3 (Fall), 345–352.

Johnsson, J. (1990). "Budget Forecasting Key for Surviving Price Competition." *Hospitals* 64:4 (February 20), 81.

Kane, R., and Kane, R. (1991). "A Nursing Home in Your Future." *New England Journal of Medicine* 324:9 (February 28), 627–629.

Kass, D. (1987). "Economies of Scale and Scope in the Provision of Home Health Services." *Journal of Health Economics* 6:1 (February), 130–146.

Kemper, P. (1990). "Case Management Agency Systems of Administering Long-Term Care: Evidence from the Channeling Demonstration." *Gerontologist* 30:6 (June), 817–824.

Kemper, P., and Murtaugh, C. (1991). "Lifetime Use of Nursing Home Care." *New England Journal of Medicine* 324:9 (February 28), 595–600.

Kirkman-Liff, B., and van de Ven, W. (1989). "Improving Efficiency in the Dutch Health Care System: Current Innovations and Future Options." *Health Policy* 13:4 (October), 35–53.

Klinkman, M. (1991). "Process of Choice of Health Care Plan and Provider: Development of an Integrated Analytic Framework." *Medical Care Review* 48:3 (Fall), 295–329.

Koren, M. (1986). "Home Care—Who Cares?" *New England Journal of Medicine* 314:14 (April 3), 917–920.

Kralewski, J., Feldman, R., Dowd, B., and Shapiro, J. (1991). "Strategies Employed by HMOs to Achieve Discounts." *Health Care Management Review* 16:1 (Winter), 9–15.

Kramer, A., Shaughnessy, P., and Pettigrew, M. (1985). "Cost-Effectiveness Implications Based on a Comparison of Nursing Home and Home Health Case Mix." *Health Services Research* 20:4 (October), 387–405.

Kurt Salmon and Associates Survey of Home Health Care (1989). "Could America Have a Home Care Glut?" *Home Health Journal* 6:3 (March), 5.

Langwell, K., and Hadley, J. (1990). "Insights from the Medicare HMO Demonstrations." *Health Affairs* 9:1 (Spring), 74–84.

Lanning, J., Morrisey, M., and Ohsfeldt, R. (1992). "Endogeneous Hospital Regulation and Its Effects on Hospital and Nonhospital Expenditures." *Journal of Regulatory Economics* 3:3 (Fall), 137–154.

Larkin, H. (1990). "HMO Ownership Pays Off for Systems That Stick with It." *Hospitals* 64:3 (February 5), 56–60.

Leutz, W., Malone, J., Kistner, M., O'Bar, T. and Ripley, J. (1990). "Financial Performance in the Social HMOs." *Health Care Financing Review* 12:1 (Fall), 9–18.

Lichtenstein, R., Thomas, W., Adams, J., and Lepkowski, J. (1991). "Selection Bias in TEFRA At-Risk HMOs." *Medical Care* 29:4 (April), 318–331.

Liu, K., Coughlin, T., and McBride, T. (1991). "Predicting Nursing Home Admission and Length of Stay." *Medical Care* 29:2 (February), 125–141.

Lubitz, J., Beebe, J., and Riley, G. (1985). "Improving the Medicare HMO Payment Formula to Deal with Biased Selection." In R. Scheffler and L. Rossiter (eds.), *Advances in Health Economics and Health Services Research*. Greenwich: JAI Press.

Luft, H. (1991). "Translating U.S. HMO Experience to Other Health Systems." *Health Affairs* 10:3 (Fall), 172–186.

———. (1981). *Health Maintenance Organizations: Dimensions of Performance*. New York: John Wiley.

Madlin, N. (1991). "EPO, Exclusive Provider Organizations: Stricter Controls Than a PPO, Cheaper to Administer Than an HMO." *Business and Health* 9:3 (March), 48–53.

Marion. (1991). *Marion Managed Care Digest on PPOs*. Kansas City: Marion Labs.

McCall, N., Knickman, J., and Bauer, E. (1991). "A New Approach to Long-Term Care." *Health Affairs* 10:1 (Spring), 164–176.

McClain, J., and Eastaugh, S. (1983). "How to Forecast to Contain Your Variable Costs: Exponential Smoothing Techniques." *Hospital Topics* 61:6 (November/December), 4–9.

McClure, W. (1978). "On Broadening the Definition of and Removing Regulatory Barriers to a Competitive Health Care System." *Journal of Health Politics, Policy, and Law* 3:3 (July), 303–327.

McGuire, T. (1981). "Price and Membership in a Prepaid Group Medical Practice." *Medical Care* 19:2 (February), 172–183.

McNerney, W. (1980). "Control of Health Care Costs in the 1980's." *New England Journal of Medicine* 303:19 (November 6), 1088–1095.

Moran, D., and Savela, T. (1986). "HMOs, Finance, and the Hereafter." *Health Affairs* 5:1 (Spring), 51–65.

Mott, P. (1986). "Hospital Utilization by HMOs: Separating Apples from Oranges." *Medical Care* 24:5 (May), 398–406.

National Association of Insurance Commissioners (NAIC). (1991). "Recommended Model Standards for the Sale of Long-Term Care Insurance Policies." Washington, D.C.

National Underwriter (NU). (1991). "Home Care." *National Underwriter* 4–4/88, 23–24.

Nelson, L., Swearingen, G., and Sing, M. (1991). "Medigap PPOs: Issues, Implications & Experience." *Health Care Financing Review* 12:4 (Summer), 87–97.

Nyberg, T. (1988). "Maxicare Selling HMOs, Reworking Finances to Return to Profitability." *Managed Care Outlook*, May 27, 2–3.

Palsbo, S., and Gold, M. (1991). *HMO Industry Profile*. Washington, D.C.: Group Health Association of America.

Phillips, R. (1984). "The Fireman's Fund Experience." In P. Feinstein, M. Gornick, and J. Greenberg (eds.), *Long-Term Care Financing and Delivery Systems: Exploring Some Alternatives*, Washington, D.C.: HCFA. 37–44.

Porell, F., and Turner, W. (1990). "Biased Selection under the Senior Health Plan Prior Use Capitation Formula." *Inquiry* 27:1 (Spring), 39–50.

Ratneshwar, S., Mick, D., and Reitinger, G. (1990) "Selective Attention in Information

Processing: The Role of Chronically Accessible Attributes." *Advances in Consumer Research* 17:1 (Spring), 547–553.

Reisler, M. (1985). "Business in Richmond Attacks Health Care Costs." *Harvard Business Review* 63:1 (January–February), 145–155.

Rice, T. (1992). "Containing Health Care Costs." *Medical Care Review* 49:1 (Spring), 19–65.

Rice, T., Thomas, K., and Weissert, W. (1991). "Effect of Owning LTC Insurance Policies on Out-of-Pocket Costs." *Health Services Research* 25:6 (February), 907–933.

Riley, G., Rabey, E., and Kasper, J. (1989). "Biased Selection and Regression to the Mean in Medicare HMO Demonstrations: A Survival Analysis of Enrollees and Disenrollees." *Medical Care* 27:4 (April), 337–350.

Riley, G., Lubitz, J., and Rabey, E. (1991). "Enrollee Health Status under Medicare Risk Contracts: Analysis of Mortality Rates." *Health Services Research* 26:2 (June), 137–163.

Rockefeller, J. (1990). "The Pepper Commission Report on Comprehensive Health Care." *New England Journal of Medicine* 323:14 (October 4), 1005–1007.

Russell, L. (1990). *Medicare's New Hospital Payment System: Is It Working?* Washington, D.C.: Brookings.

Sabatino, F. (1990). "Survey: Managed Care Led Diversification." *Hospitals* 64:1 (January 5), 56–59.

Schlesinger, M., Blumenthal, D., and Schlesinger, E. (1986). "Profits under Pressure: The Economic Performance of Investor-owned and Nonprofit HMOs." *Medical Care* 24:7 (July), 615–627.

Schmitz, V. (1990). "Better Forecasting Ensures Profitability, Quality Care." *Healthcare Financial Management* 44:1 (January), 60–66.

Seaman, L. (1990). "Preparation: The Key to Nursing Case Management." *Journal of Post-anesthesia Nursing* 5:3 (June), 177–181.

Shaughnessy, P., and Kramer, A. (1990). "Increased Needs of Patients in Nursing Homes and Patients Receiving Home Health Care." *New England Journal of Medicine* 322:1 (January 4), 21–27.

Short, P., Cunningham, P., and Mueller, C. (1991). "Standardizing Nursing-Home Admission Dates for Short-Term Hospital Stays." *Medical Care* 29:2 (February), 97–113.

Sloss, E., Keeler, E., and Brook, R. (1987). "Effect of a Health Maintenance Organization on Physiologic Health: Results from a Randomized Trial." *Annals of Internal Medicine* 106:1 (January), 130–138.

Socolar, D., Sager, A., and Hiam, P. (1992). "Competing to Death: California's High Risk System." *American Health Policy* 2:2 (March/April), 45–50.

Somers, S., and Merrill, J. (1991). "Supporting States' Efforts for Long-Term Care Insurance." *Health Affairs* 10:1 (Spring), 177–179.

Stone, R., and Short, P. (1990). "The Competing Demands of Employment and Informal Caregiving to Disabled Elders." *Medical Care* 28:6 (June), 513–526.

Sutton, H., and Sorbo, A. (1991). *Actuarial Issues in the Fee-for-Service/Prepaid Medical Group.* Denver: Medical Group Management Association.

Trauner, J. (1986). "The Second Generation of Selective Contracting: Another Look at PPOs." *Journal of Ambulatory Care Management* 9:5 (May), 13–21.

Wagner, M. (1990). "Gains in Home Infusion Therapy." *Modern Healthcare* (May 21), 87.

Wallack, S. (1991). "LifePlans Study of Long-Term Care Insurance." Washington, D.C.: HIAA.

Ware, J., et al. (1986). "Comparison of Health Outcomes at a HMO with Those of Fee-for-Service Care." *Lancet* 8488 (May 3), 1017–1022.

Weiner, J., Lyles, A., Steinwachs, D., and Hall, K. (1991). "Impact of Managed Care on Prescription Drug Use." *Health Affairs* 10:1 (Spring), 140–153.

Weissert, W., and Cready, C. (1989). "Toward a Model for Improved Targeting of Aged at Risk of Institutionalization." *Health Services Research* 24:4 (October), 485–509.

Welch, W. (1986). "The Elasticity of Demand for HMOs." *Journal of Human Resources* 21:2 (Spring), 252–266.

Welch, W., and Frank, R. (1986). "The Predictors of HMO Enrollee Populations: Results from a National Sample." *Inquiry* 23:1 (Spring), 16–22.

Welch, W., Hillman, A., and Pauly, M. (1990). "Toward New Typologies for HMOs." *Milbank Quarterly* 68:2 (Summer), 221–243.

Wilensky, G., and Rossiter, L. (1986). "Patient Self-selection in HMOs." *Health Affairs* 5:1 (Spring), 66–80.

Williams, B., Phillips, E., Torner, J., and Irvine, A. (1990). "Predicting Utilization of Home Health Resources." *Medical Care* 28:5 (May), 379–391.

Wilson, C., and Weissert, W. (1989). "Private Long-Term Care Insurance: After Coverage Restrictions Is There Anything Left?" *Inquiry* 26:4 (Winter), 493–506.

Wrightson, C. (1990). *HMO Rate Setting and Financial Strategy*. Ann Arbor, Mich.: Health Administration Press.

Yelin, E., Hencke, C., Kramer, J., Nevitt, M., Shearn, M., and Epstein, W. (1985). "A Comparison of the Treatment of Rheumatoid Arthritis in HMOs and Fee-for-Service Practices." *New England Journal of Medicine* 312:15 (April 11), 962–967.

Zwanziger, J., and Auerbach, R. (1991). "Evaluating PPO Performance Using Prior Expenditure Data." *Medical Care* 29:2 (February), 142–151.

6 Employers, Cost Sharing, and Cost Containment

> Employers were like an absentee host who paid the bill but never showed up at the table. Now they are intimately involved in planning the menu.
> —Bernard Tresnowski

> Chrysler's comparable cost per employee is $5700, or 400 percent higher health care costs than Mitsubishi. What has Chrysler gotten for its health care dollar? A health care industry that is expensive, wasteful, and inefficient.... The fee-for-service and cost reimbursement systems must be eliminated and all patients must be made more cognizant of their own health care.
> —Joseph A. Califano

Employment-based insurance is necessary to attract and retain skilled highly qualified workers and reduce sick days. However, a business that experiences excessive health costs by offering too small a dose of cost sharing in its health insurance options incurs a competitive disadvantage. Corporate health care spending exceeds after-tax total profits and is predicted to reach $186 billion in 1992. Employees are a capital asset, and health maintenance is a business cost in need of control. Corporate America is not just concerned with those currently employed; it must also be concerned with future health care costs of retirees. Union contracts often specify financial provisions for the health care expenses of retirees and their dependents that are not otherwise paid by Medicare. The sum total of the future liability of Ford and General Motors to retirees and their dependents exceeds $12 billion. A business has three basic avenues for controlling health expenses: usage reduction, management efficiency, and cost shifting (Custer 1991, Herzlinger and Schwartz 1985).

Reduction in the usage of services can be accomplished through cost sharing, wellness programs (Schwartz and Rollins 1985; Eastaugh 1991), health promotion (Warner 1986; Spilman 1986), utilization review, and alternative delivery systems such as HMOs (Whitted and Torrens 1985). The second strategy, managing costs more efficiently, can be done through self-insurance, coordination of benefit rules for phantom coverage, and negotiation of discounts (Herzlinger 1985; Eastaugh 1986).

Cost shifting takes two forms: (1) increasing the employee's premium contribution or (2) cost transfer off the insurance plan and onto the employee's pocketbook by increased cost-sharing requirements. The first method, cost shifting of premiums, fosters increased price sensitivity at the annual point of selecting an insurance plan. Unfortunately, this mechanism provides the consumer with no incentive to cooperate and does not stimulate more efficient utilization of services. However, the second method, cost sharing, affects consumption at the point of service; that is, it stimulates employees to economize and not let excess cost transfers to their pocketbooks occur. This chapter will discuss cost sharing as a cost-control strategy and the impact of heightened price sensitivity on utilization.

EXCESSIVELY LOW COST SHARING

Consider the use of cost-sharing requirements in the most costly segment of the health economy, the hospital. In Japan and Korea out-of-pocket payments represent 30 to 40 percent of hospital revenue. However, in the mid–1980s American business made such timid use of cost sharing that out-of-pocket payments declined from 5.3 percent of hospital revenues in 1983 to 4.8 percent in 1986 and a record low of 4.5 percent in 1987. The nation incurs a competitive disadvantage by offering too small a dose of cost sharing in its health coverage plans. The good news is that out-of-pocket hospital expenses are rising, from $8.8 billion in 1985 and $8.7 billion in 1987 to $11.3 billion in 1988 and a projected $15 billion in 1991 according to the federal Health Care Financing Administration Office of the Actuary. But our cost-sharing requirements would have to increase twofold to achieve parity with the Japanese and the Koreans. This author would not prefer achieving parity, since too high a level of cost sharing might deter some necessary care and erode the quality of care (in theory). But in the collective bargaining process employers should strive to increase cost-sharing requirements and should finance quality-assurance activities to protect and promote the quality of care (Siu et al. 1986). Corporations that have only slightly increased cost-sharing requirements have experienced high rates of medical cost inflation; for example, General Motors spent $3.2 billion, or $1,702 per worker, on health care in 1991 (compared to only $996 per worker in 1986).

COST TRANSFER AND USAGE REDUCTION

Cost sharing not only shifts the burden onto the employee (cost transfer), but also reduces the cost of care by deterring unnecessary services (usage reduction).

As we shall see in an example of collective bargaining, employees are highly interested in how much cost transfer is required to buy a certain amount of usage reduction. The trade-off can benefit all concerned, with the exception of the provider's pocketbook (but unions have a strong interest in asking what balance is struck between usage reduction and cost transfer). Therefore, the firm must seek to curtail, through cost sharing, what is labeled "moral hazard" in the jargon of economics (Feldstein 1981). The economist's term "moral hazard" does not imply moral turpitude. In fact, the employees' responses to increased insurance coverage are rational economic behavior, in that they demand (or have demanded for them) more service when they pay less of the price (Eastaugh 1991).

Reports to date indicate that the health status of nonpoor employees and their families does not appear to suffer measurably from increased cost sharing. There is limited evidence to suggest that the poor, especially with preexisting health problems, may have some erosion of health status under high levels of cost sharing (Shapiro, Ware, and Sherbourne 1986). Consequently, this chapter should only be considered relevant for employed populations with incomes in excess of the bottom quartile of society. Cost sharing may be a prudent strategy for the "worried well," but not for the poor and ill. According to the eight-year Rand health insurance study, individuals economize by being less prone to seek treatment or to be hospitalized for an illness that can be treated elsewhere (Manning et al. 1987; Brook 1984). Raising price sensitivity had no measurable impact on health status of the employed and their dependents. Effective prices out-of-pocket should not be expected to have much effect on necessities, but 20 to 40 percent of prevailing medical practice might not be true necessities (Eddy 1991; Brook and Lohr 1985). In the Rand study the average cost per hospitalization and per ambulatory episode was the same across a wide range of five high-low cost-sharing options. However, usage was 30 to 40 percent lower with 50 percent cost sharing versus no free care (Manning et al. 1987).

There have been many recent examples of significant increases in cost-sharing requirements. For example, Xerox instituted a 20 percent coinsurance plan for inpatient expenses, with a stopgap provision to spend no more than $4,000 or 4 percent of salary. Hewitt Associates (1991) surveyed a constant sample of half the Fortune 500 industrials, plus other firms, over the previous 12 years. The fraction of companies with substantial cost sharing, defined as requiring employees to pay more than 5 percent of their hospital bill, increased from 11 percent in 1979 to 50 percent in 1985 and to 78 percent in 1991. Until 1983 less than 18 percent of the companies required a deductible, but that percentage skyrocketed to 82% in 1991. To prevent a possible "catastrophic" fiscal impact of these increased employee cost-sharing requirements, companies instituted maximum out-of-pocket (MOOP) provisions. In 1979 only half the firms had instituted MOOP provisions, but by 1991 this figure increased to 92 percent.

Creating a Forecasting Model

Given the importance of the cost-sharing topic, it is surprising how little econometric research from the $60 million Rand health insurance experiment (Manning et al. 1987) has been translated into actuarial forecasts. In the collective bargaining process each side should ask: What is the distributional and fiscal impact under a simulated menu of cost-sharing options? Two factors, the amount of cost transfer and the resulting total expense reduction from lower utilization of services, need to be studied to answer the omnibus question on how to structure coinsurance, deductibles, and maximum out-of-pocket provisions.

The process of interpolation between a wide range of possible cost-sharing alternatives was left to an expert Delphi group of economists (including this author). In demonstrating how modeling can be beneficial in the collective bargaining process, tables will be provided from the Delphi study of an anonymous company with employees in five states. After considering two original alternatives suggested by labor and management, respectively, the Delphi group came up with a better compromise menu of cost-sharing options. The employee fraction of total health care expenses as a function of the three cost-sharing parameters is presented in table 6.1. An important consideration in bargaining is how much total expense reduction occurs as cost-sharing provisions are increased. Assuming a stable employee population, the lowest cost-sharing option in table 6.2 (free care) is 53 percent more expensive per capita than the highest cost-sharing option. The company under study had in 1990 a moderate degree of cost sharing (20 percent coinsurance, a $1,500 maximum, and a $100 deductible), but costs per family were projected to increase by 10.5 percent in 1991 (from $1,810 to $2,000). The question for the Delphi group is how we can moderate this increase without achieving diminishing returns from cost transfers. While the collective bargaining process is never such a sterile academic exercise, the projections are offered for labor and management in a spirit of ''more information is better than less'' for reaching a consensus in the name of efficiency and equity (Eastaugh 1991).

Baseline alternative zero was to leave the cost-sharing requirements unchanged and let costs increase 10.5 percent. During the process of bargaining two alternatives were developed by labor and management. Alternative A, advanced by the union, had a projected cost per family in 1991 that was 7.8 percent less than the forecast $2,000 ($1,844). The employee would pay out-of-pocket a projected 24 percent of that $1,844 ($443), instead of paying out-of-pocket 18 percent of the projected $2,000 ($360) if the preexisting cost-sharing requirements remained unchanged. The cost-transfer burden, or extra share the employee would have to pay in 1991, was $83 per family ($443 − $360) under the union alternative A, but the total expense reduction was $156 ($2,000 − $1,844). In summary, $73 of the cost reduction per family would result from utilization savings ($156 − $83), and $83 of the cost savings would be in the form of a cost transfer from company to out-of-pocket family expense.

Table 6.1
Fraction of Health Costs Paid by the Employee as a Function of Three Cost-sharing Provisions

(1) Co-Insurance	(2) Maximum Out-of-Pocket per Annum	(3) Annual Deductible					
		$0	$100	$250	$500	$1,000	4% 0f salary
0%	none	0	.08	.13	.18	.25	.29
20%	$1,500	.14	.18[a]	.21	.24	.30	.32
"	$2,000	.16	.20	.23	.26	.32	.34
"	$2,500	.18	.21	.24	.27	.33	.36
"	10% of salary	.20	.23	.26	.29	.35	.38
25%	$1,500	.17	.21	.24[b]	.27[d]	.33	.35
"	$2,000	.19	.23	.26	.29	.35	.37
"	$2,500	.21	.24	.27	.31	.37	.39
"	10% of salary	.22	.26	.29	.32	.38	.40
30%	$1,500	.21	.24	.27	.31	.36	.38
"	$2,000	.23	.26	.29	.34[c]	.39	.41
"	$2,500	.25	.28	.31	.36	.40	.42
"	10% of salary	.26	.29	.32	.37	.41	.43
40%	$1,500	.26	.29	.32	.37	.41	.43
"	$2,000	.28	.31	.35	.40	.44	.46
"	$2,500	.30	.34	.38	.43	.46	.48
"	10% of salary	.31	.35	.39	.44	.47	.49

[a]Current plan in 1990.
[b]Alternative A, first option advanced by the union: no change in maximum out-of-pocket ($1,500), moderate increase in deductible (up from $100 to $250), and small increase in coinsurance (up to 25 percent) in 1991.
[c]Alternative B, first option presented by the employer: substantial increase in deductible (to $500), moderate increases in coinsurance and maximum out-of-pocket in 1991.
[d]Alternative C, the compromise plan.

Alternative B, offered by the company (table 6.2), would reduce total cost per employee during 1991 to 16 percent less than the forecast $2,000 ($1,677). The employee would, however, be paying out-of-pocket 34 percent of that smaller dollar figure ($567), instead of paying out-of-pocket a projected $360 of $2,000 in expenses if the cost-sharing requirements remained fixed. The cost-transfer burden, or extra share the employee would have to pay, would be $207 per family ($567 − $360), but the total expense reduction would be $323 ($2,000

Table 6.2
Percentage Change in Total Health Insurance Plan Costs Relative to an Unchanged Benefit Plan (with a Projected Cost of $2,000 per Employee for 1991)

(1) Co- Insurance	(2) Maximum Out-of-Pocket per Annum	(3) Annual Deductible					
		$0	$100	$250	$500	$1,000	4% of salary
0	none	+12%	+8%	+4%	-2%	-7%	-8%
20%	$1,500	+3%	$2,000[a]	-3%	-7%	-11%	-11%
"	$2,000	+1%	-2%	-5%	-8%	-13%	-14%
"	$2,500	-1%	-3%	-6%	-9%	-14%	-14%
"	10% of salary	-2%	-4%	-7%	-9%	-14%	-14%
25%	$1,500	-3%	-5%	-8%[b]	-10%[d]	-15%	-15%
"	$2,000	-5%	-7%	-10%	-12%	-17%	-18%
"	$2,500	-6%	-8%	-11%	-13%	-18%	-18%
"	10% of salary	-7%	-9%	-12%	-14%	-19%	-19%
30%	$1,500	-8%	-10%	-13%	-15%	-19%	-20%
"	$2,000	-10%	-12%	-14%	-16%[c]	-20%	-20%
"	$2,500	-11%	-13%	-15%	-17%	-21%	-21%
"	10% of salary	-12%	-14%	-16%	-18%	-21%	-21%
40%	$1,500	-14%	-17%	-19%	-21%	-24%	-24%
"	$2,000	-15%	-18%	-20%	-22%	-25%	-25%
"	$2,500	-16%	-19%	-21%	-23%	-26%	-26%
"	10% of salary	-16%	-19%	-21%	-23%	-26%	-26%

[a]Current plan in 1990.

[b]Alternative A, first option advanced by the union: no change in maximum out-of-pocket ($1,500), moderate increase in deductible (up from $100 to $250), and small increase in coinsurance (up to 25 percent) in 1991.

[c]Alternative B, first option presented by the employer: substantial increase in deductible (to $500), moderate increases in coinsurance and maximum out-of-pocket in 1991.

[d]Alternative C, the compromise plan.

— $1,677). In summary, under the employer alternative B, $116 of the cost reduction per family would be from utilization reduction ($323 − $207), and $207 of the cost savings would be from a cost transfer of the burden from the company to the employee.

Union representatives had three basic reasons for disliking alternative B. Of special importance to the union was the increased potential financial risk of raising the maximum out-of-pocket expense cap. Second, the fraction of costs paid out-of-pocket was almost double the 1990 figure (0.18) and substantially higher than the union alternative (0.24). Third, the employees feared that too great a cost transfer to the benefit of the employer would destroy the firm's interest in cost containment through other programs (health promotion, health education).

In the process of bargaining a compromise alternative C was developed, involving 25 percent coinsurance, an unchanged $1,500 MOOP cap, and a $500 deductible (table 6.2). Management acquiesced to the request that the MOOP not be increased and that coinsurance be raised by only 5 percent; the union accepted a $400 increase in the deductible. As the reader can observe in table 6.2, costs were projected to be 10 percent less in 1991 than the forecast figure of $2,000 under this compromise altnerative C, at parity with 1990 costs of $1,810 per family. The worker would pay out-of-pocket 27 percent (table 6.1) of the $1,800 ($481), instead of paying out-of-pocket $360 of $2,000 in 1991 if no changes were made in the cost-sharing provisions. The total expense reduction, or the differential cost advantage of increasing the amount of cost sharing, would be $200 ($2,000 − $1,800). Therefore, $121 of the cost savings would be achieved by a cost transfer onto the employee, and $79 of the cost reduction per family would result from utilization reductions.

Lessons Learned

Collective bargaining need not be shrouded in excessive uncertainty. It is possible to achieve some good estimates of the expected amounts of cost transfer and usage reduction under various cost-sharing options. Cost transfer is by definition a means for shifting health care expenses away from the employer to the patient (employee or retiree). The added benefit of more cost sharing is that it stimulates cost consciousness and reduces utilization, thus reducing health care expenditures. Cost consciousness at the time the purchase decision is made moves unnecessary costs off the employee's and employer's budgets.

A second lesson learned involves the value of a scientific principle known as Occam's razor; if a simple and a complex model achieve the same predictions, one should prefer the simple model. Small changes in the cost-sharing parameters dominate moderate shifts in the demographic characteristics of the employees (family size, age) in the degree to which they have one-year impacts on health care costs. A more complex expensive model based on more than one year of claims data would buy little in terms of predictive accuracy. In the jargon of economics, the exogenous preexisting demographics of the employees are by definition worked into the baseline cost and utilization figures used for the projection. However, there is endogenous control of the degree of cost sharing, and firms should update (increase) cost-sharing provisions in an attempt to control costs without harming quality of care, access to care, health status, or the morale of the employees.

Table 6.3
Cost Sharing under Medicare, 1991

	Beneficiary Liability
Medicare Part A	
Hospital deductible	$628 per spell of illness
Hospital coinsurance	
Days 61-90	$157 per day
Days 91 on (for 60 lifetime reserve days)	$314 per day
Skilled nursing facility coinsurance	
Days 21-100	$78.50 per day
Medicare Part B	
Premium	$29.90 per month
Deductible	$100.00 per year
Coinsurance	20% of allowed charge
Balance bills	All excess up to 125% of the allowed charge, with the exception of evaluation and management services, which are limited to the lower of 140% of the allowed charge or the physician's 1990 maximum allowable actual charge (MAAC) percentage.

The microeconomic question implicit in the example offered in this chapter is who bears the burden. The two macroeconomic questions implicit in this chapter are how to constrain the rate of health care cost inflation and how to maintain the competitiveness of American firms in the global economy. Retiree health care has priced itself into the public eye. Cost sharing may help constrain the rate of increase in employee and retiree health care costs. High as the Medicare cost-sharing requirements may appear in table 6.3, the cost sharing has not kept pace with inflation.

THE COST OF RETIREE BENEFITS AND SAFETY PROGRAMS

In the early 1980s many authors promoted the concept of business coalitions to hold down health care costs. According to Brown and McLaughlin (1988) and Bradbury (1987), this concept has failed as a cost-containment strategy. However, the coalition movement might have achieved a secondary goal, stronger communication between providers, business leaders, and unions on the concept of value shopping and consumerism (McLaughlin, Zellers, and Brown 1989). We shall return to this topic in chapter 9 of this book.

Rising cost-sharing requirements will not cure all problems for the business community. Safety programs and preemployment screening are necessary approaches to reduce the growing workers' compensation burden to below 1.6 percent of payroll expense (Towers Perrin 1991). The biggest problem for large firms is that of unfunded retiree health care benefits. In 1991 half of the 449 large firms offering retiree health benefits changed current methods of funding from the pay-as-you-go approach (no funds set aside for the long run) to complete accrual funding. How prevalent is nonfederal insurance in the Medicare-eligible population? In 1991 over 24 percent of Medicare beneficiaries also had employment-related coverage, while only 23 percent lacked any form of private coverage. For budgetary reasons over the last decade the federal government has limited its share of total expenditures through high patient deductibles, cost sharing, and tightening of rules that determine when Medicare is the primary payer.

To cut costs and staff, especially during the recessions of 1982 and 1991, large companies offered continued health benefits as an inducement to retire. However, since 1989 these large employers have worried about the Financial Accounting Standards Board (FASB) proposal to establish a liability on the balance sheet to reflect the present value of anticipated future-year health benefits. Siegel (1990) and Eastaugh (1990) estimated that firms will experience in the aggregate a 10 percent reduction in profits from honestly accounting for future retiree health expenditures, with the percentage for a given firm depending on its generosity to its ex-employees. The median estimate of reduced profits to finance the retiree health care costs in 1992 is $26 billion. Many firms are considering discontinuation of such benefits. While companies will not have to add liabilities until 1993, they must begin putting information in their 1992 financial statements to the Securities and Exchange Commission (SEC). In theory, this change in the accounting rules will not affect the amount of funds a firm spends. In practice, the explicit recognition of the hidden costs of retiree health benefits will force companies to report lower profits or trim benefits. Companies will spend more cash on retiree health benefits (because of the added amounts for prefunding) even while they trim benefits and shunt more of the premium expense onto their employees. The Hewitt Associates (1991) benefit survey suggested that the median cash costs companies pay each year for retiree health benefits (as a percentage of equity) should increase from 0.5 percent in 1990 to 2.2 percent in 1992.

In 1991 most firms were passing on some of the costs of retiree health benefits to their employees. The 9,800 employees at Quaker Oats make retiring employees pay 5 to 25 percent of the premiums for insurance to supplement Medicare. Those employees with fewer years of service pick up 25 percent of the premium. Other firms make the employee pay $100 to $150 per month of the premium.

Table 6.4
Average Health Care Costs Charged to the Corporate Plan per Sick Retiree and per Capita, before and after Retirement, 1990–1991

	Regular Retiree (over age 64)	Early Retiree (under age 65)
Average expenses to the corporate plan per capita (retiree)		
1-A year after retirement	$1,393*	$2,931
1-B year before retirement	$2,661	$1,385
Average expenses to the plan per retiree utilizing the benefit**		
2-A year after retirement	$2,598	$4,239
2-B year before retirement	$4,542	$4,264

*Fewer services are charged to the plan because the retirees became eligible for Medicare.
**There are fewer retiree/users of the plan than the sum total of retirees; therefore average expenses are higher for users.

Many younger employees receive the least generous deal: the ability to purchase with after-tax wages an annuity whose proceeds can be used for medical costs after retirement. Some of these annuities offer a lifetime maximum benefit of only $75,000 to $100,000 for the retiree and spouse. Firms cannot afford to be as generous with benefits if they no longer have any tax-favored way of pre-funding the retiree plan. The complexity of projecting retiree costs is outlined in one proprietary study the author did for one corporation (table 6.4).

CONCLUSIONS

The cost-sharing strategy for reducing health care costs can work equally well for small and large firms. In contrast, management techniques for expense reduction are more dependent on business size. Self-insurance is best suited for large firms, because firms can spread the risk over many more employees. Self-insured employers, as judged by the June 1985 U.S. Supreme Court decision (53 USLW 4616) remain generally exempt from state controls and are governed instead by less constraining federal Employee Retirement Income Security Act (ERISA) requirements (Rublee 1986). Employee leasing, where an individual is leased from a company that provides benefits at lower average cost for a large pool of workers, is well suited for small businesses. The Hartford Foundation is supporting a survey of multiple employer trusts (METs), which aggregate small businesses to enlarge the population risk pool and purchase group insurance. Sufficient cost-sharing provisions are essential for keeping METs financially solvent without rejecting large numbers of high-risk applicants with poor health status. Cost sharing need not be viewed as an assault on equity. Cost sharing can help prevent risk selection, prevent unnecessary utilization (and thus provider-caused iatrogenic illness), preserve a firm's cost-competitive posture, and ultimately preserve jobs.

In 1991–92 the Health Insurance Association of America spent $5.1 million to help enact state legislation to make health insurance more affordable to small business. HIAA (1991) is attempting to get states to pass laws requiring insurers to offer coverage to employers with 3–25 workers. Small business often has to pay premiums 2–10 times higher than big business because the premiums are experience rated. HIAA is against community rating, but it does favor guaranteed availability of insurance, whole group coverage, premium pricing limits, and a reinsurance mechanism that would enable firms to cover the cost of insuring high-risk individuals. Cost sharing by the consumer is still a major strategy for cost control, by small and large business firms, and all sizes of health insurance companies (Gifford et al. 1991).

The consumer cost-sharing strategy, acting on the point of possible consumption, makes the patient the central cost container. HMOs and managed-care systems make the consumer a major cost-containment force, but act only on an annual basis at the time of selecting a health plan. The health plan is ultimately the central cost container, and to the extent that it contains costs and delivers good service, consumers will be attracted to or disenrolled from the plan. For the consumer in a prepaid plan, there is no stress concerning out-of-pocket expenses each time services are required. Some managed-care systems mix the two strategies; for example, PPOs offer annual cost-selection decisions of which plan to join, and if the consumer wishes to seek a non-PPO provider during the year, the care is paid by the plan, but cost-sharing requirements are substantial (20 to 35 percent of costs being paid out-of-pocket). These new arrangements for consumer and provider cost sensitivity are certainly an improvement on the old system: Insurers just paid bills and passed on the costs, patients consumed services with little regard for costs, and providers delivered services irrespective of the resource costs (Wells, Marquis, and Hosek 1991).

Cost-sharing options developed a kinder and gentler provision in the late 1980s. To prevent a possible catastrophic fiscal impact from employee cost-sharing requirements, many companies instituted a maximum out-of-pocket (MOOP) provision that the annual out-of-pocket expense cannot exceed a set amount, such as $2,000, per family (Gabel et al. 1990). The MOOP provision can also be set to promote equity (equal burden) between blue-collar and white-collar workers; for example, the lifetime maximum benefit limit can be set very high ($500,000), or the MOOP can be limited to 10 percent of the individual's salary. A broad array of other cost-sharing initiatives and estimated savings are presented in table 6.5.

The next chapter will outline ways to improve access. Schorr (1990) has

Table 6.5
Projected Marginal Cost Savings of Plan Design Changes for Five Insurers

Plan Design Change	Magnitude	Savings
Front-end deductible for room and board only	$700	5.2%
Coinsurance provision for surgery	70%	4.3%
(as a percentage of reasonable	80%	2.8%
and customary charges)	90%	1.2%
Coverage for mental health or nervous	50%	2.5%
disorders (as a percentage of payment with a	80%	2.2%
$1,000 annual maximum benefit)	100%	1.8%
Limit per day for mental health or nervous		
disorder	$90	.3%
Limit per day, 15-day maximum, ancillary		
usage only	$700	1.4%
Limit per day on room and board	$500	1.0%
Coinsurance provisions for lab or	70%	1.3%
X-ray (as a percentage of reasonable	80%	.8%
and customary charges)	90%	.4%
Lifetime maximum benefit limit	$500,000	.8%
	$900,000	.1%

suggested making health insurance universal, regardless of employment. The Dutch are planning to drop their employment-based insurance system soon (Netherlands Ministry of Health 1991), because they feel that an individual-based system is more equitable for the working poor and occupationally mobile people. It is unclear whether some mixed strategy of competition, reregulation, deregulation, or mandated health care benefits can best enhance access and equity.

REFERENCES

Anderson, G., Brook, R., Williams, A. (1991). "A Comparison of Cost-sharing versus Free Care in Children: Demand for Office-based Care." *Medical Care* 29:9 (September), 890–898.

Blendon, R., Donelan, K., and Thorpe, K. (1992). "The Uninsured." *JAMA* 267:8 (February 26), 1113–1117.

Bradbury, R. (1987). "A Community Approach to Health Care Competition. "*Inquiry* 24:3 (Fall), 253–265.

Brook, R. (1984). *The Effect of Coinsurance on the Health of Adults*. Santa Monica, Calif.: Rand Corporation Report to DHHS.

Brook, R., and Lohr, K. (1985). "Efficacy, Effectiveness, Variations, and Quality." *Medical Care* 23:5 (May), 710–722.

Brown, L., and McLaughlin, C. (1988). "May the Third Force Be with You: Community Programs for Affordable Health Care." In R. Scheffler and L. Rossiter (eds.), *Advances in Health Economics and Health Services Research*, vol. 9, 187–212. Greenwich, Conn.: JAI.

Califano, J. (1986). *America's Health Care Revolution: Who Lives? Who Dies? Who Pays?* New York: Random House.

Congressional Budget Office. (1991). *Rising Health Care Costs: Causes, Implications, and Strategies*. Washington, D.C.: CBO, U.S. Congress.

Custer, W. (1991). "Employer Health Care Plan Design and Its Effect on Plan Costs." *Inquiry* 28:1 (Spring) 81–86.

Eastaugh, S. (1991). "Sharing the Burden: Containing the Health Care Bill for American Industry." *Business Forum* 16:1 (Winter), 25–28.

———. (1990). "Universal Health Insurance: Equivocation throughout the Nation." *New England Journal of Medicine* 322:17 (April 26), 1239–1240.

———. (1986). "Differential Cost Analysis: Judging a PPO's Feasibility. "*Healthcare Financial Management* 40:5 (May), 44–51.

———. (1985). "Cost Sharing Forecasts Can Assist in Health Care Collective Bargaining." *Business and Health* 3:2 (December), 52–53.

Eastaugh, S., and Eastaugh, J. (1990). "Putting the Squeeze on Emergency Medicine: Pressures on Emergency Department." *Hospital Topics* 68:4 (Fall), 21–26.

Eddy, D. (1991). "What Care Is 'Essential'? What Services Are 'Basic'?" *Journal of the American Medical Association* 265:6 (February 13), 782–788.

Feldstein, M. (1981). *Hospital Costs and Health Insurance*. Cambridge, Mass.: Harvard University Press.

Fielding, J. (1984). *Corporate Health Management*. Reading, Mass.: Addison-Wesley.

Gabel, J., DiCarlo, S., Sullivan, C., and Rice, T. (1990). "Employer Sponsored Health Insurance." *Health Affairs* 9:3 (Fall), 161–175.

General Motors Corporation. (1991). *Annual Report*. Detroit, Michigan.

Gifford, G., Feldman, R., Dowd, B., and Finch, M. (1991). "A Simultaneous Equations Model of Employer Strategies for Controlling Health Benefit Costs." *Inquiry* 28:1 (Spring), 56–66.

Hall, M. (1992). "Reforming the Health Insurance Market for Small Business." *New England Journal of Medicine* 326:8 (February 20), 565–569.

Health Insurance Association of America (HIAA). (1991). *Source Book of Health Insurance Data*. Washington, D.C.: HIAA.

Herzlinger, R. (1985). "How Companies Tackle Health Care Costs: Part II." *Harvard Business Review* 63:5 (September–October), 108–120.

Herzlinger, R., and Schwartz, J. (1985). "How Companies Tackle Health Care Costs: Part I." *Harvard Business Review* 63:4 (July–August), 69–81.

Hewitt Associates. (1991). *Retiree Medical Costs*. New York: Hewitt Associates.

Levit, K., and Cowan, C. (1991). "Burden of Health Care Costs: Business, Households, and Government." *Health Care Financing Review* 12:2 (February), 103–111.

Liu, K., and Perozek, M. (1991). "Effects of Multiple Admissions on Nursing Home Use: Implications for Front-end Policies." *Inquiry* 28:2 (Spring), 140–150.

Manning, W., Newhouse, J., Duan, N., Keeler, E., Leibowitz, A., and Marquis, M. (1987). "Health Insurance and the Demand for Medical Care: Evidence from a Randomized Experiment." *American Economic Review* 77:3 (June), 251–277.

McLaughlin, C., Zellers, W., and Brown, L. (1989). "Health Care Coalitions: Characteristics, Activities, and Prospects." *Inquiry* 26:1 (Spring), 72–83.

Menefee, J. (1986). "Group Benefits Survey Results." Washington, D.C.: Wyatt Company.

Netherlands Ministry of Health. (1991). "Options for the Health Care System." Amsterdam.

Resnick, R. (1992). "Hospital Chain Teams Up with Suppliers for Quality Improvement," *Business and Health* 11:3 (March), 28–35.

Robinson, J., Luft, H., Gardner, L., and Morrison, E. (1991), "Method for Risk-adjusting Employer Contributions to Competing Health Insurance Plans" *Inquiry* 28:2 (Spring), 107–116.

Rublee, D. (1986). "Self-funded Health Benefit Plans: Trends, Legal Environment, and Policy Issues." *Journal of the American Medical Association* 255:6 (February 14), 787–789.

Schorr, A. (1990). "Job Turnover—A Problem with Employer-based Health Care." *New England Journal of Medicine* 323:8 (August 23), 543–545.

Schwartz, R., and Rollins, P. (1985). "Measuring the Cost Benefit of Wellness Strategies." *Business and Health* 2:10 (October), 24–26.

Shaller, D., and Gunderson, S. (1986). "Setting Benchmarks for Cost-Effective Care." *Business and Health* 3:10 (October), 28–32.

Shapiro, M., Ware, J., and Sherbourne, C. (1986). "Effects of Cost Sharing on Seeking Care for Serious and Minor Symptoms." *Annals of Internal Medicine* 104:2 (February), 246–251.

Shelton, J. (1985). "Private Sector Conference—Costs at Ford Motor." *Journal of the American Medical Association* 254:13 (October 4), 1788.

Siegel, J. (1990). "The FASB Exposure Draft: Issues and Implications." In *The Sourcebook on Postretirement Health Care Benefits*. Greenvale, N.Y.: Panel Publishers.

Siu, A., Sonnenberg, F., Manning, W., Newhouse, J., and Brook, R. (1986). "Inappropriate Use of Hospitals in a Randomized Trial of Health Insurance Plans." *New England Journal of Medicine* 315:20 (November 13), 1259–1266.

Spilman, M. (1986). "Effects of a Corporate Health Promotion Program." *Journal of Occupational Medicine* 11:4 (April), 34.

Tell, E., Falik, M., and Fox, P. (1984). "Private Sector Health Care Initiatives: A Comparative Perspective from Four Communities." *Milbank Memorial Fund Quarterly/Health and Society* 62:3 (Summer), 357–379.

Towers Perrin. (1991). "Responding to the Workers' Compensation Crisis: Can Employers Manage and Control Costs?" New York: Towers Perrin.

Warner, K. (1986). "Selling Health Promotion to Corporate America." *Health Education Quarterly* 13:4 (Winter), 22.

Wells, K., Marquis, M., and Hosek, S. (1991). "Mental Health and Selection of PPOs: Experience in Three Employee Groups." *Medical Care* 29:9 (September), 911–924.

Whitted, G., and Torrens, P. (1989). *Managing Corporate Health Care*. New York: Praeger.

Zabakus, E., and Mangold, W. (1992) "Adapting the SERVQUAL Scale to Hospital Services." *Health Services Research* 26:6 (February), 766–778.

IV EQUITY, ACCESS, AND THE URBAN MEDICAL CENTER

7 Access and the Uninsured

Americans are inherently pluralistic. We talk about the importance of every citizen being educated. To accomplish that ideal we have a mixed-up private/public education system. We utter general words about how everybody should have adequate health care, and create 47 overlapping arrangements to deal with the question of access. Our American tradition is to not do anything with a comprehensive single system. Although it may be very expensive and duplicative, this pluralistic approach is more dynamic and more adaptable to change.

—John T. Dunlop

Until we nationalize energy and transportation, we will not have national health insurance in this country.

—Rashi Fein

Political forces for national health insurance resemble dammed-up rivers. The pressure on the dams is enormous but unseen; it is only when the public issue attention cycle peaks because health care providers dump poor patients (or go bankrupt) that the strain is realized. A number of analysts have called for national health insurance (Etheredge 1990). Patchwork reforms with DRGs and HMOs have only exchanged old problems for new ones. Are we ready for a systematic health care system that offers (1) universal coverage, (2) universal access, (3) cost control, and (4) flexibility for steady quality-of-care improvements? Some previous studies suggest that a regulatory approach to national health insurance will simply expand bureaucracy and administrative costs (Butler and Haislmaier 1990). Pessimists argue that America is simply passing through its seventh issue attention cycle favoring, but not initiating, national health insurance. Passage of some national plan seemed forever imminent during certain periods in the past: 1979, 1973–74, 1964–66, 1947–48, 1933–34, and 1917–19.

Public hospitals are under financial stress (Altman et al. 1989). It is only when the public and nonprofit hospitals burst (dump patients or close) that the strain is realized. How does a malfunction in the indigent-care "nonsystem" manifest itself? One study of patient transfers to Cook County, Illinois, revealed that 81 percent of the patients were unemployed, only 6 percent had given informed consent for the transfer, and 24 percent were in unstable clinical condition on transfer (Schiff et al. 1986). Declines in health status may have to be horrifying and directly linked to lack of insurance coverage to engage the public interest in adequate and equitable provision of health care.

Insufficient access to primary care is the major problem in rural areas. Morrisey, Sloan, and Valvona's (1989) study of hospital markets suggested that access to rural hospital care may not be as critical an issue as is widely described in the popular press. It may be better for the rural population to drive to better-quality providers than to remain a captive to inferior, low-volume local providers. However, for many small towns, losing the hospital is like losing the local school, a source of anxiety and diminished pride.

HOW MANY AMERICANS ARE UNINSURED?

Most health care professionals are familiar with statistics that demonstrate the paradox of deprivation amid excess (e.g., excess acute-care beds and almost $2 billion per day spent on health services). Roughly 31.5 million Americans lack health insurance, even when the unemployment rate dips to 5.3 percent, and this figure includes over 8.3 million children (U.S. Congress 1991). The uninsured as a percentage of the nonaged population changed from 13.8 percent in 1977 to 14.6 percent in 1980, 16.1 percent in 1983, and 18.4 percent in 1986 (Brown 1990), declined to 15.5 percent in 1990, and increased to an estimated 17 percent during the economic downturn in 1991. In 1986, 36.5 percent of the uninsured worked in jobs earning more than $10,000 per year, and 15 percent worked in jobs earning over $25,000 per year (Brown 1990). Monheit and Short (1989) reported that 75 percent of the uninsured had jobs or were dependents of those who worked. One-third of the uninsured were children (under 18), and another one-third of the uninsured were between the ages of 18 and 24. Brown (1990) indicated that 92 percent of the firms without employee health plans had fewer than 25 employees.

The Kennedy proposal to guarantee basic health benefits for all Americans would extend health insurance coverage to the 70 percent of the uninsured working more than 20 hours per week (Nexon 1990). The benefits of such a plan may be overstated because 13 million people would have to stop receiving coverage from their spouses' employment insurance plans and begin to receive coverage from their current employers.

On average, Medicaid spending is financed 57 percent by the federal government and 43 percent by state governments. Medicaid spending is the most rapidly inflating budget item for federal and state governments. From 1987 to 1990 annual Medicaid spending inflated at 17 percent per year, reaching $72 billion in 1990. From 1990 to 1992 Medicaid spending is expected to inflate at 23 percent per year (reaching $105.3 billion in 1992). There is substantial inefficiency in the Medicaid system, yet the prices paid to providers are substantially lower than average prices in most states. Half of the cost inflation is good news: It is the result of more uninsured individuals becoming eligible for Medicaid and willing to utilize Medicaid. Medicaid participation jumped from 23.5 million citizens in 1989 to an estimated 28.8 million in 1992, but one in seven citizens is still uninsured (Congressional Budget Office 1992).

Point-in-time data on the uninsured population are skewed toward the demographic traits of those individuals who have periods of being temporarily uninsured. Swartz and McBride (1990) reported that over half of the uninsured periods last less than five months. If only uninsured spells at a point-in-time survey are reported, 59 percent last longer than two years, and only 13 percent end within four months. From the more realistic longitudinal viewpoint, observing people over time, only 15 percent of uninsured periods last longer than two years. Employed people and higher-income people are more likely to experience uninsured spells than point-in-time data on the uninsured indicate. One in every five uninsured individuals has family income exceeding $3,100 per month. Two-thirds of the people who lose employer coverage, but do not lose employment, have uninsured spells that end within four months. The majority of this employed/uninsured group lack insurance while serving as probationary employees on new jobs. The hard-core uninsured/unemployed population, lacking insurance for over two years and not eligible for Medicaid, may represent less than 5.4 million Americans. An expanded Medicaid program could help these 5.4 million citizens. Can we afford to allow one in seven nonelderly Americans to want for lack of health insurance? Are we our brothers' keepers with respect to health care?

Hospitals and physicians provide a substantial volume of charity care (Blumenthal and Rizzo 1991; Dunham 1991; Holleman et al. 1991, Kilpatrick et al. 1991). Indigent care is service provided to those who are incapable of paying for all or part of their medical bill and do not qualify for medical assistance programs. Care for the medically indigent includes charity care and some fraction of the bad debts. Sloan, Blumstein, and Perrin's (1988) analysis of American Hospital Association data found that billed charges to "self-pay" patients are likely to be uncompensated care. In their Tennessee sample the self-pay patients were most likely to be maternity or accident cases. At their local Vanderbilt teaching hospital most uncompensated-care patients had incurred small bills. However, patients with hospital bills over $25,000 accounted for 35 percent of total hospital expenses (and only 2 percent of the patients).

A number of analysts (Ohsfeldt 1985; McDaniel 1986; Eastaugh 1990a) have pointed out that the terms "uncompensated" or "indigent" care lump both charity care and bad debt into a single category. It is hard to get any accurate national estimate as to what fraction of bad debt involves poor people financially incapable of paying their bills, in contrast to nonpoor people unwilling (because they are dissatisfied) to pay some fraction of their bill. In affluent suburban markets bad debt might involve less than 10 percent charity care, whereas in the ghetto bad debt is 95 percent charity care. In 1991 an estimated $4.4 billion of charity care was provided by hospitals, and there was $8.6 billion of bad debt (1.6 and 3.15 percent of hospital gross revenues, respectively). While $13 billion of free care to the poor may seem an insignificant amount in macroeconomic terms within a nation that spends over $14 billion per week on health care, it represents an ethical and financial problem for one-third of the hospitals (Eastaugh and Eastaugh 1990).

Uncompensated care is one of the forgotten stepchildren of our increasingly competitive medical marketplace (Brook 1991; McCue 1991). Hospitals compete for market share of the paying-patient business, but no one competes for nonpaying patients (Bazzoli 1986; Kinzer 1984). The debate over indigent care will lead nowhere until we reach some consensus on whether our top priority is institutional financial support or providing access to a minimum standard of care for underinsured citizens. Institutional managers argue in terms of minimizing uncompensated care and mainstreaming the poor to all hospitals, no matter how costly and inefficient. The tenet of faith among managers and some researchers (Hadley and Feder 1985) that equity, efficiency, and access are a zero-sum equation is certainly open to question. Moreover, one could question whether we can promote affordable managed-care systems for the uninsured and still maintain the dream of mainstreaming all people into "best-quality" service-delivery systems. We hear reports on how the poor are dumped from hospitals. Policy makers insist that indigent care is a vexing problem and demand that providers do "it" better—with hardly any consideration of the "it" we want improved. Good care for our population is the answer. But what is the question?

WANTED: STABLE FINANCING AND BETTER MANAGEMENT

A stable, sufficient source of financing indigent care is critically needed, but better management among the "suffering" providers is also a necessity. These two issues are linked, but a public policy solution for one problem will not assure the resolution of the other. The hospital sector, disturbed to varying degrees by the absence of revenue for providing service for the uninsured, is the major advocate of improved public insurance programs. The uninsured poor, often described as the medically indigent, are financially unable to pay their hospital bills. The hospital sector, in response to price competition and revenue controls, has been accused of limiting the care that it will provide to the poor (Relman 1986; Schiff et al., 1986) or of exhibiting signs of financial distress (National Association of Public Hospitals [NAPH] 1991). However, financial distress can be reduced or eliminated by better management and cost-reduction techniques (Eastaugh 1985). Because the poor are often more severely ill, they may be presumed to cost more per case treated. Hospitals serving a high volume of uninsured individuals, however, have the twin problems of inadequate revenues and inefficient levels of productivity.

The best hospital managers will improve efficiency per department while continuing the public effort to lobby for better reimbursement per patient. One cannot finance indigent care with productivity improvements alone; but without better productivity and increasing reliance on ambulatory care, the money invested in indigent care merely props up inefficient institutions. Policy analysts should be concerned with how resources raised for indigent care can be most effectively allocated. Then we can ask for increasing stewardship of public funds and a stable sufficient level of financing for indigent care.

The problem of indigent care is not simply a hospital finance and cost-shifting issue (Rosko 1990). Indigent service provision is a much broader social problem. The delivery of appropriate and effective medical care for the poor encompasses ethical issues such as the right to care, systemic issues such as access and new modes of service delivery (managed care), and financial issues such as who will pay for uncompensated care. Competition has made indigent care an important endemic "priority problem" for policy makers, rather than simply another "back-burner" issue of concern for the public health community. Hospital executives have a valid point when they note that managing a facility in a system of set prices and prospective contracts for 50 to 70 percent of the patients threatens their ability to provide service to nonpaying patients. Nonpayment for charity care is already seriously limiting the ability of some hospitals to continue to provide their historic share of indigent care (American Hospital Association [AHA] 1989).

Hospital lobbyists call for a "level playing field" and argue that the current situation is like telling Bloomingdale's and Sears to compete for customers and capital with the proviso that Sears must give away its goods to the poor, while Bloomingdale's is allowed to transfer its poor customers to Sears. There is no "free lunch"; if the poor cannot pay for their own care, and government will not, then someone else must bear the burden. Who else but the payers of the premium, businesses and the employed, and insurers with insufficient market share (and bargaining leverage) can bear this implicit burden of cost shifting? The problem is that this implicit burden priced itself into the public eye and so became a more explicit burden. As pointed out by Reinhardt (1985), the much-deplored "cost shifting" for indigent care was effectively a cosmetic quick fix to assure the poor a level of access to quality care. Now that payers are increasingly opting not to pay the cost-shifting factor for indigent care—inflated charges over actual costs—the question is how we shall pay the health care bill of the poor.

The conventional wisdom among inner-city hospital managers can best be described with an imperfect syllogism: Financially distressed hospitals do a disproportionate amount of indigent care; therefore, hospital income redistribution through a "sin" tax (e.g., alcohol and tobacco) or a patient surcharge will reduce the "unfair" financial distress; and redistributing income to the financially distressed institutions will address the problem of indigent care.

It would be prudent to note that our current problems are past solutions; therefore, more needs to be done than simply to channel public or private funds. The major premise of the syllogism is flawed. Increasing the volume of indigent care does not cause financial distress, nor does financial distress result mainly among the institutions disproportionately serving the indigent. In fact, a number of indigent measures are poor contributors in explaining more than 1.5 to 15 percent of the variance in financial ratios (Sloan, Blumstein, and Perrin 1988; Rundall and Lambert 1985). Moreover, the minor premise in the syllogism is also flawed. While improved cash flow can ameliorate distress in the short run, it has the unfortunate side effect of keeping the pathology in the system. The pathology includes operational inefficiencies, poor-quality managers, unbusinesslike trustees, and excess hospital beds. Not closing beds and maintaining a low occupancy rate harms profitability. Gapenski (1991) reported in a study of 169 Florida hospitals that if the occupancy rate increased from 53 to 80 percent, the operating margin would increase from 0.12 percent to 3.1 percent, and the after-tax return on assets would increase from 0.32 percent to 6.4 percent, if the other 23 factors in his equations were held the same.

IDEALS AND POSSIBLE ACTION

What seems new about the 1990s is that corporate America, including all three automotive companies in Detroit, has endorsed the concept of national health insurance. What do health policy analysts make of the current situation? Some of us "old dogs" draw an analogy between what we thought about HMOs in 1970 and what we think about national health insurance lobbying efforts in 1990. Advocates of prepaid HMO care in 1970 resided in one of two groups: idealists in search of equity or managers in search of HMO cost-efficiency (and "soft rationing"). Analogously, advocates of national health insurance fall into categories: idealists in the health professions in search of health care as a right, managers of hospitals interested in getting paid for uncompensated care, or managers of large corporations interested in decreasing their insurance expenses (Griffith 1989; Eastaugh 1991; Employee Benefits Research Corporation [EBRC] 1991).

During this time of health-sector turbulence, many hospital managers encapsulate the policy issue under one label: "uncompensated care." This language signifies the direction, context, and vigor of the hospital lobby in generating improved cash flow for its sector. Alas, in a political world few people will fight for the cause of cash flow. What matters is not uncompensated care in and of itself. What matters is "uncovered people" not getting the required level of care of having to settle for substandard care. Protection of equity and access in the delivery of health services will make a better election-year issue than fighting to get better cash flow for hospitals. One would hope that the current preemption of concern for access by economic priorities will erode, especially as careful studies demonstrate that short-run cost savings in ignoring the poor produce long-run life-cycle cost explosions for society 8 to 20 years in the future (Shapiro 1986). Deterioration in health status among those poor or uninsured may not show up in annual survey data (Brook et al. 1983), but the untreated health care problems can become very significant over decades. The 1986 law that made Texas the first state to put into effect regulations intended to minimize patient "dumping" states explicitly in the basic preamble that a businesslike hospital should be an ethical hospital (Relman 1986). Patients are to be transferred only with their informed consent (when possible) and for valid medical, not economic, reasons.

Necessity may be the mother of invention, but lack of necessity impedes innovation. Many hospitals are financially distressed because they avoid work-load-driven staffing, operate with excess staff, pay excessive prices for equipment and supplies, and eschew initiating employee incentives for improving productivity (Eastaugh 1985). A major portion of the financial problems of the hospital may be the result of poor decision making and not an excess volume of nonpaying or poorly paying patients. Pouring more money into such facilities will not cure bad management. It will only delay the day of reckoning. Winston Churchill said, "Give us the tools and we will finish the job." Many indigent-care facilities lack the tools, the toolmakers, and the aggressive modern managers to act as troubleshooters and enhance quality and productivity. Moreover, politicians as a general rule disallow public-enterprise accounting, destroy the incentive to operate with efficiency by decreasing budgets, disallow employee incentive compensation, and frustrate good managers. In the case of public hospitals, the solution involves elimination of civil-service "protections" for unproductive, antiproductive, or incompetent employees. The choices for many hospitals are either closing, converting, selling, contract managing, or getting their internal house in order so as to foster efficiency and quality of care. This may involve breaking a little crockery, but if the goal is to maintain autonomy, the facility that survives will be the one that rewards its "best employees." If public hospitals and poorly managed teaching hospitals are not up to this challenge, they may go the way of the American buffalo. All three institutions had their golden eras, and now the two kinds of hospitals face extinction at the hands of entrepreneurs out to serve a public demand for less cost shifting and more cost-efficiency. The public policy problem may be finding enough points of access for the poor throughout the restructured hospital industry. A greater dose of unpalatable demarketing medicine could, under a worst-case scenario, include "dumping" poor patients, reducing services covered, and restricting eligibility. The medical needs of the poor would become the big loser in such a competitive environment (Lurie et al. 1986, 1984).

MONEY DOES NOT CURE ALL ILLS

A hospital experiencing substandard financial performance should not confuse poor results with destiny. Just because a facility serves a large volume of non-paying patients does not mean that it should also exhibit poor financial health. Indeed, in the Rundall and Lambert study (1985) utilizing California data, three indigent-care variables could only capture 12 to 15 percent of the variance for a range of liquidity and leverage financial ratios. Only one financial ratio, total operating margin, had a significant fraction (.34) of variance explained by the indigent-care measures. The Sloan, Blumstein, and Perrin study (1988) was even more unsuccessful in trying to explain institutional financial ratios. The vast majority of the variation in financial health can perhaps best be explained by differences in management that lead to better productivity and more aggressive diversification. Diversification and productivity incentive systems have been found to be much more significant predictors of financial standing than the volume of indigent care provided (Eastaugh 1985, 1984). Contrary to one study of New York hospitals from 1979 to 1981 (Brecher and Nesbitt 1985), financial decay is not the predetermined destiny of hospitals that serve a higher-than-average volume of indigent-care patients. Such hospitals require both better management and a stable, "sufficient" source of financing. We shall discuss the definition of "sufficient" in the next section. It is clear that the old cost-shifting game has almost been played out, and somebody or some group of bodies (federal, state, and local) must explicitly finance indigent care. Given that state governments are in better financial shape than the federal government, most of the action in indigent-coverage reform has been at the state level in the past 10 years (Lewin and Associates 1983; Colorado Task Force 1984; NAPH 1991, 1985).

DEFINING A STABLE SUFFICIENT MODE OF FUNDING

One should at the minimum reimburse indigent-care delivery at marginal cost with either a sin tax, a sick tax (x percent paid by all hospitals), or a fair-share pool (different rates of x put up by all hospitals "underserving" the indigent, so that net, all contribute equally to such care). The incentives could be set asymmetrically, so as to reward hospitals serving an increased volume of the indigent and penalize hospitals that demarket or discriminate against the indigent. For example, if a hospital increases the volume of indigent patients by more than 5 percent over the baseline-year figure, it would be paid at 10 percent above marginal cost (.66 of average cost). However, if the facility decreased indigent care by more than 5 percent, it would be paid only half of average cost. If the volume of indigent services was relatively stable from year to year, the hospital would be paid at marginal cost (taken as 0.6 of average cost).

Two caveats are in order. First, numerous studies have been done to measure the marginal costs of hospital and hospital educational programs (Berry 1986). The literature on the subject can be used to justify estimates of marginal cost as a fraction of average cost ranging from 0.5 to 0.7. The 0.6 figure represents the most frequently cited midrange figure, and it was also the figure adopted by Medicare to make outlier payments. Hospital-industry representatives dislike the cost-containment rationale for paying indigent care at marginal cost rather than at actual costs or full charges. Davis et al. (1990) and Blendon, Aiken, and Freeman (1986) suggested a more generous payment system for an expanded federalized Medicaid program. However, given that the medical care system is being leeched for dollars to compensate in some way for years of free spending under blank-check retrospective cost reimbursement, a stringent formula would be the most politically feasible. In other words, the hospital sector should be happy with 0.6 of a loaf in lieu of no loaf or payment at all for the nonpaying patients. Consequently, by only receiving marginal-costs payments, we as a society are recognizing the burden on nonindigent patients to cover the fixed costs of operating a hospital. The next three sections will survey state programs to expand access.

THE RIGHT TO CARE: REAFFIRMATION THROUGH MANAGED CARE AND FUND POOLS

The most prevalent change in the delivery system for the medically indigent has been the rise in managed-care networks or systems—for example, in California, Massachusetts, Arizona, and Oregon (Iglehart 1983; Shelton 1989). Managed-care programs with primary-physician gatekeepers can assure that dollars for indigent care are better channeled to ambulatory and preventive care. There has been some shortfall between program plans and performance, but in general, policy makers are pleased with the cost-containment aspects of such programs (Seidman and Pollack 1991; Kirkman-Liff, Christianson and Hillman 1985). For example, Arizona governor Bruce Babbitt defended his state's managed-care program at the 1986 annual meeting of the Association of American Medical Colleges. The governor indicated that not only did the program save money, but it provided increased case coordination and better-quality medical treatment. Kirkman-Liff (1985) reported that during Louis Harris interviews 4 percent of the poor households in Arizona self-reported some degree of direct provider refusal to provide care for an individual with a serious health problem. The emergence of managed-care networks has allowed the poor to be served with more continuity of care and has assured that inpatient imperatives for cash flow do not come to dominate the health agenda (Temkin and Winchell 1991).

Managed care is one of a number of large-scale strategies to finance care for the uninsured. Other strategies include rate programs reallocating resources to the uninsured (New Jersey, Maryland; six additional states require an ''add-on'' to be paid by third-party payers). For example, New Jersey reallocated $771 million of resources from 82 fiscally healthy hospitals to 36 hospitals serving a disproportionate share of poor patients in 1990. In 1991 the legislature let lapse a state trust that collected a surcharge on all hospital bills and distributed the proceeds among hospitals that cared for nonpaying patients. The surcharge, which had reached 19 percent, was blamed for pushing up insurance costs, forcing growing numbers of employers to drop health coverage for their work forces, and making individual policies too expensive.

A state may create revenue pools raised from surcharges on hospital revenues (states must circumvent section 514 of the Employee Retirement Income Security Act [ERISA] by imposing the tax on hospital net or gross revenues). If the state attempts to tax employee insurance benefits, the growing number of self-funded insurance plans can invoke ERISA 514 to avoid making any contributions. In 1991, 10 states had a tax on hospital revenues. For example, the South Carolina "sick tax" on hospital revenues is equally matched by tax receipts from the state's counties. Weak financial incentives to provide a minimum level of un-compensated care at each hospital have been adopted in six states. Other states have considered a hospital property tax to raise money for the poor (O'Donnell and Taylor 1990; Tuckman and Chang 1991). Six additional piecemeal strategies are often advocated to assist the uninsured or the underinsured:

1. State risk-sharing pools to allow "uninsurable," high-risk individuals to obtain affordable health insurance coverage (16 states).

2. Catastrophic public insurance (the Wisconsin program will provide vouchers for those whose incomes are not 75 percent higher than the poverty line).

3. More comprehensive federalized Medicaid expansion to select target populations.

4. Proposed direct federal subsidies to overburdened "financially distressed" providers.

5. Mandated temporary continuation of employer insurance coverage for the employee and family after unemployment or a change in marital status (available after six to nine months if the former employee can continue to pay the full premium cost).

6. Group-insurance purchasing for small businesses through multiple employer trusts (METs) that aggregate firms to enlarge the risk pool.

In summary, managed care can assure more efficient use of limited resources by balancing primary care and preventive medicine on an "equal playing field" with the highly expensive inpatient care. Other keys to success are exclusive selection of clinicians and a reasonable use of cost-sharing arrangements.

State Medicaid program directors realize that lack of affordable private health insurance is a statistically significant determinant of welfare reentry. Many families without private health insurance have remained off welfare with some short-term assistance through continued Medicaid coverage the first few months back on the job. Some state Medicaid programs have expanded their scope, like the Washington State basic health plan (Kobler 1990). This plan has funding to cover only 29,000 of the 410,000 people who are eligible for this managed-care demonstration project. Other states focus their strategy on selective contracting and competitive pricing (Shelton 1989; Heinen, Fox, and Anderson 1990). Other states focus on the inability of small employers to purchase insurance. In Kentucky the state has helped small companies to provide health benefits by setting up area development districts to act as insurance brokers. The districts create an insurance trust for companies of 50 employees or less and then find the best-value insurance plan available. Companies joining the MET in the 1990s receive a 20 percent state income-tax credit the first year and a 15 percent credit the second year.

MANDATING HEALTH BENEFITS: A SMALL AND COSTLY APPROACH

A number of state and federal officials are studying proposals to mandate health insurance coverage to assist the 22 million uninsured Americans that are employed or are dependents of those who work. Berki (1989) advanced the traditional economic argument against mandating firms to purchase health insurance: It would increase labor costs and so result in increasing unemployment, particularly among small businesses. The one counterexample that perhaps proves the rule is the Korean economy, which mandated employee health care benefits for large firms in 1977, medium-size firms in 1981, and small firms in 1989 (Eastaugh 1991). Korea could mandate health insurance without raising unemployment because of its very high growth rates during this period (6 to 9 percent growth in GNP annually). The same conditions were true for the Hawaii state economy in the mid-1970s. Mandating health insurance benefits for the employed still does nothing to mainstream services at public hospitals serving Medicaid and uninsured patients, and it does nothing for the unemployed. Mandating benefits also does nothing to promote cost containment or restructure the delivery system (Summers 1989; Swartz 1990).

Two states have some limited experience trying to mandate that employers purchase health insurance for their employees. Hawaii since 1974 and Massachusetts in 1988 (but with implementation delayed to 1993) shared the same general approach: (1) to strengthen the existing employer-based insurance system, (2) to mandate that every employed worker be able to obtain health insurance, and (3) to counteract the tendency of small business firms to save money by underinsuring their work force. Differences do exist between the two states. Massachusetts has been slow to start the program supported by Governor Michael Dukakis in 1988. The Hawaii program specifies both a defined benefit package (e.g., at least 120 days of hospitalization) and defined contribution "guidelines" (i.e., employers pay at least half the premium, and employees cannot pay more than 1.5 percent of gross income on health insurance premiums). The Massachusetts program does not define a minimum benefit package, but instead mandates a defined contribution requirement of at least $1,680 per worker by the employer.

All firms in Massachusetts employing six or more workers may someday have to pay a 12 percent tax on the initial $14,000 of wages (up to a maximum of $1,680) for eligible employees not insured. This "pay or play" strategy means that the state of Massachusetts would operate an insurance fund for the uninsured (or provide service directly through managed-care contracts) with the taxes collected. An eligible employee must work at least 30 hours per week for three months, or only 20 hours for heads of households or employees on the payroll for more than six months. A former interest group supporting the Dukakis approach was the state hospital association, which viewed 10 to 15 percent bad-debt rates for teaching hospitals as a major problem. Massachusetts has the highest density of medical students and residents per capita of any state in the nation. The prevalence of bad debt, teaching costs, and low hospital productivity explain the high hospital costs in the state. Hospital spending per capita in Massachusetts, highest in the nation, was 38 percent above the national average in 1991. Hospital executives' support for mandating employer-based coverage has declined as they have come to view this law as being an insufficiently focused hospital financing mechanism (Goldberger 1990).

Due to the state fiscal crisis and a downgrading of the Massachusetts credit rating, newly elected Republican Governor William Weld had to delay implementation of the 1988 Health Security Act to some future date (1993). The question remains as to whether employers in the state will be able to afford $580 million in 1993 to provide insurance for 345,000 uninsured workers (only 51 percent of the total uninsured population in the state). Will a mandatory contribution cause the loss of 10,000 jobs or 25,000 jobs in a state with high unemployment?

In contrast to the recent experience in this one northeastern state, the Hawaii program has worked reasonably well. Hawaii is a small state with very low levels of unemployment. The insurance industry supported the concept of mandatory benefits (Kim 1991). It enjoyed the small increment of new business in an insurance market dominated by only two players (Blue Shield and Kaiser). The president of the Hawaii Blue Shield plan estimated that the mandated-benefits law assisted only 5,000 to 10,000 workers to gain insurance coverage, and that 30,000 citizens received improved coverage because of the improved benefits package. The law still left 51,000 citizens without health insurance in 1991. It is disappointing that the Hawaii program helps only 15 percent of the previously uninsured, and that Massachusetts demonstration projects with managed care in 1991 may have assisted only 1.5 percent of the uninsured. The most successful and least successful mandatory state-mandated insurance programs do nothing to help the vast majority of the uninsured. More could be done for the working poor at less expense to the state economy if we would sufficiently fund public health clinics to provide the working poor with inexpensive basic care. This approach would upgrade the public health system and not increase the local unemployment rate.

AVOIDING THE PROBLEM OF "YOUR JOB OR YOUR HEALTH"

American industry opposes the ideological concept of mandating any fringe benefits and estimates, according to the *Wall Street Journal* (October 2, 1990), that a Kennedy-Waxman mandatory insurance bill would cost 3.5 million jobs. The microeconomic theorem is easily summarized: Make labor more expensive by mandating that health premiums be paid by the employer, and the firms will utilize less labor. However, the author estimates that the Chamber of Commerce overestimates the job loss at 3.5 million jobs, and liberals underestimate the national job loss at only 50,000 jobs. Some 300,000 to 400,000 jobs might be lost, with a compensating gain of 45,000 jobs in the health industry serving 5 to 6 million newly accessed consumers of health service. The net loss of jobs to the general economy should be weighed against the positive benefits of improved health status, including enhanced productivity on the job and less job turnover and absenteeism (workers can stay working longer rather than attending to an undertreated illness in their family). In the language of economics, health insurance is an investment in human capital, not just an expense. Considering the expense side of the benefit-cost equation, employers will be crafty at passing on the cost of new health coverage to the employees by depressing future wages and reducing the work force. As Needleman (1990) and Friedman (1990) have pointed out, mandating benefits is a very regressive secret payroll tax on the workers. Of the $14 billion of additional expense that small businesses would have to finance under a Kennedy-Waxman plan, 90 percent would eventually be transferred onto the employee through forgone wages, cuts in other fringe benefits, direct payments (e.g., cost-sharing hikes), or loss of jobs.

With a low level of political support, the Kennedy-Waxman mandated-benefits package will not become law in the near future. Too few people would benefit. Many providers might benefit, but efficiency might be reduced. Allocation efficiency might be harmed—for example, if mandating health insurance coverage reduced hospital bad debt from $11.6 billion to $8.0 billion, would the net $3.6 billion go to (1) reducing health care costs, (2) improved hospital financial reserves (and retirement of some long-term debt), or (3) new high-cost hospital technologies? Only a fool would suggest that the majority of the $3.6 billion would be given to the public as a rebate for reduced hospital bad debt (option 1). It might be more efficient to spend a fraction of that $3.6 billion on public health clinic services, with low copayments, for the working poor. The federal government may have to do more to assist local governments in funding basic primary care (Chang and Holahan 1991; Berwick and Hiatt 1989).

The one positive externality of the federal budget crisis debate for FY 1991 was the add-on to state finances by mandating medical services for children of the poor. Even an additional $550 million over the period 1991–95 will help. Children are often the forgotten group in American society; for example, the Hawaii program does not require coverage of dependents. The progressive aspect of the child-coverage bill is that each year the age will move up until children have full health protection to age 18. States are also required to act as the "medigap" insurer for the elderly poor, paying deductibles, copayments, and Medicare Part B premiums that Medicare does not pay. For the elderly above the poverty line, only Part B premiums will be covered by state funds.

FISCAL PROBLEMS FOR STATE AND LOCAL GOVERNMENTS

Uncompensated hospital care, adjusted for inflation, increased from $6.6 billion (in 1991 dollars) to $13 billion between 1981 and 1991. During the same decade, unsponsored care (the costs of uncompensated care that are not offset by payments from state and local governments) increased from $4.7 billion in 1981 to $10.4 billion in 1991. Unsponsored care rose more rapidly than uncompensated care over the decade because only 20 percent of uncompensated care was offset by state and local governments in 1991, compared with 27 percent in 1980 (Congressional Budget Office [CBO] 1991).

State governments have less capacity to expand Medicaid programs (NAPH 1991). The provision of the federal budget bill mentioned in the last section requires states to expand Medicaid funds to pay Medicare premiums of 2.53 million low-income and disabled persons. Starting in 1991, Congress required states to phase in coverage of children through age 18 in poor families, beginning with children under age 6 prior to October 1990 and with the age limit of the law rising to age 18 by the year 2003. While this federal law is progressive, federal dollars do not finance the burden. Federal mandates are crippling the ability of state governors to finance public education, streets, sewers, and other infrastructure support. Medicaid represented 13.1 percent of the average state budget in 1991 ($33.4 billion), but this figure will rise to 16 percent or $52 billion by 1995. Given that a state government cannot run a deficit or print currency, where should the governors cut spending to finance the growing needs of the elderly (including chronic nursing care)? Some Oregon politicians have an answer to this question (Tresnowski 1991).

A physician, John Kitzhaber, president of the Oregon Senate, advocated confronting the reality of limits by defining an adequate level of care to which all should have access. In chapters 11–13 we shall discuss cost-benefit analysis and the limits on medical technology enhancing quality of life. Oregon Medicaid program management is trying to allocate funds by linking service costs to expected benefits within the context of available revenue. The plan is expected to be implemented by 1993. The list of conditions under study now exceeds 1,800. The issue of defining services that are sufficiently effective and beneficial compared to other basic health services is a problem for all third-party payers. For example, we spend $4.2 billion on neonatal intensive-care units, but millions of pregnant women do not receive prenatal care. The nation spends $70 billion annually on patients in their last six months of life, but pediatric clinics in poor neighborhoods are being closed for lack of funding. Antidumping laws are little help for facilities in financial trouble (Laddaga and Haynes 1991; Eastaugh and Eastaugh 1990), and more leaders call for some form of rationing. A list of 1,800 procedures, rank ordered by "crude cost-effectiveness" is a new form of explicit economic rationing. The ad hoc nature of the Oregon Health Services Commission attempt to guess at relative cost-effectiveness rankings may impugn the reputation of true cost-effectiveness and cost-benefit studies as done by economists (see chapters 11–13; Eddy 1991).

The American tradition of implicit rationing is becoming more explicit (Granneman 1991; Frank, Salkever, and Mitchell 1990). State Medicaid directors are in some cases defining classes of individuals that should receive certain types of transplants. Is the expenditure of $200,000 justified by 5 expected extra years of life or by 10 years? Should the decision be different if the person is wealthy and can pay for the treatment as compared with the payment being made from public funds? Medical technology will continue to improve in that area and has the potential to spend vast sums of money.

Until and unless someone in a decision-making position is willing to address these types of questions, health care will continue to absorb an ever-increasing proportion of the gross national product. It is not the job of biomedical researchers, physicians, or hospital administrators to make these sorts of global resource-allocation decisions. It is the job of the elected officials to decide the trade-offs between health care and alternative uses of the available funds. The state of Oregon is attempting to make just this type of decision for its Medicaid program (outlined in chapter 11), and it will be interesting to see how these laudable efforts are distorted or thwarted by the legal system.

EFFICACY, SOCIAL WELFARE, AND VALUES

Kelly (1985) reported that charity patients in tax-exempt urban hospitals were less likely to have surgery and had fewer diagnostic and therapeutic procedures than privately insured patients. In addition, charity patients were discharged after only 5.8 days, in comparison to an average duration of stay of 6.7 days for private patients. These relative comparisons might provoke some to claim that charity patients are underserved. However, the test of history seems to belie any assertion other than to say that both groups were "overserved" and that the efficiency and efficacy of much of this inpatient care were suspect.

More recently, Wenneker, Weissman, and Epstein (1990) reported that the privately insured patients received 80 percent more cardiac angiography, 40 percent more coronary bypass operations, and a 28 percent higher rate of angioplasty in Massachusetts. Hadley, Steinberg, and Feder (1991) in a national study reported that the uninsured receive fewer high-discretion high-cost procedures: 75 percent fewer total knee replacements, 45 percent fewer hip replacements, and 29 percent fewer coronary bypass operations. The question for public policy makers is whether these utilization differentials represent (1) overmet needs of the insured, (2) unmet needs of the uninsured, or (3) some combination of (1) and (2). Many corporate benefit managers fear that the insured population is receiving too much unnecessary care (Siegel 1990; Eastaugh 1990b; Simmons 1990). In 1991 the average length of stay for charity and private patients converged to 4.7 days. The health of both groups does not appear to have suffered.

This supports Feldstein's (1973) assertion that there is a multibillion-dollar "social welfare loss to all society from having excess insurance" producing too much care (inpatient days, tests, procedures, and operations).

One might assume that in an "age of plenty," with so much savings from forgone unnecessary utilization and a glut of beds and doctors, policy makers would not hasten to address the problem of indigent care. After all, with so many empty beds and underutilized doctors, indigent care is something they could perform in their spare time (as part of a social contract; the public could reimburse at marginal cost for their services). We have not faced up to the shared obligation of indigent care between both the private and public sectors, because there is little consensus as to whether health care is a desired commodity (like a college education) or a necessary commodity (like food). If health care is a desired commodity, then providers will produce service along multiple levels of amenities and technical quality. Most citizens would not begrudge the rich first-class amenities in what Reinhardt (1985) referred to as "Yuppie boutique" medicine. However, public policy might consider some assurance that technical quality is not "substandard" for the medically indigent. "Boutique medicine" would involve not just better amenities, but better quality of care. Society would provide boutique medicine for those who can pay, just as we have "boutique education" at Harvard and Stanford. Those people who buy the myth that providers are roughly equivalent might be equally gullible in believing that Stanford is equivalent to the local community college. The analogy breaks down in a number of ways: The poor who merit it have some chance to get into Stanford, and the Mayo Clinic can afford to franchise itself in four locations (whereas Stanford has agreed to stay at one location). This may be an unfortunate circumstance, but it is not an unfair circumstance.

If health care is a necessary basic commodity like food, society should underwrite a minimum basic-needs coverage policy for all. We have attempted to mainstream the Medicaid-eligible "covered poor" into the great majority of hospitals, so that equity is better served than in the market for education. However, as with the food stamp program, there has been little social pressure to federalize Medicaid in an egalitarian spirit. Federal policy making has always operated on the "big-wheel principle"—he who is now first will later be last, and he who is last will be first. Consequently, the winds of change may make the egalitarians powerful again in a few years. Then we may have an equitable federal indigent-care policy, even if national health insurance is judged too expensive. Americans have the highest aspirations for the right of access to the best care for everyone, but we never have the necessary amount of resources to do this on a fee-for-service basis. Managed care is one strategy whereby we institutionalize the right to care with an efficient mode of service delivery.

DOES A ONE-PAYER NATIONALIZED APPROACH MAKE SENSE?

A number of analysts have suggested a statewide one-payer approach to statewide insurance coverage (Beauchamp and Rouse 1990). Physicians for a National

Health Program have advocated abolishing all private and public insurance plans to create a one-payer plan to cover everyone, financed entirely by taxes, with a system of state and regional boards negotiating with providers on compensation (Himmelstein and Woolhandler 1989). The benefits of such a one-payer system are obvious to many: less paperwork, less administrative expense, and fewer financial barriers to access. Himmelstein and Woolhandler may have been over-optimistic in assuming that administrative expense could be trimmed from 15 to 20 percent of health spending to 3 to 4 percent.

Other progressive/left-wing groups have attacked the administrative expense implicit in our current multipayer patchwork system of health insurance coverage. Citizen Action claimed in October 1990 that the 200 commercial insurance firms covering 70 million Americans spent 25 percent of expenses on administration and marketing. Carl Schramm, president of the Health Insurance Association of America, claimed that the more appropriate fair-cost comparison for small-scale organizations was 13 percent. However, Citizen Action went on to say that the comparable figure was 2.4 percent for Medicare and 3.0 percent for Canada.

The problem with the Canadian approach is that the local government can ration care through inconvenience: long waits for elective surgery, tests, and checkup visits (Grumet 1989). Many managed-care health plans have been cited for having these same problems, but to a lesser degree. Rather than copy the Canadian model, Enthoven and Kronick (1989) advocated preserving an employer-based approach, offering tax incentives, and mandating "universal coverage for all" through a competition health care plan approach. The many health plans, contracting with both employers and statewide "public sponsors," would compete for enrollees based on price and quality. A third alternative, advocated by the National Leadership Commission on Health Care (Simmons 1990) would keep Medicare and the present health insurance system, but spend an additional $15 billion in public funds to guarantee a basic adequate benefits package. To avoid the unpopular word "taxes," the commission advocated premiums and fees in the form of income-tax surcharges. The Pepper Commission report (Rockefeller 1990) was a little bit more realistic in scaling the price tag to the $60 to $90 billion range, depending on how much new access is financed in the long-term-care arena.

Levey and Hill (1989) coined a phrase to neatly summarize why no national health plan can be passed (or done cheaply): The inertia surrounding the issue is the product of a long American tradition of equivocation on health policy. "Equivocation triumphs" each decade because the public is willing to pay 5 to 10 percent more in administrative expense to maximize the diversity of health plans available. The lack of widespread discontent with our expensive medical system seems to ensure slow marginal change in existing programs. On the other hand, optimists can point out that progressive reforms were passed by Congress despite a diffuse 1980s mood of skepticism and barebones reimbursement. It was a Congress plagued by deficits that passed the Hospice Act in 1982 and the Catastrophic Health Benefit Act for the elderly in 1988 (Davis et al. 1990). A cost-effective national system is easy to outline on paper: access reform ("buy in'' for the working poor), supply reform (''competition'' between providers), and information reform (''buy-right'' consumerism based on value shopping for providers based on technical quality, amenities, and cost). Many nations have retrenched from this ideal and have encouraged their citizens to purchase more customized private insurance (New Zealand, Korea, Japan, and the United Kingdom).

REFERENCES

Altman, S., Brecher, C., Henderson, M., and Thorpe, K. (1989). *Competition and Compassion: Conflicting Roles for Public Hospitals.* Ann Arbor, Mich.: Health Administration Press.

American Hospital Association (1989). *The Cost of Compassion.* Chicago: American Hospital Association.

Bazzoli, G. (1986). ''Health Care for the Indigent.'' *Health Services Research* 21:3 (August), 353–393.

Beauchamp, D., and Rouse, R. (1990). ''Universal New York Health Care: A Single-Payer Strategy Linking Cost Control and Universal Access.'' *New England Journal of Medicine* 323:10 (September 6), 640–644.

Berki, S. (1989). ''Michigan Health Plan: Universal Health Security.'' Lansing, Mich.: Report of the Governor's Task Force on Access to Care.

Berry, R. (1986). ''Cost Functions and Production Functions in a Sample of 45 Hospitals.'' Final Report of the Arthur Young Graduate Medical Education Study, vols. 2 and 3, DHHS Contract 100–80–0155 ASPE (October).

Berwick, D., and Hiatt, H. (1989). ''Who Pays?'' *New England Journal of Medicine* 321:8 (August 24), 541–542.

Blendon, R., Aiken, L., and Freeman, H. (1986). ''Uncompensated Care by Hospitals or Public Insurance for the Poor: Does It Make a Difference?'' *New England Journal of Medicine* 314:18 (May 1), 1160–1163.

Blendon, R., and Edwards, J. (1991). ''Caring for the Uninsured: Choices for Reform.'' *Journal of the American Medical Association* 265:19 (May 15), 2563–2566.

Blumenthal, D., and Rizzo, J. (1991). ''Who Cares for Uninsured Persons? A Study of Physicians and Their Patients Who Lack Health Insurance.'' *Medical Care* 29:6 (June), 502–519.

Brecher, C., and Nesbitt, S. (1985). ''Factors Associated with Variation in Financial Condition among Voluntary Hospitals.'' *Health Services Research* 20:3 (August), 267–300.

Brook, R. (1991). ''Health, Health Insurance, and the Uninsured.'' *Journal of the American Medical Association* 265:22 (June 12), 2998–3002.

Brook, R., Ware, J., Rogers, W., and Newhouse, J. (1983). ''Does Free Care Improve Adults' Health?'' *New England Journal of Medicine* 309:22 (December 8), 1426–1434.

Brown, L. (1990). ''The Medically Uninsured: Problems, Policies, and Politics.'' *Journal of Health Politics, Policy, and Law* 15:2 (Summer), 413–426.

Butler, S. (1991). ''Tax Reform Strategy to Deal with the Uninsured.'' *Journal of the American Medical Association* 265:19 (May 15), 2541–2545.

Butler, S., and Haislmaier, E. (1990). *A National Health System for America*. Washington, D.C.: Heritage Foundation.

Chang, D., and Holahan, J. (1991). *Medicaid Spending in the 1980s: The Access-Cost Containment Trade-off Revisited*. Washington, D.C.: Urban Institute Press.

Chang, C., and Tuckman, H. (1991). "The Single-hospital County: Is Its Hospital at Risk?" *Health Services Research* 26:2 (June), 207–221.

Children's Defense Fund (1991). *The Health of America's Children*. Washington, D.C.: Children's Defense Fund.

Chulis, G. (1991). "Assessing Medicare's Prospective Payment System for Hospitals." *Medical Care Review* 48:2 (Summer), 167–206.

Cohodes, D. (1986). "America: The Home of the Free, the Land of the Uninsured." *Inquiry* 23:3 (Fall), 227–235.

Colorado Task Force on the Medically Indigent. (1984). "Colorado's Sick and Uninsured: We Can Do Better." Report volume 1 (January).

Congressional Budget Office. (1992). *Selected Options for Expanding Health Insurance Coverage*, Washington, D.C.: U.S. Congress.

———. (1991). *Trends in Health Expenditures for Medicare and Medicaid*. Washington, D.C.: CBO, U.S. Congress.

Cornelius, L. (1991). "Access to Medical Care for Black Americans with an Episode of Illness." *Journal of the National Medical Association* 83:7, 617–626.

Davidson, G., and Moscovice, I. (1989). "Health Insurance and Welfare Reentry." *Health Services Research* 24:5 (December), 599–614.

Davis, K., Anderson, G., Rowland, D., and Steinberg, E. (1990). *Health Care Cost Containment*. Baltimore: Johns Hopkins University Press.

Dunham, N., Kindig, D., and Ramsey, P. (1991). "Uncompensated and Discounted Care Provided by Physician Group Practices." *Journal of the American Medical Association* 265:22 (June 12), 2982–2986.

Dunlop, J. (1986). "Business' Interest in Health Care Won't Wane." *Hospitals* 60:13 (July 5), 103–104.

Eastaugh, S. (1991). "Sharing the Burden: Containing the Health Care Bill for American Industry." *Business Forum* 16:1 (Winter), 25–28.

———. (1990a). "Health Insurance Reform in the 1990s." *Journal of the American Academy of Physician Assistants* 3:5 (July/August), 384–395.

———. (1990b). "Universal Health Insurance: Equivocation throughout the Nation." *New England Journal of Medicine* 322:17 (April 26), 1239–1240.

———. (1985). "Improving Hospital Productivity under PPS: Managing Cost Reductions without Quality and Service Reductions." *Hospital and Health Services Administration* 30:4 (July/August), 97–111.

———. (1984). "Hospital Diversification and Financial Management." *Medical Care* 22:8 (August), 704–723.

Eastaugh, S., and Eastaugh, J. (1990). "Putting the Squeeze on Emergency Medicine: Competition and Indigent Care." *Hospital Topics* 68:4 (Fall), 21–26.

Eddy, D. (1991). "Oregon's Methods: Did Cost-effectiveness Analysis Fail?" *Journal of The American Medical Association* 266:15 (October 16), 2135–2141.

Employee Benefits Research Corporation (EBRC). (1991) *Assessing the Access Problems*. Washington, D.C.: Employee Benefits Research Institute.

Enthoven, A., and Kronick, R. (1989). "A Consumer-Choice Health Plan for the 1990s." *New England Journal of Medicine* 320:1 (January 5), 26–30.

Etheredge, L. (1991). "Negotiating National Health Insurance." *Journal of Health Politics, Policy and Law* 16:1 (Spring), 157–167.

———. (1990). "Universal Health Insurance: Lessons of the 1970s, Prospects for the 1990s." *Frontiers of Health Services Management* 6:4 (Summer), 1–35.

Feder, J., Hadley, J., and Mullner, R. (1984). "Falling through the Cracks: Poverty, Insurance Coverage, and Hospital's Care for the Poor." *Milbank Memorial Fund Quarterly* 62:4 (Fall), 640–660.

Fein, R. (1991). "Health Security Partnership: A Federal-State Universal Insurance and Cost Containment Program." *Journal of the American Medical Association* 265:19 (May 15), 2555–2559.

Feldstein, M. (1973). "The Welfare Loss of Excess Health Insurance." *Journal of Political Economy* 81:2 (March/April), 251–280.

Frank, R., Salkever, D., and Mitchell, J. (1990). "Market Forces and the Public Good: Competition among Hospitals and Provision of Indigent Care." in *Advances in Health Economics and Health Services Research*, edited by Scheffler, R., Greenwich, Conn.: JAI Press, 159–183.

Friedman, E. (1990). "Health Insurance in Hawaii: Paradise Lost or Found?" *Business and Health* 8:4 (June), 52–59.

Gapenski, L. (1991). "Determinants of Hospital profitability." Paper presented at AUPHA annual meeting, Washington, D.C., March 24.

Garner, M. (1992). "Reporting Charity Care: New Accounting Rules." *Health Progress* 73:1 (January-February), 58–63.

Ginzberg, E. (1991). "Beyond Universal Health Insurance to Effective Care." *Journal of the American Medical Association* 265:19 (May 15), 2559–2563.

Gleicher, N. (1991). "Expansion of Health Care to the Uninsured and Underinsured Has to Be Cost Neutral." *Journal of the American Medical Association* 265:18 (May 8), 2388–2390.

Goldberger, S. (1990). "The Politics of Universal Access: The Massachusetts Health Security Act of 1988." *Journal of Health Politics, Policy, and Law.* 15:4 (Winter), 857–885.

Grannemann, T. (1991). "Priority Setting: a sensible approach to medicaid policy?", *Inquiry* 28:3 (Fall) 300–5.

Griffith, J. (1989). "The Struggle Is the Essence." *Frontiers of Health Services Management* 6:2 (Winter), 31–34.

Grumbach, K., Himmelstein, D., and Woolhandler, S. (1991). "Liberal Benefits, Conservative Spending." *Journal of the American Medical Association* 265:19 (May 15), 2549–2555.

Grumet, G. (1989). "Health Care Rationing through Inconvenience." *New England Journal of Medicine* 321:9 (August 31), 607–611.

Hadley, J., and Feder, J. (1985). "Hospital Cost Shifting and Care for the Uninsured." *Health Affairs* 4:3 (Fall), 67–80.

Hadley, J., Steinberg, E., and Feder, J. (1991). "Comparison of Uninsured and Privately Insured Hospital Patients: Condition on Admission, Resource Use, and Outcome." *Journal of the American Medical Association* 265:3 (January 16), 374–379.

Heinen, L., Fox, P., and Anderson, M. (1990). "Findings from the Medicaid Competition Demonstrations." *Health Care Financing Review* 11:4 (Summer), 55–69.

Himmelstein, D., and Woolhandler, S. (1989). "A National Health Program for the

United States: A Physician's Proposal." *New England Journal of Medicine* 320:2 (January 12), 102–108.

Holahan, J., Moon, M., Welch, W., and Zuckerman, S. (1991). "American Approach to Health Systems Reform." *Journal of the American Medical Association* 265:19 (May 15), 2537–2541.

Holleman, M., Loe, H., Selwyn, B. (1991). "Uncompensated Outpatient Medical Care by Physicians." *Medical Care* 29:7 (July), 654–660.

Hultman, C. (1991). "Uncompensated Care Before and After PPS: The Role of Hospital Ownership and Location." *Health Services Research* 26:5 (December), 585–601.

Hyman, H. (1986). "Are Public Hospitals in New York City Inferior to Voluntary, Nonprofit Hospitals? A Study of JCAH Hospital Surveys." *American Journal of Public Health* 76:1 (January), 18–23.

Iezzoni, L. (1992). "Purpose of Admission and Resource Use," *Health Care Financing Review* 13:2 (Winter), 29–40.

Iglehart, J. (1983). "Medicaid Turns to Prepaid Managed Care." *New England Journal of Medicine* 308:16 (April 21), 976–980.

Inspector General. (1990). Inspector General v. Burditt, Health and Human Resources Federal Departmental Appeals Board, Civil Remedies Division Case no. C–42 (January 28).

Johns, L. (1989). "Selective Contracting in California: An Update." *Inquiry* 26:3 (Fall), 345–352.

Kelly, J. (1985). "Charity Care by Nonprofit Hospitals in 1977." In *Hospitals and the Uninsured Poor: Measuring and Paying for Uncompensated Care* (Summer). New York: United Hospital Fund of New York.

Kilpatrick, K., Miller, M., Dwyer, J., and Nissen, D. (1991). "Uncompensated Care Provided by Private Practice Physicians." *Health Services Research* 26:3 (August), 277–289.

Kim, H. (1991). "Hawaii: Life after Mandatory Insurance." *Modern Healthcare* 21:7 (February 18), 21–25.

Kinzer, D. (1984). "Care of the Poor Revisited." *Inquiry* 21:1 (Spring), 5–16.

Kirkman-Liff, B. (1985). "Refusal of Care: Evidence from Arizona." *Health Affairs* 4:4 (Winter), 15–24.

Kirkman-Liff, B., Christianson, J., and Hillman, D. (1985). "An Analysis of Competitive Bidding by Providers for Arizona Indigent Medical Care Contracts." *Health Services Research* 20:5 (December), 549–578.

Kobler, T. (1990). "Implementation of the Washington State Basic Health Plan." *Henry Ford Hospital Medical Journal* 38:3 (Fall), 125–127.

Kronick, R. (1991). "Can Massachusetts Pay for Health Care for All?" *Health Affairs* 10:1 (Spring), 26–43.

Laddaga, L., and Haynes, J. (1991). "Anti-dumping Law." *Healthcare Financial Management* 45:3 (March), 84–88.

Levey, S., and Hill, J. (1989). "National Health Insurance: The Triumph of Equivocation." *New England Journal of Medicine* 321:25 (December 21), 1750–1754.

Lewin and Associates, Inc. (1983). *Health Care Financing for the Medically Indigent in Florida: A Proposed System*. Final Report to the Florida Task Force on Competition and Consumer Choices in Health Care (January), Washington, D.C.

Lundberg, G. (1991). "National Health Care Reform." *Journal of the American Medical Association* 265:19 (May 15), 2566–2569.

Lurie, N., Ward, N., Shapiro, M., and Brook, R. (1984). "Termination from Medi-Cal: Does It Affect Health?" *New England Journal of Medicine* 311:7 (August 16), 480–484.

Lurie, N., Ward, N., Shapiro, M., Gallego, C., Vaghaiwalla, R., and Brook, R. (1986). "Termination of Medi-Cal Benefits: A Follow-up Study One Year Later." *New England Journal of Medicine* 314:9 (May 8), 1266–1268.

McCarthy, C. (1986). "Coping with the Constant Challenge of Change." *Hospitals* 60:18 (September 20), 104.

McCue, M. (1991). "Use of Cash Flow to Analyze Financial Distress in California Hospitals." *Hospital and Health Services Administration* 36:2 (Summer) 223–241.

McDaniel, J. (1986). "Charity Care: A Proposal for Reform." *Hospital and Health Services Administration* 31:2 (March–April), 124–134.

Mitchell, J. (1991). "Physician Participation in Medicaid Revisited." *Medical Care* 29:7 (July), 645–653.

Monheit, A., and Short, P. (1989). "Mandating Health Coverage for Working Americans." *Health Affairs* 8:4 (Winter), 22–37.

Morrisey, M., Sloan, F., and Valvona, J. (1989). "Defining Geographic Markets for Hospitals and the Extent of Market Concentration." *Law and Contemporary Problems* 51:2 (September), 222.

Mundinger, M. (1985). "Health Service Funding Cuts and the Declining Health of the Poor." *New England Journal of Medicine* 313:1 (July 4), 44–47.

National Association of Public Hospitals. (1991). "Financing and Provision of Health Care to the Medically Indigent." Updated status report.

———. (1985). "Texas Public Hospitals and Care for the Poor." Report to the Texas Association of Public Hospitals (May).

Needleman, J. (1990). "Mandating Employee Health Benefits? A New Look." *Bulletin of the New York Academy of Medicine* 66:1 (January–February), 80–93.

Nexon, D. (1990). "Senator Kennedy's Proposal to Guarantee Basic Health Benefits for All Americans." *Henry Ford Hospital Medical Journal* 38:3 (Fall), 110–113.

Nutter, D., Helms, C., Whitcomb, M., and Weston, W. (1991). "Restructuring Health Care in the U.S." *Journal of the American Medical Association* 265:19 (May 15), 2516–2524.

O'Donnell, J., and Taylor, J. (1990). "The Bounds of Charity: Current Status of the Hospital Property-Tax Exemption." *New England Journal of Medicine* 322:1 (January 4), 65–68.

Ohsfeldt, R. (1985). "Uncompensated Medical Services Provided by Physicians and Hospitals." *Medical Care* 23:12 (December), 1338–1344.

Pallarito, K. (1990). "Problems Prompt Second Thoughts about Mass. Universal Health Plan." *Modern Healthcare* (September 24), 34.

Pauly, M., Danzon, P., Feldstein, P., and Hoff, J. (1991). "A Plan for Responsible National Health Insurance." *Health Affairs* 10:1 (Spring), 5–25.

Politzer, R., Harris, D., and Gaston, M. (1991). "Primary Care Physician Supply and the Medically Underserved." *Journal of the American Medical Association* 266:1 (July 3), 104–108.

Reinhardt, U. (1985). "Economics, Ethics, and the American Health Care System." *New Physician* 9:10 (October), 20–28.

Reiser, S. (1992) "Consumer Competence and the Reform of American Health Care." *JAMA* 267:11 (March 18), 1511–1515.

Relman, A. (1986). "Texas Eliminates Dumping: A Start toward Equity in Hospital Care." *New England Journal of Medicine* 314:9 (February 27), 578–579.

Rieselbach, R., and Jackson, T. (1986). "In Support of a Linkage between the Funding of Graduate Medical Education and Care of the Indigent." *New England Journal of Medicine* 314:1 (January 2), 32–35.

Rockefeller, J. (1990). "The Pepper Commission Report on Comprehensive Health Care." *New England Journal of Medicine* 323:14 (October 4), 1005–1007.

Roper, W. (1989). "Financing Health Care: A View from the White House." *Health Affairs* 8:4 (Winter), 97–102.

Rosko, M. (1990). "All-Payer Rate-setting and the Provision of Hospital Care to the Uninsured in New Jersey." *Journal of Health Politics, Policy, and Law* 15:4 (Winter), 815–831.

Rundall, T., and Lambert, J. (1985). "Analysis of Emerging Strategies: Hospital Behavior in Competitive Markets." Report to the Western Consortium for Health Planning under Contract to DHHS, 232–82–0006 (March).

Saywell, R., Zollinger, T., and Chu, D. (1989). "Hospital and Patient Characteristics of Uncompensated Hospital Care." *Journal of Health Politics, Policy and Law* 14:2 (Summer), 287–307.

Schiff, R., Ansell, D., Schlosser, J., Idris, A., Momson, A., and Whitman, S. (1986). "Transfers to a Public Hospital: A Prospective Study of 467 Patients." *New England Journal of Medicine* 314:9 (February 27), 552–557.

Schlenker, R. (1991). "Nursing Home Costs, Medicaid Rates, and Profits under Alternative Medicaid Payment Systems." *Health Services Research* 26:5 (December), 606–626.

Seidman, R., and Pollack, S. (1991). "Trends in Hospital Deductions from Revenue in California." *Hospital Topics* 69:1 (Winter), 19–26.

Shapiro, M., Ware, J., and Sherbourne, C. (1986). "Effects of Cost Sharing on Seeking Care for Serious and Minor Symptoms." *Annals of Internal Medicine* 104:2 (February), 246–251.

Shelton, N. (1989). "Competitive Contingencies in Selective Contracting." *Medical Care Review* 46:3 (Fall), 271–292.

Sherlock, D. (1986). "Indigent Care in Rational Markets." *Inquiry* 23:3 (Fall), 261–267.

Shorr, L. (1990). "Successful Health Programs for the Poor and Underserved." *Journal of Health Care for the Poor* 1:3 (Winter), 271–277.

Siegel, J. (1990). "The FASB Exposure Draft: Issues and Implications." In *The Sourcebook on Postretirement Health Care Benefits*. Greenvale, N.Y.: Panel Publishers.

Simmons, H. (1990). *Report of the National Leadership Commission on Health Care: The Health of the Nation—A Shared Responsibility*. Ann Arbor, Mich.: Health Administration Press.

Sloan, F., Blumstein, J., and Perrin, J. (1988). *Cost, Quality, and Access in Health Care: New Roles for Health Planning in a Competitive Environment*. San Francisco: Jossey-Bass.

Stern, R., Weissman, J., and Epstein, A. (1991). "Emergency Department as a Pathway to Admission for Poor and High-cost Patients." *Journal of the American Medical Association* 266:16 (October 30), 2238–2243.

Summers, L. (1989). "Some Simple Economics of Mandated Benefits." *American Economic Review* 79:2 (May), 177–183.

Swartz, K. (1990). "Why Requiring Employers to Provide Health Insurance Is a Bad Idea." *Journal of Health Politics, Policy, and Law* 15:4 (Winter), 779–791.

Swartz, K., and McBride, T. (1990). "Spells without Health Insurance: Distributions of Durations and Their Link to Point-in-Time Estimates of the Uninsured." *Inquiry* 27:3 (Fall), 281–88.

Temkin, H., and Winchell, M. (1991). "Medicaid Beneficiaries under Managed Care: Provider Choice and Satisfaction." *Health Services Research* 26:4 (October), 509–530.

Thorpe, K. (1991). "The RUG System: Its Effect on Nursing Home Case Mix and Costs." *Inquiry* 28:4 (Winter), 357–365.

Tresnowski, B. (1991). "Oregon's Initiative Promises Wealth of Experience to Guide Health Care Reform." *Inquiry* 28:3 (Fall), 207–208.

Tuckman, H., and Chang, C. (1991). "Proposal to Redistribute the Cost of Hospital Charity Care." *Milbank Quarterly* 69:1 (Spring), 113–142.

U.S. Congress. (1991). *Medicaid Source Book: Background Data and Analysis*. House Committee on Energy and Commerce, Subcommittee on Health. Washington, D.C.: U.S. Government Printing Office.

Vladeck, B. (1992) "Health Care Leadership in the Public Interest." *Frontiers of Health Services Management* 8:3 (Spring), 3–25.

Wenneker, M., Weissman, J., and Epstein, A. (1990). "Association of Payer with Utilization of Cardiac Procedures in Massachusetts." *Journal of the American Medical Association* 264:10 (September 12), 1255–1260.

8 The Cost of Teaching Hospitals

Increased subspecialization is an acute problem in major teaching hospitals. The doctor says to the patient: I hope you got what I treat. The patient retorts: I hope you treat what I got.

—Isadore Levine, M.D.

He who pays the piper can call the tune.

—Old English Proverb

Future research that explicitly recognizes variations in medical staff characteristics and organizations may be fruitful in discovering reasons underlying variations in hospital performance in response to regulation. Put another way, is "control" of medical staff a necessary condition for containment of hospital costs?

—Frank A. Sloan

On an annual basis a number of physicians complain to Congress that teaching hospitals are an endangered species. Payers have to offer teaching hospitals higher reimbursement for a number of reasons, as outlined in this chapter. Economists and quality-assurance reviewers are concerned that all the additional care paid for may not be medically necessary. Mecicine is far from monolithic in style, and therefore preferred practice pattern (PPP) efficiency profiles vary widely across the country. For example, Burns and Wholey (1991), in a study of 55,000 discharges, reported that the medical school attended by the physician influences the patient's length of stay.

Patient care in teaching hospitals will always require some legitimate extra costs, such as (1) the surgical resident spending an extra 20 to 90 minutes in the operating room learning to do a technique from the more experienced mentor attending surgeon or (2) the apprentice resident ordering a liberal large number of tests to avoid making a mistake or missing a rare interesting condition (that is, before learning how to better balance risk aversion and wasted effort and not follow every "wild goose chase"; Eeckhoudt, LeBrun, and Sailly 1985; Eastaugh 1979). These so-called learning effects are legitimate costs of training the next generation of competent, high-quality clinicians. The indirect cost of education requires more than simply an additional increment of variable patient-care costs. Teaching hospitals require additional fixed costs beyond the additional space required to house biomedical research projects. For example, because the teaching function requires additional space in the patient's room for groups of residents and medical students, builders typically allocate 30 to 50 percent more square feet of space per bed to accommodate the traffic.

The educational component of medical care costs is frequently given adequate earmarked support via funds from departments of education in Canada and Europe (Relman 1984; Eastaugh 1980a). The American tradition is to subsidize such costs indirectly through the "back door" of patient hospital bills. For example, the 1991 survey of the Association of American Medical Colleges (AAMC) reported that 85 percent of residents' stipends and fringe benefits were derived from hospital patient revenues. The Commonwealth Task Force on Academic Health Centers report (1985), a two-year project by a 16-member national task force of teaching hospital professors and managers, suggested that a tax on all hospital admissions should be collected to reimburse hospitals for doing graduate medical education. This is a rather attractive payment "solution" for teaching hospitals because it involves minimum disruption of business as usual ("don't look at what we do, just pay us"). Such a proposed tax on hospital admissions, a sort of "sick tax" for education, has the administrative advantage of distributing the costs of teaching hospitals across all inpatients without disaggregating how much of this cash flow underwrites (1) appropriate treatment of a more severely ill case mix (Newhouse 1983), (2) charity care for the poor (Epstein 1986; Rieselbach and Jackson 1986), or (3) inappropriate high-cost care (Keeler 1990).

The initial DHHS adjustment formula for the indirect cost of graduate medical education was based on a multiple regression analysis by two researchers at HCFA. Pettengill and Vertrees (1982) analyzed 1980 Medicare cost reports from 5,071 hospitals and concluded that costs rose 5.795 percent for each increase of 0.1 in the ratio of residents to beds after adjusting for DRG mix and local wage levels. Pressure from the Council of Teaching Hospitals led Congress to double this adjustment rate to 11.59 percent. The stated reason was that this extra payment factor would help underwrite uncompensated care and increased severity of illness not captured by the DRG categories (U.S. Senate Finance Committee 1983). Nonteaching hospitals in the shadow of major teaching hospitals with 0.8 residents per bed would receive half the Medicare payment for the same DRG case treated. Because this payment formula was excessively generous to the 136 hospitals that provide 55 percent of the residency slots in the nation, payment rates for the indirect cost of graduate medical education were reduced in 1986. As part of the Consolidated Omnibus Budget Reconciliation Act (COBRA) effective April 7, 1986, the indirect teaching adjustment was reduced to 8.1 percent for FY 1986 and FY 1987. This reduction was made in part because the DRG rates would recognize, for the first time, hospitals serving a disproportionate share of poor patients. The Bush administration has proposed cutting the indirect teaching adjustment to 4.4 percent ($2.5 billion) by 1993.

Medicare reimbursement for residents stimulated more hospitals to initiate residency programs. The number of residency programs accredited by the Council for Graduate Medical Education increased by 21 percent from 1983 to 1991. But while the number of programs increased, the number of residents declined to below 85,000 in 1991 because of a decline in the number of graduates from American medical schools. The residents are distributed unevenly: 74.9 percent work for the 330 largest Council of Teaching Hospital (COTH) programs, and 25.1 percent work in 925 other teaching hospitals.

State hospitals are most dependent on residents to provide patient care. Forty COTH state hospitals have 47.3 residents per 100 beds, whereas the 20 non-COTH state teaching hospitals have 12.55 residents per bed. The 33 COTH county or municipal hospitals have 34.4 residents per bed, while the 119 non-COTH county or municipal hospitals have 7.3 residents per bed. The 277 private tax-exempt COTH hospitals have 21.3 residents per bed, whereas non-COTH tax-exempt private hospitals have 3.2 residents per bed. In 1991 an estimated 54,000 residents and interns received $2.6 billion in salary and $468 million in fringe benefits (AAMC 1991).

Anderson and Lave (1986) presented a good explanation of why resource costs increase at a slower rate as teaching programs get larger. A curvilinear formula takes into account the basic fact that teaching costs less than double as R doubles (e.g., R increases from 0.3 to 0.6). For example, under the old linear formula, two teaching hospitals in the same location were receiving quite different payment rates if they had different levels of R—even though they were both experiencing approximately the same factor markets, comparable severity of illness and elderly case loads, and equivalent amounts of charity care.

In addition to the Medicare payment rate adjustments for graduate medical education, many teaching hospitals benefit from the disproportionate-share adjustment. The disproportionate-share adjustment was designed in 1985 to compensate hospitals that serve a very high fraction of low-income patients. According to the Congressional Budget Office (CBO 1991), this disproportionate-share adjustment accounts for $1.6 billion of the estimated $51.7 billion in Medicare prospective payments. The 42 teaching hospitals with disproportionate-share indexes of 55 percent or more receive an average adjustment of $1,190 per patient, representing 20 percent of their payments from Medicare.

MEDICARE PAYMENT FOR TEACHING

The original Medicare payment bonus of 11.59 percent for each 0.1 increment in the resident-per-bed ratio was considered biased (prejudiced) in favor of teaching hospitals because the coefficient was set at twice the level of the regression coefficient (Pettengill and Vertrees 1982). The overpayment for teaching has been confirmed by Custer and Willke (1991). Many rural hospitals were paid by Medicare half the price that some local teaching hospital received for the same patient DRG in the mid–1980s. In America, if one group gets a great deal under the system of price controls, the losers scream. The corollary of the regulatory squawk theory (Hilton 1972) is that the losers seek parity. Rural hospitals won their point with Congress in the late 1980s. The indirect graduate medical education teaching adjustment was decreased from 11.59 percent to 7.7 percent, and the urban-rural payment gap was scheduled to be closed by 1995 (ProPAC 1991). This is a textbook example of the reaction of a countervailing power, the rural hospitals winning one back from the big urban teaching hospitals.

One is still left with the more basic question of what the teaching-adjustment payment factor should be. Some of the extra cost might be unnecessary or inappropriate (Eastaugh 1987). Thorpe (1988) redid the regression analysis with more recent data and concluded that the fair payment rate might be 3.15 percent for each 0.1 increment of the resident-to-bed ratio. In the current cost-cutting climate Medicare will probably trim the indirect graduate medical education adjustment. ProPAC (1991) has proposed trimming the adjustment to 5.5 percent in 1992 and lowering it steadily to 3.2 percent in 1996. Congress is also narrowing the urban-rural gap, to the benefit of many financially distressed rural hospitals. If teaching hospitals enjoyed a prejudiced position in their favor during the mid–1980s, the prejudice of the Medicare payment formula may be against them in the 1990s.

Managers of residency programs will be under pressure to provide residents a superior educational experience based on a reasonable workload supervised by senior attending physicians. Continued requests for more federal aid could lead to massive intervention in medical education. The federal government would want more control over the quantity, quality, and type of residency slots (e.g., more primary-care and fewer surgical residency positions). This trend has already been noted by Petersdorf (1985), Eastaugh (1987), and a number of politicians. Faculty and hospital managers may have to face the trade-off of some loss of autonomy for stabilization of revenue sources. Nonfederal payers of inpatient care seem less willing to generously underwrite residency training; therefore, teaching hospitals' revenue may decline without an expansion in competitive-bidding schemes. Manpower-training-program decisions may increasingly be made by federal or state governments rather than by institutional decision makers. Smaller and leaner teaching programs may soon be mandated by legislation (Ginzberg 1990).

The need for better cost analysis in an era of fluctuating payment policies should be obvious to all managers and providers in teaching settings. One of the basic problems with the aforementioned cost studies is that true cost-accounting systems at the institutional level are lacking. The Arthur Young and

Policy Analysis, Inc. (1986) study offered the analytical advantages of a good cost-accounting framework, uniform accounting across 36 teaching hospitals and 9 control (nonteaching) hospitals, and uniform measurement of severity of illness, disease stage, and quality of care. The next four sections will survey joint production activities, standard costing, results of the Arthur Young study, and the role of severity-of-illness measures.

JOINT PRODUCTS AND TOTAL COST PER CASE

Lave and Frank (1990) and Pfordresher (1985) reported that it is very difficult to partition joint activities such as teaching, research, and patient care. *Joint activity* is a phrase used to describe the simultaneous production of multiple outputs during a given activity. Joint activity is most obvious when multiple individuals are involved in multiple tasks at the patient's bedside. However, joint activity also occurs in instances in which a single individual is involved in multiple tasks or activities. Here a joint product may be indicated by comparative amounts of time taken to perform a task. If an attending physician acting alone, for example, performs a patient-care task in an average of 12 minutes and a second-year resident takes an average of 18 minutes, then the resident's time may be attributed in part to patient care and in part to education. The attending physician's average time in this example is presumed to have no educational content. Thus, if the task is performed in that given period of time, whether by attending physicians or second-year residents, it is taken entirely as an input to patient care. But if the time taken is greater, then a portion becomes an input to education, on the normative premise that the individuals performing the task are not yet as skilled, on average, as the attending physicians and therefore must still be learning.

The most basic question to consider is why joint-production institutions exist. Joint production most often derives from economies of simultaneous production. Joint production may also arise from joint factor supply, especially in a profession like medicine. For example, if a factor required to produce instructional outputs, like faculty members, is to be made available only if allowed to produce research, a phenomenon labeled joint factor supply exists. One should see the folly in postulating the existence of a godlike dean who is capable of determining the minimum amount of research time to buy if the only objective is hiring a teaching faculty (Reuschel and Earle 1991).

Fortunately, deans in the real world are concerned with the quality and quantity of patient care, research, and education. Deans must consider issues such as how much additional faculty practice-plan effort on patient care must be requested to restrain tuition rate increases, secure adequate faculty resources, optimize the prestige of the research program, and still produce the level of educational output that the residency program is committed to produce.

Two caveats are in order. First, the sum of pure time spent on each of the three activities has to be less than total time effort, and the sum of pure and joint time has to be more than total hours worked. Second, one could optimize the production of one activity and erode the quality of the other two activities. It is obviously not desirable to reduce research and patient care to the minimum levels actually required for educational purposes. Consequently, we shall include measures of the quality of patient care in the cost functions for teaching hospitals.

MEASURING TOTAL COST PER CASE

Unbiased cost analysis of teaching hospitals must focus on total costs: physician costs plus inpatient costs per illness episode. It has often been stated that residents and interns save money on their patients' physician fees even as they raise hospital costs (Cameron 1985). In teaching hospitals these salaried residents and interns are paid by the hospital and provide many services that could otherwise be performed and billed separately by an attending senior physician. On the other hand, services are sometimes largely performed by the resident and also billed by the attending physician, so the payer is stuck with the problem of "paying twice" (Garg et al. 1982). If net total cost per patient episode is higher among teaching hospitals, this higher price might in turn purchase an added benefit. Perhaps patients receive better-quality care through continuous 24-hour availability of residents and the immediacy of their responses to patient-care problems. Irrespective of whether any quality-enhancing activities turn out to be cost-saving or cost-increasing, regulatory forces and business will continue their vigilant attempts to minimize double billing.

Some evidence points to greater utilization of ancillary services at teaching hospitals without any obvious improvement in quality of care (Frick, Martin, and Schwartz 1985; Garg et al. 1982; Eastaugh 1987; Bradbury et al. 1991). It has also been argued that graduate medical education programs introduce operational inefficiencies into the activities of senior attending physicians. The teaching hospital as a complex organization may exhibit cost-decreasing or cost-increasing behavior. On the positive side, teaching facilities may be the first to question "tenet-of-faith" habits—for example, the evening-before-surgery shave has proven to be harmful and costly (Brown, Ehrlich, and Stehman 1984). On the downside, Beck (1986) has suggested that teaching hospitals have a cost-increasing bias to employ overly expensive nonclinicians, wasting millions of dollars by using highly trained, expensive labor to perform tasks that require only moderate or minimal skill.

Determining the costs (and benefits) of graduate medical education is complicated by all these confounding factors. Moreover, our sample of 36 hospitals selected from a national sample of four strata of teaching facilities and nine nonteaching hospitals (rather than only 9) would have substantially more statistical power. However, the Arthur Young analysis has the advantage over Cameron (1985) of measuring hospital costs as accurately as possible. In contrast, previous studies from Salkever (1970) to Cameron (1985) have had to create "costs" from patient-charge-claim data for each case. Charges are not an accurate approximation of costs. In addition, our sample was not restricted to Medicare and Medicaid patients only. Our analysis also collected severity-of-illness and cost information for a population sample of patients (Eastaugh, chapter 2 in Arthur Young 1986).

STANDARD COSTING METHODS IN THE ARTHUR YOUNG STUDY

There is no uniform system for hospital cost allocation and standard cost accounting. Cost-reimbursement systems of the major third-party payers, most notably Medicare and Medicaid, have a substantial influence on how hospitals define, accumulate, and allocate costs (Eastaugh 1980b). Commercially available software programs were designed to maximize reimbursement by defining the statistical basis for the allocation of overhead costs through sensitivity analyses. Therefore, we found different allocation bases among hospitals for the same overhead department costs with great variability in the final costs allocated to each department. These differences presented a standardization problem in comparing patient costs among different facilities at both the hospital and departmental levels.

Four basic types of data are needed to produce a uniform and accurate comparison of hospital costs: (1) hospital expense data, (2) hospital revenue and statistical data, (3) nonhospital financial data from other institutions within a medical complex, and (4) estimated and imputed physician cost data. In order to accurately compare these four types of financial data across all hospitals in the study sample, two uniform matrices were developed. The first was a standard matrix of 26 ancillary-service and 21 general-service cost centers. A cost center was defined as the basic unit of cost aggregation on the hospital's records. The cost data were then allocated to programs and departments using a standardized statistical basis across all study hospitals. The second matrix necessary for the study was a uniform hospital chargemaster. Because the hospital case costs were developed using a bottom-up approach from actual patient-service profiles, a standard chargemaster was necessary to ensure comparability between hospitals at the case and departmental levels.

The second type of financial data collected was hospital revenue and statistical data. Hospital revenue was identified as patient revenue, nonpatient operating revenue, and other revenue. Patient revenues were standardized by the 26 ancillary-service cost centers and by payer. The third type of financial data collected consisted of those costs or services provided and those revenues received from nonhospital components of a medical complex. An example of this type of fund-flow analysis would be derived from an associated medical school and/or university affiliation relationship. For example, the hospital could receive free computer support in exchange for picking up administrative staff labor expenses. Faculty members may be paid by the medical school. Administrative services may be provided by a university. In more complex teaching hospitals any one of a number of other related-party cost flows may occur.

The fourth type of financial data collected was "imputed" physician cost data. Various services performed for the hospital may not be paid for by the hospital. A significant portion of the teaching effort in smaller teaching institutions is performed by volunteer physicians. It is necessary to collect sufficient data to be able to impute a reasonable cost to the time spent by those volunteers. Cameron (1985) and other previous studies did not have the resources to incorporate the necessary adjustments for funds flow and voluntary physician time, thus biasing the results for major teaching hospitals. The Arthur Young study included data from 45 hospitals and cost over $6 million under federal contract. These data were collected both from primary sources within the hospital and from various secondary sources, such as the DHHS Regional Charge Screens on regional and local levels. At each of the 36 teaching hospitals, the department chairpersons provided source data on the number of faculty hours replaced by volunteer faculty and estimated salary levels of equivalent faculty at various ranks. In addition to this site-specific data, Association of American Medical Colleges (AAMC) data on faculty salaries by position by region, AMA data on physician earnings by specialty by region, and local intermediary physician price data were collected. For each individual voluntary physician the salary equivalent was calculated— that is, hours times salary estimate. The department chairperson's salary estimate was the preferred figure, although this was tested against other payment data.

Faculty salaries are a major expense to both graduate and undergraduate medical education programs. Although faculty salaries are usually paid by medical schools, some clinical faculty members receive a portion of their salaries directly or indirectly from a teaching hospital in return for administration, teaching, and supervisory services. Since Medicare and Medicaid patient-service payments are the largest source of funding for graduate medical education programs, federal reimbursement for these services has become a major source of medical school faculty salaries.

As medical school funding levels become difficult to maintain and teaching hospitals face more difficult financial times, the search for alternative means of funding faculty salaries intensifies. Professional fees associated with patient-care activities have become an increasingly important source of alternative funding. Physicians do not, in general, share compensation data. Even within organized group practices, the department chairperson and group-practice administrator frequently will be the only individuals who have access to individual physician compensation levels. To physicians, compensation levels are a measure of "success." Physicians and physician groups were assured that information provided would not be used in a punitive way and that confidentiality would be maintained.

Hospital cost allocation is a politically less sensitive task than physician cost allocation. Indeed, from the institutional perspective, the cost-finding and accounting expertise of Arthur Young and Company offered a major incentive for participation in this study. One crucial intermediate step necessary in determining both cost per case and cost per unit of service is to assign to various procedures weighted values representative of their consumption of resources. In order to do this, we standardized the output measurement by cost center in all hospitals in the study sample. The relative value units (RVUs) by procedure were based, for the most part, on standard unit-of-service criteria used by the state of Maryland. For example, laboratory units were weighted by RVUs for test complexity. After we assigned weighted units by quantity of procedures performed, procedures with high relative value unit per procedure were matched. The assignment processes, as a minimum, assigned 80 percent of the relative value or other weighted unit-of-service measurement to any given cost center. All other procedures were assigned an average weight. These units were then keyed into a tape that included units of service weighted by procedures at 26 graduate medical education (GME) cost centers.

ARTHUR YOUNG GME RESULTS

Our focus was on average unit cost per episode: hospital plus physician costs. We were not concerned with the typical HCFA specification for how inpatient total costs of production vary among hospitals. The dependent variable in our regressions was total cost per case. Average cost was measured as a function of nine independent variables (Arthur Young 1986): R (resident and intern full-time equivalents per bed); DRG cost weight (1.0 national average); Horn et al.'s (1985) severity-of-illness index; other case variables (length of stay and whether the individual was covered by Medicaid or was self-paying); a department-level quality index (using percentage of adverse patient outcomes divided by at-risk potential adverse patient occurrence opportunities [the APO rate done by the same raters across the sample hospitals]); and three input price wage indexes for physicians, nurses, and technicians. To avoid problems of multicollinearity in our cost-estimation procedure, we did not include resident wage rates (because they were already captured through the 0.91 correlation with nurse wage rates), and we excluded capital prices (because they had a 0.8 correlation with technician wage rates).

The last three variables were included in the analysis to separate the cost-of-education effect from input-price effects driving up the costs of care. Better quality of care could be cost-increasing or cost-decreasing. For example, Haley, Schaberg, and Crossley (1981) reported that the surgical department saves the hospital seven days of variable cost for every wound infection APO avoided. Length of stay was included in the analysis because patients within a DRG category have a wide variation in length of stay (Lave and Frank 1990; U.S. Senate Finance Committee 1983) not captured by the DRGs, case severity, or acuity. DRG conditions that have higher cost weights are by definition more complex and expensive to treat than those with lower weights (e.g., bypass surgery has a weight thirteen times as high as that of lens procedure DRG 39). The Medicaid/self-pay variable was included in the analysis because poor people often have inadequate prior medical care, deficient nutritional status, more complications, and secondary health problems (i.e., a net level of additional acuity not captured by severity of illness or length of stay).

To capture at least part of the effect that the teaching function has on case costs, independent variable R interns and residents per bed, was included. To improve the econometric fit of this variable in the regression model, we multiplied the observed value in each facility by 1,000. Table 8.1, column 1, presents the regression results for a random sample of 300 to 375 patients at each of the 45 hospitals. Columns 2 through 9 in table 8.1 present the results from patients in the eight tracer diagnoses under study. The maximum tracer sample size within each group was 25 cases per hospital (e.g., if only 14 cases of tracer 2 could be found at a given hospital in the year 1984, then only 14 cases would be included for analysis). The impact on average cost of increasing residents per bed by 0.1 ranged from zero to 4.1 percent for benign prostatic hypertrophy to 10.5 percent for nonsurgical treatment of acute myocardial infarction. The value for the random sample was a 7.2 percent increase in cost.

Quality of care had a negative, but statistically insignificant, impact on patient costs. One would not want to read too much into this finding, but perhaps the net cost to society of investing in quality-enhancing activities is self-financing. Superior-quality care may cost a little bit more, but it avoids the costly consequences of fixing poor-quality care through prolonged duration of stay. The cost of treating Medicaid and self-pay patients was only 1 to 2 percent higher, given that the equation already included a measure of severity of illness. This could best be described as a proxy measure of "social acuity."

The Horn et al. (1985) severity-of-illness index had the expected positive and significant impact on average cost. A 0.1 unit increase in the index was associated with a 2 to 5 percent higher cost per case. If severity of illness has a case-mix and cost effect within DRGs, rather than across DRGs, this suggests that Horn et al.'s measure may be a fine-tuning mechanism to add onto or supplement the DRGs. In the context of an inventory-control problem, DRGs may capture broad-based product lines, but severity measures a second dimension (degree or amount). We will survey some competing measures of patient severity in the next section. We will not be able to answer the critical question of how much the reduction in variance of unexplained cost has to be to justify the data collection. However, by 1991 Horn had already marketed a less expensive alternative measure, the computerized severity index (CSI), to over 100 hospitals.

SEVERITY-OF-ILLNESS MEASURES

The concept of severity of illness encompasses many dimensions. For the purposes of payment, the fundamental concept underlying each system is translated into resource demand. But each severity system originated as an attempt to classify cases according to a particular notion of severity or to measure a particular parameter chosen to serve as a proxy for resource demand. Attempting

Table 8.1
Cost per Case Regressions for a Random and Tracer Sample at 45 Hospitals (Arthur Young Study, 1986)

	Random Sample	1. Acute Myocardial Infarction	2. Upper G.I. Hemorrhage	3. Asthma	4. Gastroenteritis Acute Colitis	5. Complicated Delivery	6. Gallbladder	7. Hysterectomy[a]	8. Benign Prostatic Hypertrophy
# Patients	n = 13,436	n = 857	n = 827	n = 821	n = 704	n = 793	n = 951	n = 833	n = 848
Average Cost	$4,150	$8,407	$5,633	$2,040	$1,693	$4,001	$7,890	$6,329	$6,818
• Variable (units of measurement)									
Residents per bed (1 per 10 beds)	7.2	10.5	5.7	2.5	0[ns]	0[ns]	5.4	4.2	4.1
Severity (.1 change in 4 point SOI)	3.2	4.0	3.6	2.5	2.4	2.7	5.2	3.3	3.2
DRG Cost Weight (.1 change)	7.7	11.7	6.2	1.5[b]	4.9	8.4	1.7	-3.4[b]	3.7
Length of stay (1 Day)	5.0	21.1	22.2	8.9	24.2	4.5	14.1	20.0	17.3
Medicaid or self-pay patients	.1[ns]	.41	-.2[ns]	.43	.89	1.7	-.02[ns]	.21[ns]	-.16[ns]
Quality of care (APO actual/at risk)	-.01[ns]	—	—	—	—	—	—	—	—
RN wage (1% change)	1.1[ns]	18.2	5.6	4.2	2.3[ns]	-8.3[b]	-4.4[b]	5.6[b]	1.5[ns]
Physician wage (1% change)	5.1	7.6	3.7	1.9[b]	-1.1[ns]	10.0	7.4	.6[ns]	2.4
Technician wage (1% change)	12.0	31.3	-.5[ns]	5.7[ns]	14.6	52.1	35.3	10.1	11.2
R-squared (fraction of variance explained)	.541	.523	.585	.438	.735	.628	.606	.508	.680

NOTES: Coefficients are mean elasticity estimates. APO = Adverse Patient Occurrence 15-item inventory. All variables significant at the .01 level, except those marked b and c.

[a]Surgical cases; b = .05 level of significance; c = not significant at 0.1 level.

to distinguish between several concepts related to severity serves to illustrate the subtleties:

1. *Severity*, in the strictest sense, has usually been used to describe extent of disease (deviation from normal physiology, extent of organ failure) or risk of death or morbidity.
2. *Acuity* describes the urgency with which intervention is required.
3. *Complexity* describes effects due to interaction of multiple diseases or conditions.
4. *Intensity* is associated with the level of care required and is the term most consistently associated with (legitimate) demand for hospital services.
5. *Treatment difficulty* is associated with the extent and rate of the patient's response to therapy.

In case-mix systems designed to span the spectrum of cases in acute-care hospitals, the link between the underlying concept on which a severity system is founded and resource demand may be inconsistent across disease categories. Moreover, advanced clinical stages of disease are not always associated with increased resource consumption, for example, admission of a cancer or AIDS patient for terminal care. While well justified by the intensity of supportive care required, this admission may still impose far less resource burden than would an admission at an earlier stage of the same disease, when aggressive experimental intervention was indicated.

A fundamental objective is to base the classification on characteristics of the patient rather than on the services that were provided, in an attempt to reflect legitimate resource demand rather than to include excessive or inappropriate resource consumption. Typically this is done by focusing on physiologic parameters, objective clinical findings, or the final diagnosis, combined with patient characteristics such as age and sex. In many systems, including DRGs, the quantum jump in resource demand associated with the need for an operating-room procedure is reflected by considering surgical procedures in the classification scheme, relying on PRO utilization controls to ensure that procedures performed were necessary.

As a result of this attempt to avoid defining resource categories in a circular fashion, most systems are unable to indicate the degree of diagnostic challenge that some patients pose. No classification scheme based on the final diagnosis can possibly reflect the resources required by a "complex rule-out," an uncommon manifestation of a disease (a "zebra") whose diagnosis and treatment are usually straightforward. A high prevalence of "zebra" cases has a significant impact on teaching hospitals specializing in tertiary services, who see a disproportionate number of zebra patients requiring extensive workups due to unusual presentations of common diseases.

A suitable severity adjustment to the DRGs would provide all hospitals with an equitable incentive to become more efficient (Eastaugh 1990; Steinwald and Dummit 1989). Currently, hospitals that admit an atypically high proportion of high-severity patients and are paid the DRG average have an "excessive" in- centive to become more efficient. However, they might never be able to lower costs to the DRG average payment levels without harming the quality of care. Consequently, teaching hospitals with a higher severity of illness might be faced with the choice of eroding either their financial health or the quality of care provided. Conversely, hospitals that presently admit an atypically high proportion of low-severity patients and are paid the DRG average have little incentive to become more efficient.

There are a number of systems in use, based on discharge abstract data, that provide hospitals with measures of case mix and severity, including DRGs and the PAS-A list from the Commission on Professional and Hospital Activities (CPHA). In the PAS-A list system, severity is quantified by the existence of secondary diagnoses (the complications and comorbidity conditions) that are thought to cluster isoresource cases. Moreover, DRGs differentiate types of operating-room procedures in different DRGs, rather than just noting the exis- tence or nonexistence of an operating-room procedure.

Two newer systems are analyzed here: disease staging and the manual severity- of-illness (SOI) index (Horn et al. 1985). The key attribute of the manual SOI system is that it attempts to capture how ill a patient is within a specific disease condition—not just that the patient has the specific condition. As a result, it predicts resource use somewhat better than DRGs alone (Horn, Horn, and Moses 1986). The SOI index is a more complex measure and captures more patient information than disease staging. Advocates of the disease-staging approach would disagree (Gonnella, Hornbrook, and Louis 1984). The only inputs to disease staging are ICD–9-CM diagnosis and procedure codes, whereas the SOI system uses information based on laboratory values, radiologic findings, vital signs, and other data found in the medical record but not captured in the current five-digit discharge abstract data base. In addition, disease staging has no mech- anism to combine all of a patient's diseases together to form a single overall stage for a patient. Disease staging as a case-mix measure has been found to be substantially less predictive of resource utilization per case than DRGs. Even when combined with DRGs, disease staging has added little predictive power (Coffey and Goldfarb 1986).

Several new severity measurement systems have appeared in recent years, including the computerized severity index six-digit coding system (CSI; Horn 1986), Western Pennsylvania Blue Cross PMCs (patient management 800 cat- egories; Young 1986) and MEDISGRPS (Brewster et al. 1985). Brewster et al.'s MEDISGRPS system goes beyond traditional five-digit discharge abstract data. This parallels the two Horn systems (SOI, CSI) and PMCs. It uses about 500 "key clinical findings" to designate the severity of a patient on a scale of 0 to 4. These key clinical findings are recorded by trained hospital personnel on the third day of hospitalization (the MEDISGRPS authors refer to this as "on ad- mission"), and the information is processed by a computer program that deter- mines the severity of the patient on admission to the hospital. The MEDISGRPS system designates one rating for the severity of the patient on admission and another with data collected at ten days if the patient is still in the hospital. In this section we shall examine the relative ability of disease staging and SOI to enhance the resource-consumption predictive power of DRGs, but no assessment will be made of the MEDISGRPS, PMC, or CSI systems.

The Horn SOI Measure

The severity-of-illness (SOI) measure was developed by a panel of physicians and nurses who were asked to define patient severity and develop the requisite list of parameters that would be necessary to implement the definition. The panel suggested 32 variables, which were ultimately reviewed and collapsed into seven dimensions, each having four levels of increasing severity. The decision to include certain parameters was based on the relationship of the parameter to patient severity. Parameters not directly related to the patient, such as those related to the skill or experience of the physician, were excluded. Four levels of severity were chosen for each variable and for the overall severity index (rather than five or some other odd number) to avoid the problem of having most responses fall naturally at the middle level. An even number of levels forces the rater to choose decisively between two middle points and hence provides more distinction among patients. Raters require careful initial training (and periodic follow-up) to become proficient in coding SOI. Horn, Horn, and Moses (1986) reported that almost all raters scored 90 percent or greater agreement with blind reratings of the same records, with an average agreement of 93.5 percent across 90 raters in 18 hospitals. The seven SOI dimensions are the following:

1. The stage of the principal diagnosis at admission, including the greatest extent of organ involvement.
2. Complications that developed during the hospital stay due to the principal disease or as a direct result of the therapy or hospitalization.
3. Preexisting problems other than the principal diagnosis and its complications (e.g., diabetes in a patient admitted with acute myocardial infarction).
4. The degree to which the patient requires more than the minimal level of direct care expected for the principal diagnosis. A dependency score above level 1 indicates that the stage of illness, complications, or preexisting diseases require extra monitoring or care.
5. Diagnostic and therapeutic procedures performed outside of the operating room. The highest level of procedure, such as those required for life support, rather than the total number of procedures performed, determines the score for this dimension. The need for such a procedure also should be reflected in one or more of the first three dimensions (stage, complications, and/or preexisting problems).
6. The patient's response to hospital treatment for the principal diagnosis, complications, and interactions. This relates to treatments for acute illness or acute manifestations of chronic illness that one expects to manage during a hospital stay. It does not relate

to improvement in underlying chronic conditions for which there is no expectation of either cure or significant progress during the hospitalization.

7. The extent to which a patient shows residual evidence of the acute injury or illness at the time of discharge.

Disease Staging

The SOI measure uses a generic instrument that can be applied to all cases and generates a four-level measure of severity. In contrast, disease staging covers most cases in our sample but not all conditions. SysteMetrics (Louis et al. 1983), under contract to the National Center for Health Services Research, developed stages for 480 specific disease conditions. The recent efforts by SysteMetrics include the development of the staging process using not only data drawn from the medical records, but also ICDA codes from computerized discharge data sets. Staging is a system of categorizing patients into one of four levels of severity based on pathophysiological parameters primarily obtained from the medical record abstract (computer software has been developed to enable staging to be done using discharge abstract data). Disease staging has three basic limitations in the context of the Arthur Young study:

1. Stage-one conditions are by definition patients with a single uncomplicated diagnosis, and often the hospitalization is questionable. Since teaching hospitals might only rarely deal with such patients, the remaining levels of staging may be inadequate for measuring severity for a particular condition.

2. Garg et al. (1978) suggested that the construct validity of staging is supported because an increased stage correlates with increased cost. However, there is little evidence to determine whether the various stages have statistically significant differential charges and whether these differences would remain when charges are adjusted to costs.

3. While the method is sensitive to complications of the principal diagnosis, it is insensitive to patients in whom multiple diseases (not related to the principal diagnosis) interact in an additive, multiplicative, or other way.

One central conceptual strength of disease staging is that the severity measure is independent of provider behavior (e.g., treating a condition medically or surgically). By utilizing only diagnostic information to define stages of specific diseases and neglecting procedure classification, disease staging does not confound treatment preference with case-mix severity. In only three situations are procedures used to form stage classifications, and only because this identifies the diagnoses more precisely (e.g., cesarean deliveries). This conceptual strength of the disease-staging process, however, leads to a practical problem. Because the technique does not distinguish surgical from nonsurgical patients, costs within the same diagnosis and stage vary widely.

We shall limit our literature review to the familiar DRGs. The new 486 DRGs, like the old DRGs, utilize length of stay as the primary dependent variable to reflect resource use. DRGs as a case-mix measure differentiate surgical from nonsurgical cases and consequently exhibit significant differences in case complexity between teaching and nonteaching hospitals. The Goldfarb and Coffey (1987) retrospective regression study of 144 teaching hospitals and 226 nonteaching hospitals reported that teaching institutions admitted 1.4 times as many surgical candidates as nonteaching hospitals after differences in disease staging between hospitals were controlled. A more extensive commitment to teaching (e.g., membership in COTH or a medical-school-based hospital) did not significantly increase surgical intensity (.46 versus .33 of cases). The intent of the calculation was to get away from the surgery/nonsurgery distinction embedded in the DRGs and to standardize for disease stage of the patient population. Goldfarb and Coffey also reported no differences between hospital types in case-mix-standardized fatality rates, despite the greater use of resources in teaching hospitals. This result concerning patient outcomes is surprising given the conventional wisdom that the continuous all-day availability of residents and the immediacy of their responses to problems should result in increased quality of service. One could speculate that a more sensitive measure, such as an inventory of adverse patient occurrences (APOs), would better detect differences in the quality of care than a crude measure (fatality). APO items include iatrogenic adverse reactions, complications, incomplete clinical management, unexpected cardiac or respiratory arrest, unplanned return to the operating room, nosocomial infection, iatrogenic neurological deficit, death, and other dysquality events, infections, and so on (Panniers and Newlander 1986). In our study we collected APO data on the random case sample to provide a measure of quality of care at the case level. The APO measure will be used in the following analysis due to the unavailability of the disease-specific (tracer sample), quality-of-care measures assessed by the Rand Corporation.

Methodological Concerns

One of the basic conceptual problems with the SOI index is the inclusion of treatment decisions in the measure—that is, if more is done, the case must be more severe. Some components of the severity score reflect higher ancillary utilization by providers, and the researcher cannot tell how much of this is independent of the medical status of the patient. The SOI index is less effective than disease staging in providing a case-mix measure attributable purely to patient differences and independent of provider practices due to the treatment standards of the hospital's medical staff. Medical staff selects the workload, draws on hospital inputs to provide care consistent with peer standards, and generates positive outputs (live discharges, education, research, and so on). One difficulty in analyzing the effects of the SOI index is that it comingles the case mix and the provider practice behavior into one measure (labeling it "severity"), confounding the separation of patient-driven treatment actions from medical-staff-driven decisions about the treatment process that might be affected by demand for graduate medical education (Goldfarb and Coffey 1987; Eastaugh 1990).

It would be difficult to collapse the seven-dimension SOI measure into a scale that is independent of treatment preferences of attending physicians, residents, and interns. For example, dimension 4, the dependency score, is a measure of illness requiring extra monitoring or care. We have no independent verification of whether that extra care is medically appropriate if assessed by some unbiased peer reviewer. One study suggested that teaching hospitals do not have a more severe case mix if the severity measure is itself independent of resource consumption (Goldfarb and Coffey 1987). Using 1977 data, the authors reported that severity was no higher in teaching hospitals in a national sample of 9 medical-school-based hospitals, 44 other COTH member hospitals, 91 community teaching hospitals, and 226 nonteaching hospitals. While the sample size is impressive, the data were more limited than in our study (they were based on eight-year-old discharged record abstracts), and the measure of severity was crude. The health-services researcher is firmly placed on the horns of a dilemma: The measure of severity must by definition be increasingly crude as it is made unbiased for provider practices (independent of physician resource decisions driven by GME needs or by the idiosyncratic preferences of the medical staff unrelated to GME). In a multiple analysis of variance, the SOI measure has a clear identification of the patient's idiosyncratic factor (individual response to therapy), but how much of the residual behavior is the provider's idiosyncratic behavior and not truly patient severity?

There is ample evidence that provider taste can dominate treatment behavior patterns (Brook, et al. 1984; Wennberg, Freeman, and Culp 1987). For example, if a patient resides in a community teaching hospital intensive-care unit (ICU), does that prove that the patient is more severely ill? If the Medicare PP3 has created a tendency to treat more cases in less costly channels of service distribution (outside of the ICU or even outside of the hospital), does that mean that these patients are suddenly less severely ill because they command fewer resources relative to habits under pre–1984 treatment practices? One should note that a nonteaching hospital might have wide latitude to eschew a more conservative style of medicine and so be able to report a more severe case mix. In the Horn et al. (1985) study, contrary to expectations, the one nonteaching hospital had severity scores that exceeded those of the two community teaching hospitals. It is difficult to state how much of the extra severity was attributable to (1) poor medical practices; (2) physician preferences to avoid the new and untried, without harm to quality-of-care outcomes; or (3) differences in actual patient severity.

Regression analysis was used to examine the relative power of the three case-mix measures available to the study (DRGs, SOI, and disease staging) in explaining variation in total (combined hospital and physician) cost. The results of the regression analysis showed that DRGs as a case-mix measure were more effective in explaining variation in cost than either of the other measures alone. In the random case sample of all hospitals in the study, DRGs explained approximately 15 percent of total cost per case, versus 4.7 percent for SOI and 2.0 percent for disease staging. One might suggest that DRGs and disease staging are measuring much the same construct (product-line categories), whereas the SOI measure offers a more substantial improvement in explained variation in costs (i.e., it measures a second construct—acuity amount of illness within a product line).

Further analysis of DRGs showed a marked difference in explanatory power by hospital department. Table 8.2 presents a summary of the reduction in unexplained variance in cost for DRGs as a case-mix measure and for the two severity measures in combination with DRGs. The result if surgical cases are compared to nonsurgical cases is pronounced. For surgical cases (all cases in the random sample assigned to the department of surgery), the DRG accounted for more than 25 percent of the total variation in cost, but it explained only 2.1 percent for the nonsurgical cases. (The difference in explanatory power of the DRGs between any of the four nonsurgical departments was minimal. For this reason, the results are presented as surgical versus nonsurgical cases, rather than by department.) While this result is not surprising, given the inputs to the algorithm used to construct DRGs, it does support the findings of previous studies that suggest that DRGs might not be an effective measure for differentiating resource utilization and, by extension, cost for cases that do not involve extensive surgical intervention.

RECENT DEVELOPMENTS IN SEVERITY SYSTEMS

The early 1990s have been a time of steady improvement and competitive testing of severity systems (Miller, Cuddleback, and Gallo 1991). Eight new or refined severity systems will be surveyed in this section. Some abstract-based systems using elements of the Uniform Hospital Discharge Data Set (UHDDS) have not performed well, for example, CPHA Body Systems Count, and therefore are not surveyed here. Other abstract-based systems like refined diagnosis related groups (RDRGs), acuity index method (AIM), and patient management categories (PMC) are surveyed. The systems that are chart based, requiring additional data collection (CSI, APACHE III), tend to do a better job in explaining outcome or quality variations between providers.

The "free" (no license fee) system of refined diagnosis related groups was developed by the Health Systems Management Group of Yale University in the 1980s for HCFA. It was designed to account for severity within existing DRGs by differentiating patients on the basis of complications and comorbidities specific to the principal diagnosis or procedure. A patient is first assigned to a major diagnostic category (MDC) on the basis of principal diagnosis; the MDCs are identical to the 23 MDCs used in the current DRG system. Patients with temporary tracheostomies and early deaths (within two days of admission) are assigned to separate groups. All other patients are assigned to one of 317 categories referred to as adjacent DRGs (ADRGs) on the basis of their principal diagnoses

Table 8.2
Percentage Improvement in Explained Variation of Cost per Case, Sample of 300–375 Cases per Hospital

(% listed are R^2, percent variance explained)		DRGs	DRGs and Severity of Illness	DRGs and Disease Staging	DRGs Severity of Illness and Disease Staging
Sample					
45 hospitals	- all cases	15.3%	18.9%	16.9%	19.8%
	- surgical cases	28.7%	32.9%	30.9%	34.6%
	- non-surgical cases	2.1%	6.0%	3.3%	6.7%
Nonteaching hospitals ($n = 9$)	- surgical cases	36.8%	45.1%	37.2%	45.8%
	- non-surgical cases	4.4%	8.8%	5.7%	9.6%
Minor teaching ($n = 3$)	- surgical cases	28.0%	34.5%	32.7%	35.9%
	- non-surgical cases	2.9%	4.8%	5.9%	6.9%
Moderate teaching ($n = 4$)	- surgical cases	34.5%	37.1%	40.0%	41.1%
	- non-surgical cases	.1%	5.9%	1.5%	6.9%
Major teaching hospitals ($n = 16$)	- surgical cases	26.7%	31.5%	31.2%	35.0%
	- non-surgical cases	1.9%	4.9%	2.8%	5.5%
COTH medical centers ($n = 12$)	- surgical cases	22.8%	27.4%	25.7%	29.2%
	- non-surgical cases	2.8%	6.7%	4.2%	7.8%

or surgical procedures. Within these categories the patient's secondary diagnoses determine the appropriate RDRG. The RDRG system classifies secondary diagnoses as major, moderate, or minor, according to their effect on resource demand. Ohio has mandated the use of RDRGs since 1989. Except for MDC 15, neonates, for whom a separate grouping methodology was developed, RDRGs were derived on the basis of data from adult populations. As a first step in creating the RDRGs, all possible principal diagnoses (those diagnoses that describe the chief reason for a patient's hospitalization) were divided into 23 mutually exclusive categories known as major diagnostic categories or MDCs. Generally, all diagnoses within a MDC correspond to a single organ system (e.g., respiratory system, circulatory system, digestive system) and are associated with a particular medical specialty. Because not all diagnoses are organ-system based, a number of residual MDCs were created (e.g., systemic infectious diseases, myeloproliferative diseases, and poorly differentiated neoplasms). The system has not been thoroughly evaluated on pediatric and adolescent populations. In this study, RDRGs were tested both with and without an age split. First, all patients were considered together to develop one set of resource-consumption weights. Then patients age 18 and over were considered separately from those under 18 to develop a second set of weights. Excluding MDC 15, there are a total of 1,126 RDRGs (Fetter and Freeman 1991). HCFA uses a simplified list of 430 basic RDRGs pilot tested in New York State. The RDRG system was developed from analysis of more than four million discharges in Maryland and California. An important goal of this effort was to ensure that RDRGs would be applicable to all types of patients, not just Medicare patients. Thus the discharges analyzed included all payer data, including pediatric cases.

RDRGs utilize specific sets or classes of comorbid conditions (CCs, secondary diagnoses) for each ADRG rather than a list of substantial CCs for all DRGs (McGuire 1991). By utilizing specific CC classes, the RDRGs are better able to predict hospital costs and are able to accomplish a 50 percent improvment in the R-squared (over DRGs alone) from 0.28 to 0.42 without costly additional data collection from the medical chart. The medical ADRGs have three severity ratings (refinement classifications): baseline (class 0, e.g., otitis media), moderate (class 1, e.g., diabetes, gastrointestinal obstruction), and major (class 2, e.g., meningitis). The surgical RDRGs have a fourth class (class 3, e.g., stroke, myocardial infarction). ADRGs try to capture the complexity of care, which may be more relevant than the medical severity of illness in explaining cost per patient. Using a chart-based severity system typically rates coronary bypass surgery patients as modestly ill (level 1 or 2) at admission; but RDRGs place over 55 percent of the bypass patients into the most complex ADRG class.

The acuity index method (AIM, developed by Iameter) severity score is derived from information contained in the UHDDS. Each DRG is subdivided, based on secondary diagnoses and operating-room procedures related to the principal diagnosis and procedure. The patient's age and sex are also considered. The clinical judgment of medical and surgical subspecialists was used to assign "comparative severity" rankings to pathologic and therapeutic processes represented by ICD–9-CM codes. Each DRG has its own unique algorithm, with an acuity rating from 1 (least sick) to 5 (most sick). Severity-adjusted norms for length-of-stay charges and mortality rates may then be compared with actual case experience.

Patient management categories (PMCs, developed by the Pittsburgh Research Institute) were initially designed as a basis for comparative hospital cost analyses and hospital payment systems. The categories were defined to represent clinically specific groups of patients, each requiring a distinct diagnostic and treatment strategy for effective care. Patient categories were initially identified by physician panels, independent of patient data. The resulting classification scheme comprises more than 880 PMCs, encompassing all patients in general, acute-care hospitals, including psychiatric patients and neonates. The categories defined by physicians were mapped onto ICD–9-CM codes. Assignment of patients to PMCs is accomplished using UHDDS data (diagnoses, procedures, age, and sex). Related PMCs are grouped into "modules" and considered together. Patients with co-morbid conditions may be assigned to a maximum of five PMCs. In addition to the clinical classification scheme, the system includes weights based on the relative cost of the diagnostic and therapeutic services typically required for each patient type, as defined by physician panels. This contrasts with the empirical methods of deriving category weights used by other systems, which rely primarily on hospital charges for services actually provided to particular patients. The software that assigns cost weights includes adjustments for patients who fall into multiple PMCs.

APACHE III (APACHE Medical Systems): The original APACHE system (the acronym stands for acute physiology and chronic health evaluation) was designed to predict the intensity of services required and the risk of death for intensive-care patients. It was also designed to provide a basis for evaluating the quality of care provided. The system requires 12 physiologic values that are routinely collected within a patient's initial 24 hours in an intensive-care unit (e.g., heart rate, mean blood pressure, temperature, hematocrit, white blood cell count, serum creatinine, arterial blood gases, and Glasgow coma scale). The values are derived through weights, adjusted for age and chronic disease, that are designed to reflect the degree of physiological variance from a norm. APACHE III and II-b scores are independent of physician practice patterns, therapeutic choices, and invasive diagnostic procedures. This George Washington University Hospital system does not attempt to distinguish complications and comorbidities from the underlying (acute) disease. The developers of APACHE argued for limiting the scope of the system to those clinical areas where physiologic hypotheses relating clinical indicators to outcome or resource demand can be formulated and tested. To the extent that these clinical areas are responsible for a significant proportion of the overall variance, this more limited strategy would not necessarily compromise the overall result. APACHE II-b is a hospitalwide evaluation system that builds on APACHE II, reflecting severity of illness in four specific disease classes—stroke, congestive heart failure, pneumonia, and acute myocardial infarction. Additional clinical data elements are required, depending on the 16 disease groups. APACHE III is utilized for intensive-care patients (Knaus, Wagner, and Draper 1991).

The computerized severity index (CSI, developed by Health Systems International) is designed to be used together with DRGs to explain differences in resource use among patients. The system attempts to quantify the patient's total burden of illness by incorporating the clinical problem (severity of the principal diagnosis) and the clinical environment (severity of the complications and comorbidities) the patient experiences during hospitalization. The severity measures are based on the patient's laboratory test results, vital signs, and history and physical findings abstracted from the medical record. The severity of individual diseases is measured on a scale ranging from 1 (normality or mild disease) to 5 (death). Relying on standard five-digit ICD–9-CM codes to indicate the presence of disease, CSI generates a sixth digit that reflects the severity of the principal and most severe secondary diagnoses. The vendor makes the system's logic available to clients, and Susan Horn seeks input on potential refinements. The individual disease severity scores identify the complications or comorbidities that make the greatest contributions to the patient's overall severity. An overall severity score is generated by considering the interaction of the principal diagnosis with the patient's secondary diagnosis, as well as the severity of each secondary diagnosis. CSI's severity score can be computed at any time during the hospital stay, but it is generally determined within the first and/or last 48 hours. A unique feature of the implementation of CSI is interactive abstracting (Thomas and Ashcraft 1991). Beginning with the ICD–9-CM codes for diagnosis and procedures, the system requests only the specific additional data needed to make relevant distinctions. This helps keep CSI 50 percent less expensive than disease staging.

MedisGroups (medical illness severity grouping system) (MediQual) classifies patients into one of four severity groups based on clinical data. The system employs approximately 260 key clinical findings (KCF) that are abstracted from the medical record. A proprietary classification scheme assigns patients to severity groups, independent of diagnosis or procedure data (except insofar as the KCFs are obtained as results of diagnostic procedures). The four severity groups are designed to reflect increasing levels of physiologic instability or risk of organ failure. Three states mandate the usage of MedisGroups—Pennsylvania (1987), Iowa (1991), and Colorado (1992). An admission severity score is assigned within the first 48 hours of an inpatient stay. The classification is repeated by separately abstracting current values of KCFs on the eighth day of the hospital stay or on the sixth postoperative day. In addition to computing empirical measures of resource consumption by admission severity score, MedisGroups is unique in its emphasis on the change in severity score over the course of the patient's hospitalization as an indicator of the effectiveness of therapy or the presence of complications of care. Patients who fall into the two highest severity categories upon the second evaluation are characterized as "major morbidity."

MediQual has encouraged the use of rates of major morbidity, alone or in combination with rates of in-hospital mortality, as an indicator of quality of care (Iezzoni et al. 1991). The system is marketed as a clinical management information system, rather than just a patient classification system or a method of measuring the severity of patients' illnesses. UHDDS and UB–82 data are also collected and incorporated into the MedisGroups data base.

The fundamental concept behind illness outcome groups (IOGs), developed since 1987 by MediQual, is to create groups of clinically related DRGs or RDRGs that have been shown, in a large data base created by combining the experience of 102 MedisGroups client hospitals, to present similar risk of mortality or major morbidity. By aggregating DRGs or RDRGs with similar clinical behavior, it may be possible to achieve almost the same explanatory power with a much smaller number of categories, while avoiding the statistical problems associated with small numbers of cases in low-volume DRGs.

CURTAILING INAPPROPRIATE UTILIZATION

One of the conceptual problems that economists have had in the area of utilization in hospitals is understanding the wide range of heterogeneous products that physicians identify in the teaching hospital setting. In teaching hospitals physicians simultaneously produce the joint products of education, research, and patient care. Even within the category of patient care, the care "produced" is quite diverse, due to the great variance in the complexity of cases handled. Thus physicians have largely ignored medical economics studies because they do not capture the diversity of patient care within hospitals or across different hospital types. For example, the product of a hospital cannot be captured with just four figures: inpatient days, operative cases, outpatient visits, and number of residents on staff.

Payment incentives can have a downward impact on hospital utilization and cost (Prince 1991; Campbell 1991). New Jersey was the first state to experiment with a DRG payment system and the first all-payer DRG system (1980–87). In 1991 some 19 state Medicaid programs operated a prospective case-mix system, and Connecticut was the only state to drop use of the DRG approach within the 19 programs. Since New Jersey has the longest duration of experience with DRGs over the widest possible population cohort, the impact of its DRGs on hospital utilization has been widely studied. Broyles (1990) reported that the New Jersey DRG system reduced length of stay and cut radiological procedures per diem (and per case). On the other hand, the DRG system was associated with an increase in laboratory procedures per diem and a slight rise in laboratory use per case. This last result is a surprise, because it was thought that DRGs offered the incentive to trim utilization per case, but perhaps would collapse most of the same care (90 to 95 percent of the same work) into a shorter period of hospitalization (so utilization per diem would rise).

Carter and Melnick's (1990) study of 300,000 Medicare patients concluded

Table 8.3
Trends in Average Expense per Admission, Staff Productivity, and Labor Costs per Day in 28 Large Teaching Hospitals, 1976–1990

	Expense per Adjusted Inpatient Stay	FTE Staff Adjusted Inpatient Day	Expense for Personnel per Adjusted Inpatient Day
1976	$2,476.61	4.04	$204.47
1978	3,239.09	4.34	250.29
1980	4,286.84	4.57	314.02
1982	5,975.21	4.86	423.51
1984	7,650.78	5.23	532.14
1986	9,464.82	5.97	651.32
1988	11,476.59	6.29	765.19
1990	13,824.90	6.56	857.84
Total % Growth, 1976-1990	458.2	62.4	319.5

that to the extent that cost per admission is greater in major teaching hospitals, length of stay is the primary cause, not intensity of service provided per day. This result may not hold for other patient age groups, but there is some anecdotal evidence that this generalization may prove true. This author has tracked expenses in 28 large nonfederal teaching hospitals since 1976 as cohorts in a National Research Council (1977) study. The expenses per case and per day utilizing the standard American Hospital Association adjustment process for workload, are displayed in table 8.3. Whereas the inflation per diem is nearly double the consumer price index cited in chapter 1, the cost per case is inflating at triple the rate of the general economy. This suggests that teaching hospitals need to trim length of stay to contain cost per case.

In this context, Finkler, Brooten, and Brown (1988) studied neonatal care for a group of patients not subject to reimbursement and concluded that strong reductions in length of stay can save money without harming quality. They indicated that proportional reductions in service utilization were even greater than declines in length of stay, with no detrimental patient outcomes. In length of stay, more is not necessarily better, especially when the hospital is a dangerous and costly place for a prolonged visit. The 25 percent lowest-cost teaching hospitals in table 8.3 have seen their average length of stay for myocardial infarction cases decline from 15.7 days in 1976 to 8.6 days in 1987 and 3.2

days in 1991, and no member of the medical staff would suggest that the quality of care has declined.

Excessively long lengths of stay are a source of public concern not only because they are costly, but also because such care is often unnecessary. It has even been suggested that reduction of unnecessary or excessive amounts of care could raise the general health status of the population by decreasing the likelihood of iatrogenic complications. Reducing the length of stay minimizes the chance of exposure to antibiotic-resistant bacteria peculiar to hospitals; thus the number of difficult-to-treat infections may be lessened. Shortened lengths of stay are a morale builder for adult patients; and in the case of children, the trauma of separation from their parents is minimized, even when there are liberal visiting privileges (Innes, Grant, and Beinfield 1968). One study suggested that the marginal benefit of excessive days of hospitalization is negative, with 20 percent of the patients being exposed to some hazardous episode (Schimmel 1974). Clearly, the problems of cost and iatrogenic disease played a major part in the congressional commitment to the Professional Standard Review Organization (PSRO) program enacted in 1972 and the PRO program of the 1980s and 1990s.

Brown, Ehrlich, and Stehman (1984) demonstrated that significant cost savings can be obtained by reducing the time involved in preoperative skin preparation. Beck (1986) suggested an annual variable cost savings of $700,000 per 10,000 surgeries per year. He went on to critique a number of aseptic "fetishes that continue to be used despite repeated proof of their lack of value."

Utilization patterns are not merely a function of patient characteristics and the requirement of "good medicine." Medical care requirements can be met with different amounts of resources and lengths of hospitalization. How these requirements of good medicine are met depends in some part on the physician characteristics and the hospital environment. Surgical utilization is affected by hospital characteristics such as the laboratory turnaround time, the availability of hospital beds, the availability of a surgical suite, and the type of hospital ownership (federal, voluntary, municipal) (Eastaugh 1987). Utilization patterns are critical areas for further study in a number of areas, including ambulatory care (Weiner et al. 1991) and long-term care (Kenney and Holahan 1991).

If utilization review has not trimmed the lengths of stay of teaching hospitals as substantially as nationwide declines in length of stay (National Center for Health Statistics [NCHS] 1991), at least certain insurance companies are reaping the benefits of utilization review. Wickizer, Wheller, and Feldstein (1990) studied 223 insured groups and found that utilization review in the two-year period reduced inpatient days 11 percent, routine inpatient services by 7.0 percent, and ancillary services by 9.0 percent. Medical staff should work at trimming unnecessary admissions, tests, and procedures, a topic to which we shall return in chapters 11 and 12. In an attempt to assess the impact of chart reviews, feedback, and lectures on residents' ordering behavior, Manheim et al. (1990) randomized residents into two groups: the cost-conscious program-review group and a control group. The authors concluded that a reduction of $391 in charges per patient resulted from lower lengths of stay, and charges were $106 lower in radiology (both statistically significant at the 0.01 level). The lower-cost experimental group's style of care achieved lower patient impairment ratings at discharge, indicating that more efficient care may be quality-enhancing at the one university hospital.

ALTERNATIVE MEASURES OF THE TEACHING HOSPITAL DEPENDENCY LINK

One additional question is whether there are not some more relevant behavior variables involving the hospital and the sources of education (residency directors, deans) that better measure graduate medical education. These more complex variables might not be as administratively simple or appropriate as a single scalar measure (resident-to-bed ratio), but they may be more indicative of the mutual dependency between the hospital and the education program. A number of studies used the following measure of teaching-staff characteristics (National Research Council 1977; Eastaugh 1980a, 1979):

1. Fraction of the attending physicians on the surgical service with actual teaching faculty appointments at the local medical school who receive salary from the school (intended as an index of the hospital's dependence on the medical school for physicians)
2. Fraction of the affiliated medical school's students who did their required core clinical clerkship on the hospital surgical service (intended as an index of the school's dependence on the hospital as a training ground)
3. Fraction of surgeons (excluding anesthesiologists) at the facility who are foreign medical graduates (FMGs)

The fraction of the medical school's students depending on the individual hospital as a source of clinical education is intended as a proxy measure of the school's dependency on the hospital. One might suggest that if the school is highly dependent on a hospital for teaching cases, the students, interns, residents and attending physicians, acting as agents of the school's interest, would have added reason to increase length of stay or tests ordered in order to maximize the number of teaching days available and to maximize tests and cost per case in order to serve a technological interest in maximizing revenues for new equipment (Eastaugh 1987).

The basic premise of the economic model emerging from cost analysis is that physicians are influenced in patient-management decisions by the economic advantage of actions to them or their hospital, or perhaps to their medical school. We should guard against overutilization that results from physician pursuit of less explicit forms of economic advantage than income-maximization tendencies under a fee-for-service system of reimbursement. The subtle incentives to overutilize are much more insidious and affect salaried and private entrepreneur physicians equally.

Physician background characteristics are determinants of physician behavior. The duration of stay and number of tests per patient are likely to be affected by the educational background of the surgeon and the strength of the affiliation with the local medical school (Eastaugh 1979). The process outlined in figure 8.1 implies a causal sequence. Differing combinations of physician and hospital characteristics lead to different styles of medicine, which in turn lead to different utilization patterns (Twaddle and Sweet 1970). For example, one might presuppose that medical school faculty members involved in patient care have a professional interest in curtailing inappropriate prescriptions, but it might not always be in the faculty members' interests to curtail all types of excessive utilization. Faculty members and attending physicians might have an interest in maximizing their revenues.

Hospital-based specialists are interested in maintaining distribution channels that ensure "interesting" product assortment, efficiency (whenever possible), and progressiveness (including the ability to foster technological change). Elimination of a service or department should be analyzed in light of risks and benefits, response from the competition, and alienation of internal hospital-based vested interests. The hospital-based physicians frequently lobby for revitalization rather than elimination.

If we presume that the surgeon wishes to maximize prestige or popularity within the profession, rather than overutilize for the sake of overutilization, then the problem for policy makers becomes one of framing a set of incentives that makes prestige maximization incompatible with overutilization. Underutilization that has a detrimental effect on quality would injure the physician's prestige and image among his or her peers.

Future research might consider whether physicians operate under the norms hypothesis (Wennberg 1990), making length-of-stay decisions based on the average or modal staff characteristics within their hospital and their region, rather than handling these decisions on an individual basis. In particular, a fair test of the norms hypothesis would be to take a sample from teaching and nonteaching hospitals and compare staff characteristics for one surgeon to characteristics of everyone who made decisions about a given patient. From there, the study would proceed to characteristics of surgeons in the surgical service of a given hospital and to characteristics of all surgeons in the health-service area for a sample of both teaching and nonteaching hospitals.

NATIONAL PRICES ARE NOT YET HARMING QUALITY

Goodall (1990) and Pope (1990) both argued that the transition from hospital-specific Medicare costs to adjusted national DRG Medicare prices since 1988 has been inequitable. Both of these health economists argued that Medicare should return to a blend of hospital-specific costs and national prices, as was done in the prospective payment system phase in the period from 1984 to 1988. There is a wide variety of cost per case, but the question is what proportion of

Figure 8.1
Interdependence of the Medical School, the Physician Staff, and the Hospital Staff in the Production of Patient Care

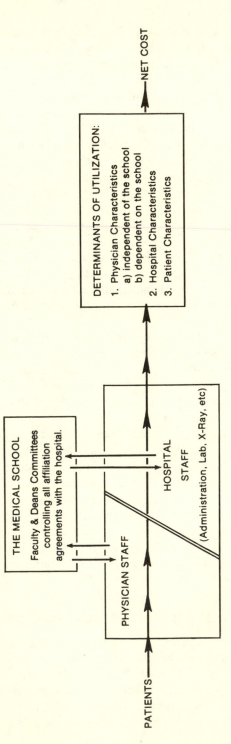

the cost differences is justified (and what is due to inefficiency, excess length of stay, and so on). Keeler (1990) took the position of the ethical regulator and identified cost due to sickness at admission as a clearly justifiable expense. He measured severity using the APACHE II acute physiological score variables (see Knaus et al. 1991, Knaus et al. 1985, Wong and Knaus 1991) and concluded that the national DRG prices are adequately connected to costs. Some of the remaining variance in cost per case is noise, some comes from differences in efficiency and treatment intensity, and some comes from justifiable factors that are yet to be measured in a severity index. There is no evidence that underpayments to high-cost hospitals and profits earned by low-cost hospitals have had any detrimental impact on the quality of patient care. Witsberger and Kominski (1990) supported the position that less utilization may not harm quality, especially for the five surgical conditions with the fastest annual declines in length of stay (inguinal hernia repair, transurethral prostatectomy, mastectomy, exploration of the spinal canal, and knee and ankle arthroplasty). They also concluded that some of the extra outpatient surgery may not be appropriate care.

Payment system changes are affecting the way we educate future doctors. The Harvard Medical School New Pathways Program, pioneered in a number of places from New Mexico to Boston, suggests a number of innovative case-study and computer-driven teaching methods for the 1990s (Tosteson 1990). It is difficult for medical school educators to allocate sufficient time to procedural skills, medical technology, and general knowledge acquisition and save enough time for respect and caring (Humanity 101). Younger physicians seem more receptive to computers, economic analysis (chapters 11–13), and consumerism. Patient utility judgments count more in the modern world because patients are rightfully becoming more assertive about their own bodies. Certain subjects have to be trimmed to make room for the new material (e.g., cuts in microbiology or pharmacology lab hours). A number of medical educators have called for fundamental changes in teaching programs (Cator et al. 1991; Tosteson 1991).

Some medical educators have suggested an expansion of the training period to absorb the rapidly expanding body of medical knowledge. While these suggestions are made in good faith, a number of subspecialists outside of the university environment would welcome a decrease in the production of competitors for all the reasons suggested in chapters 3 and 4. Would the future residents put up with longer training periods? McKay (1990) reported that residents are quite unresponsive to changes in the length of a training program (they will stick with it and not switch to a residency with a shorter training period).

REFERENCES

Alemi, F. (1992). "Improving the Accuracy of Severity Indexes." *Medical Decision Making* 12:1 (January–March), 8–14.

Alemi, F., Rice, J., and Hankins, R. (1990). "Predicting In-Hospital Survival of Myocardial Infarction: A Comparative Study of Various Severity Measures." *Medical Care* 28:9 (September), 762–775.

Ament, R., Breachslin, J., Kobrinski, E., and Wood, W. (1982). "The Case Type Classifications: Suitability for Use in Reimbursing Hospitals." *Medical Care* 20:5 (May), 460–467.

Anderson, G., and Lave, J. (1986). "Financing Graduate Medical Education Using Multiple Regression to Set Payment Rates." *Inquiry* 23:2 (Summer), 191–199.

Arthur Young and Policy Analysis, Inc. (1986). *A Study of the Financing of Graduate Medical Education: Final Report.* 3-volume study of 45 hospitals, DHHS 100–86–0155 (October). Washington, D.C.: U.S. Government Printing Office.

Association of American Medical Colleges (AAMC). (1991). Data on Medical Students and Medical School Finances. Washington, D.C.: AAMC.

Barer, M. (1991). "Controlling Medical Care Costs in Canada." *Journal of the American Medical Association* 265:18 (May 8), 2393–2394.

Beck, W. (1986). "Asepsis and DRGs." *Infections in Surgery* 8 (August), 425, 448.

Beran, R. (1979). "The Rise and Fall of Three-Year Medical School Programs." *Journal of Medical Education* 54:3 (March), 248–249.

Blumberg, M. (1991). "Biased Estimates of Expected Acute MI Mortality Using MEDISGR0UPS Admission Severity." *Journal of the American Medical Association* 265:22 (June 12), 2965–2970.

Bradbury, R., Stearns, F, and Steen, P. (1991). "Interhospital Variations in Admission Severity-adjusted In-hospital Mortality and Morbidity." *Health Services Research* 26:4 (October), 407–424.

Brewster, A., Karlin, B., Jacobs, C., Hyde, L., Bradbury, R., and Chae, Y. (1985). "MEDISGROUPS: A Clinically Based Approach to Classifying Hospital Patients at Admission." *Inquiry* 22:4 (Winter), 377–387.

Brook, R., Lohr, K., Chassin, M., Kosecoff, J., Fink, A., and Solomon, D. (1984). "Geographic Variations in the Use of Services: Do They Have Any Clinical Significance?" *Health Affairs* 3:2 (Summer), 63–73.

Brown, T., Ehrlich, C., and Stehman, F. (1984). "A Clinical Evaluation of Chlorhexidine Spray as Compared with Iodophor Scrub for Preoperative Skin Preparation." *Surgery, Gynecology, and Obstetrics* 158:4 (April), 363–366.

Broyles, R. (1990). "Efficiency, Costs, and Quality: The New Jersey Experience Revisited." *Inquiry* 27:1 (Spring), 86–96.

Burns, L., and Wholey, D. (1991) "Effects of Patient, Hospital, and Physician Characteristics on Length of Stay and Mortality." *Medical Care* 29:3 (March), 251–271.

Cameron, J. (1985). "The Indirect Costs of Graduate Medical Education." *New England Journal of Medicine* 312:19 (May 9), 1233–1238.

Campbell, C., Gillespie, K., and Romeis, J. (1991). "Effect of Residency Training Programs on the Financial Performance of VA Medical Centers." *Inquiry* 28:3 (Fall), 288–299.

Carter, G., and Melnick, G. (1990). *How Services and Costs Vary by Day of Stay for Medicare Hospital Stays.* Washington, D.C.: ProPAC.

Cator, J., Cohen, A., Baker, D., and Shuster, A. (1991). "Medical Educators' Views on Medical Education Reform." *Journal of the American Medical Association* 265:8 (February 27), 1002–1006.

Chase, R., and Hayes, R. (1991). "Beefing Up Operations in Service Firms." *Sloan Management Review* 33:1 (Fall), 15–26.

Chin, D., Hopkins, D., Melmon, K., and Holman, H. (1985). "The Relation of Faculty Academic Activity to Financing Sources in a Department of Medicine." *New England Journal of Medicine* 312:16 (April 18), 1029–1034.

Cleary, P., Greenfield, S., and Mulley, A. (1991). "Variation in Length of Stay and Outcomes for Six Medical and Surgical Conditions." *JAMA* 266:1 (July 3), 73–79.

Coffey, R., and Goldfarb, M. (1986). "DRGs and Disease Staging for Reimbursing Medicare Patients." *Medical Care* 24:9 (September), 814–829.

Commonwealth Task Force on Academic Health Centers. (1985). *Future Financing of Teaching Hospitals: A Framework for Public Policy* (October). New York: Commonwealth Fund.

Congressional Budget Office (CBO). (1991). *Medicare's Disproportionate Share Adjustment*. Washington, D.C.: CBO.

Custer, W., and Willke, R. (1991). "Teaching Hospital Costs: The Effects of Medical Staff Characteristics." *Health Services Research* 25:6 (February), 831–857.

Detsky, A., McLaughlin, J., Abrams, H., Abbe, K., and Markel, F. (1986). "Do Interns and Residents Order More Tests Than Attending Staff?" *Medical Care* 24:6 (June), 526–534.

Eastaugh, S. (1990). "Financing the Correct Rate of Growth of Medical Technology." *Quarterly Review of Economics and Business* 30:4 (Winter), 34–60.

———. (1987). *Financing Health Care*. Dover, Mass.: Auburn House, 323–377.

———. (1981). *Medical Economics and Health Finance*. Dover, Mass.: Auburn House.

———. (1980a). "Organizational Determination of Surgical Lengths of Stay." *Inquiry* 17:2 (Spring), 85–96.

———. (1980b). "Financial Ratio Analysis and Medical School Management." *Journal of Medical Education* 55:12 (December), 983–992.

———. (1979). "Cost of Elective Surgery and Utilization of Ancillary Services in Teaching Hospitals." *Health Services Research* 14:4 (Winter), 290–308.

Eeckhoudt, L., LeBrun, T., and Sailly, J. (1985). "Risk-Aversion and Physicians' Medical Decision-making." *Journal of Health Economics* 4:3 (September), 273–281.

Epstein, A. (1986). "Socioeconomic Characteristics and Utilization for Hospitalized Patients: Do Poor People Cost More?" *Clinical Research* 84:1 (January), 360–373.

Fein, R. (1967). *The Doctor Shortage*. Washington, D.C.: Brookings Institution.

Fein, R., and Weber, G. (1971). *Financial Medical Education: An Analysis of Alternative Policies and Mechanisms*. New York: McGraw-Hill.

Feinglass, J., Martin, G., and Sen, A. (1991). "Financial Effect of Physician Practice Style on Hospital Resource Use." *Health Services Research* 26:2 (June), 183–205.

Fetter, R., and Freeman, J. (1991). *DRG Refinement with Diagnostic Specific Comorbidities and Complications: A Synthesis of Current Approaches to Patient Classification*. Washington, D.C.: Health Care Financing Administration.

Finkler, S., Brooten, D., and Brown, L. (1988). "Utilization of Inpatient Services under Shortened Lengths of Stay: A Neonatal Care Example." *Inquiry* 25:2 (Summer), 271–280.

Foley, J., and Mulhausen, R. (1986). "The Cost of Complexity: The Teaching Hospital." *Hospital and Health Services Administration* 31:5 (September/October), 96–109.

Frick, A., Martin, S., and Schwartz, M. (1985). "Case-Mix and Cost Differences between Teaching and Nonteaching Hospitals." *Medical Care* 23:4 (April), 283–295.

Garg, M., Elkhatib, M., Kleinberg, W., and Mulligan, W. (1982). "Reimbursing for Residency Training: How Many Times?" *Medical Care* 20:7 (July), 719–726.

Garg, M., Louis, D., Gleibe, W., Spirka, C., Skipper, J., and Parekh, R. (1978). "Evaluating Inpatient Costs." *Medical Care* 16:3 (March), 191–201.

Ginzberg, E. (1990). *The Medical Triangle: Physicians, Politicians, and the Public.* Cambridge, Mass.: Harvard University Press.

Glandon, G., and Counte, M. (1992). "Measurement of Hospital Financial Position: Continuity of Indicators." *Public Budgeting and Financial Management* 4:1 (Spring) 57–82.

Goldfarb, M., and Coffey, R. (1987). "Case-Mix Differences between Teaching and Nonteaching Hospitals." *Inquiry* 24:1 (Spring), 68–84.

Goldschmidt, Y., and Gafni, A. (1991). "A Managerial Approach to Costing Fixed Assets: The Role of Depreciation and Interest." *Health Care Management Review* 16:4 (Fall), 55–66.

Gonnella, J., Hornbrook, M., and Louis, D. (1984). "Staging of Disease: A Case-Mix Measurement." *Journal of the American Medical Association* 251:5 (February 3), 637–641.

Gonnella, J., Louis, D., and Zelenik, C. (1990). "The Problem of Late Hospitalization." *Academic Medicine* 65:5 (May), 314–319.

Goodall, C. (1990). "A Simple Objective Method for Determining a Percent Standard in Mixed Reimbursement Systems." *Journal of Health Economics* 9:3 (November), 253–271.

Haley, R., Schaberg, D., and Crossley, K. (1981). "Extra Charges and Prolongation of Stay Attributable to Nosocomial Infection." *American Journal of Medicine* 70:1 (January), 51–58.

Hilton, G. W. (1972). "The Basic Behavior of Regulatory Commissions." *American Economic Review* 62:2 (May), 47–54.

Horn, S. (1986). "Measuring Severity: How Sick Is Sick? How Well Is Well?" *Healthcare Financial Management* 40:10 (October), 21–32.

Horn, S., Buckley, G., Sharkey, P., Chambers, A., Horn, R., and Schramm, C. (1985). "Inter-Hospital Differences in Patient Severity: Problems for Prospective Payment Based on DRGs." *New England Journal of Medicine* 313:1 (July 4), 20–24.

Horn, S., Horn, R., and Moses, H. (1986). "Profiles of Physician Practice and Patient Severity of Illness." *American Journal of Public Health* 76:5 (May), 532–535.

Hough, D., and Bazzoli, G. (1985). "The Economic Environment of Resident Physicians." *Journal of the American Medical Association* 253:12 (March 22), 1758–1762.

Hsia, D., Krushaat, W., Fagan, A., Febbutt, J., and Kusserow, R. (1988). "Accuracy of Diagnostic Coding for Medicare Patients under the Prospective-Payment System." *New England Journal of Medicine* 318:4 (January 22), 352–355.

Iezzoni, L., Ash, A., Coffman, G., and Moskowitz, M. (1991). "Admission and Mid-Stay MEDISGROUPS Scores as Predictors of Hospital Charges." *Medical Care* 29:3 (March), 210–220.

Innes, A., Grant, A., and Beinfield, M. (1968). "Experience with Shortened Hospital

Stay for Postsurgical Patients." *Journal of the American Medical Association* 204:8 (May 20), 647–652.

Jolly, P. (1991). "U.S. Medical School Finances." *Journal of the American Medical Association* 266:12, 55–66.

Keeler, E. (1990). "What Proportion of Hospital Cost Differences Is Justifiable?" *Journal of Health Economics* 9:3 (November), 359–365.

Kenney, G., and Holahan, J. (1991). "Nursing Home Transfers and Mean Length of Stay in the Prospective Payment Era." *Medical Care* 29:7 (July), 589–609.

Kirz, H., and Larsen, C. (1986). "Costs and Benefits of Medical Student Training to an HMO." *Journal of the American Medical Association* 256:6 (August 8), 734–739.

Knaus, W., Draper, E., and Wagner, D. (1985). "APACHE II: A Severity of Disease Classification System." *Critical Care Medicine* 13:12 (December) 818–827.

Knaus, W., Wagner, D., Draper, E., Zimmerman, J. (1991). "APACHE III Prognostic System: Risk Predictor of Hospital Mortality." *Chest* 100:6 (December), 1501–1565.

Kovener, A. (1991) "Case of the Unhealthy Hospital." *Harvard Business Review* 69:5 (September-October) 12–26.

Lave, J., and Frank, R. (1990). "Effect of the Structure of Hospital Payment on Length of Stay." *Health Services Research* 25:2 (June), 325–347.

Louis, D., Barnes, C., Jordan, N., Moynihan, C., Pepitone, T., Spirka, C., Sredl, K., and Westnedge, J. (1983). *Disease Staging: A Clinically Based Approach to Measurement of Disease Severity.* Final Report to DHHS (NCHSR 233–78–3001), Rockville, Maryland (August). Washington, D.C.: U.S. Government Printing Office, NTIS-PB83–254649.

Louis, D., and Gonnella, J. (1991). *Q-Stage: Q-Scale.* New York: SysteMetrics/McGraw-Hill.

Malenka, D., Roos, N., Fisher, S., and Wennberg, J. (1990). "Further Study of the Increased Mortality Following Transurethral Prostatectomy." *Journal of Urology* 144:8 (August), 224–228.

Manheim, L., Feinglas, J., Hughes, R., Martin, G., Conrad, K., and Hughes, R. (1990). "Training House Officers to Be Cost Conscious: Effects of an Educational Intervention on Charges and Length of Stay." *Medical Care* 28:1 (January), 29–41.

McGuire, T. (1991). "An Evaluation of Diagnosis-related Group Severity and Complexity Refinement." *Health Care Financing Review* 12:4 (Summer), 49–60.

McKay, N. (1990). "Economic Determinants of Specialty Choice by Medical Residents." *Journal of Health Economics* 9:3 (November), 335–357.

McMahon, L., Wolfe, R., and Tedeschi, P. (1989). "Variation in Hospital Admissions among Small Areas: A Comparison of Maine and Michigan." *Medical Care* 27:6 (June), 623–631.

Mennemeyer, S. (1978). "Really Great Returns to Medical Education?" *Journal of Medical Education* 13:1 (January) 73–90.

Miller, M., Cuddleback, J., and Gallo, J. (1991). *Severity of Illness Measures for Hospitals.* Tallahassee, Fla.: Florida Health Care Cost Containment Board.

Mooney, G., Hall, J., and Donaldson, C. (1992). "Utilization as a Measure of Equity." *Journal of Health Economics* 10:4 (March), 465–470.

National Center for Health Statistics. (1991). Vital and Health Statistics: Data from the National Health Interview Survey. Hyattsville, Md.: DHHS.

National Research Council. (1977). *Health Care for American Veterans.* Washington, D.C.: National Academy of Sciences.

New York State. (1991). *Products of Ambulatory Care (PACs) and Products of Ambulatory Surgery (PAS) Reimbursement Project.* New York: New York State Ambulatory Care Case Mix Demonstration Project.

Newhouse, J. (1983). "Two Prospective Difficulties with PPS of Hospitals, or, 'It's Better to Be a Resident Than a Patient with a Complex Problem.' " *Journal of Health Economics* 2:3 (September), 269–274.

Oleske, D., Glandon, G., Giacomelli, G., and Hohmann, S. (1991). "Cesarean Birth Rate: Influence of Hospital Teaching Status." *Health Services Research* 26:3 (August), 325–338.

Nutt, P. (1992). "Contract Management and Institutional Cost Control." *Hospital and Health Services Administration* 37:1 (Spring), 115–130.

Panniers, T., and Newlander, J. (1986). "Adverse Patient Occurrences (APO) Inventory: Validity, Reliability, and Implications." *Quality Review Bulletin* 12:9 (September), 311–315.

Perry, D., and Challoner, D. (1979). "A Rationale for Continued Federal Support of Medical Education." *New England Journal of Medicine* 300:22 (January), 66–71.

Petersdorf, R. (1985). "A Proposal for Financing Graduate Medical Education." *New England Journal of Medicine* 312:20 (May 16), 1322–1324.

Pettengill, J., and Vertrees, J. (1982). "Reliability and Validity in Hospital Case-Mix Measurement." *Health Care Financing Review* 4:2 (December), 101–128.

Pfordresher, K. (1985). "Clinical Research and Prospective Payment." Report of the Council of Teaching Hospitals, monograph (January). Washington, D.C.: American Association of Medical Colleges.

Pope, G. (1990). "Using Hospital-specific Costs to Improve the Fairness of Prospective Reimbursement." *Journal of Health Economics* 9:3 (November), 237–251.

Prince, T. (1991). "Assessing Financial Outcomes of Not-for-Profit Community Hospitals." *Hospital and Health Services Administration* 36:3 (Fall), 331–348.

Prospective Payment Assessment Commission (ProPAC). (1991). *Medicare Prospective Payment and the American Health Care System: Report to Congress.* Washington, D.C.: ProPAC.

Rapoport, J., Teres, D., Lemeshow, S., Avrunin, J., and Haber, R. (1990). "Explaining Variability of Cost Using a Severity of Illness Measure for ICU Patients." *Medical Care* 28:4 (April), 338–348.

Reinhardt, U. (1975). *Physician Productivity and the Demand for Health Manpower.* Cambridge, Mass.: Ballinger.

Relman, A. (1984). "Who Will Pay for Medical Education in Our Teaching Hospitals?" *Science* 226:1 (October 5), 20–23.

Reuschel, J., and Earle, D. (1991). "Measuring Productivity in the Academic Setting." *Medical Group Management Journal* 38:5 (September/October), 52–55.

Rieselbach, R., and Jackson, T. (1986). "In Support of a Linkage between the Funding of Graduate Medical Education and Care of the Indigent." *New England Journal of Medicine* 314:1 (January 2), 32–35.

Rosko, M. (1988). "DRGs and the Severity of Illness Measures: An analysis of Patient Classification Systems." *Journal of Medical Systems* 12:2 (Spring) 257–266.

Salkever, D. (1970). "Studies in the Economics of Hospital Costs." Ph.D. diss., Economics Department, Harvard University.

Schimmel, E. (1974). "Hazards of Hospitalization." *Annals of Internal Medicine* 60:1 (January) 100–110.

Schwartz, W., Newhouse, J., and Williams, A. (1985). "Is the Teaching Hospital an Endangered Species?" *New England Journal of Medicine* 313:3 (July 18), 157–162.

Sloan, F. (1976). "A Microanalysis of Physicians' Hours of Work Decisions." In M. Perlman (ed.), *Economics of Health and Medical Care*, 302–325. New York: John Wiley.

Starfield, B., Weiner, J., Mumford, L., and Steinwachs, D. (1991). "Ambulatory Care Groupings." *Health Services Research* 26:1 (April), 53–74.

Steinwald, B., and Dummit, L. (1989). "Hospital Case-Mix Change: Sicker Patients or DRG Creep?" *Health Affairs* 8:2 (Summer), 35–47.

Stevens, C. (1971). "Physicians Supply and the National Health Care Goals." *Industrial Relations* 10:5 (May), 119–144.

Thomas, J., and Ashcraft, M. (1991). "Measuring Severity of Illness: Six Severity Systems and Ability to Explain Cost." *Inquiry* 28:1 (Spring), 39–55.

Thorpe, K. (1988). "Use of Regression Analysis to Determine Hospital Payment: The Case of Medicare's Indirect Teaching Adjustment." *Inquiry* 25:2 (Summer), 219–231.

Tosteson, D. (1991). "New Pathways for Medical Education." *Journal of the American Medical Association* 265:8 (February 27), 1022–1023.

———. (1990). "New Pathways in General Medical Education." *New England Journal of Medicine* 322:4 (January 25), 234–238.

Twaddle, A., and Sweet, R. (1970). "Characteristics and Experiences of Patients with Preventable Hospital Admissions." *Social Science and Medicine* 4:1 (July), 141–145.

United States Senate Finance Committee. (1983). *Social Security Amendments of 1983*. Report 98–23 (March 11), 52.

Weiner, J., Starfield, B., Steinwachs, D., and Mumford, L. (1991). "Development and Application of a Population-oriented Measure of Ambulatory Care Case-Mix," *Medical Care* 29:5 (May) 452–472.

Wennberg, J. (1990). "Status of the Prostate Disease Assessment Team." *Health Services Research* 25:5 (December), 709–716.

Wennberg, J., Freeman, J., and Culp, W. (1987). "Are Hospital Services Rationed in New Haven or Over-utilized in Boston?" *Lancet* 1:8543, 1185–1187.

Wickizer, T. (1992). "Estimating the Effects of Utilization Review on Hospital Use and Expenditures." *Health Services Research* 27:1 (April), 95–106.

Wickizer, T., Wheller, J., and Feldstein, P. (1989). "Does Utilization Review Reduce Unnecessary Hospital Care and Contain Costs?" *Medical Care* 27:6 (June), 632–647.

Witsberger, C., and Kominski, G. (1990). *Recent Trends in Length of Stay for Medicare Surgical Patients*. Washington, D.C.: HCFA, R–3940.

Wong, D., Knaus, W. (1991). "Predicted Outcome in Critical Care: APACHE." *Canadian Journal of Anesthesiology* 38:3 (April) 374–83.

Young, W. (1986). *Measuring the Cost of Care Using Patient Management Categories*. HCFA Publication Number 86–03228 (June). Washington, D.C.: U.S. Government Printing Office.

Young, W., and Maciose, D. (1992). ''Product Line Analysis using PMCs versus DRGs.'' *Public Budgeting and Financial Management* 4:1 (Spring), 83–106.

V CONSUMER EDUCATION, SERVICE QUALITY, AND HEALTH MANPOWER

9 Quality Measurement, Consumer Information, and Value Shopping

"Cost control should not mean remote control medicine by utilization review from a distance. We must educate to enhance quality and efficiency by peer review."

—C. Everett Koop, M.D.

Physicians doing unnecessary care for reasons of added income is not the problem. We are startled to find how poor the level of medical knowledge is oftentimes. There are a lot of doctors out there who really need help.

—John Davis, M.D.

The state medical society is essentially a trade union. They have a very narrow outlook, viewing utilization profiles or quality reports as information that should be kept from the public.

—Benjamin Barnes, M.D.

The quality-of-care issue can be approached from a supplier's point of view (e.g., using the Deming method for improvement; Veney and Kaluzny 1991; Lynn and Osborn 1991) and from a consumerist point of view (the quality-disclosure method; Health Care Financing Administration [HCFA] 1991). A number of issues remain moot. Should the health sector place more emphasis on physician reeducation, credentials, PRO review, or public disclosure of quality scorecards? Quality is a difficult-to-measure attribute that has only recently pushed itself into the public eye. In 1981 the Public Citizen Health Research Group issued a policy statement calling on the federal government to assist Medicare beneficiaries in avoiding high-priced physicians. Consumerism should extend beyond simple price-disclosure activities to include expanded information on quality and availability of care. The libertarian conservatives in the Bush administration should be supportive of any efforts designed to promote informational equality between providers and patients. Improved informational equality is a necessary condition for stimulating competitive markets. However, the traditional conservatives in organized medicine may resist any efforts to supply patients with more information concerning cost, quality, and access (Morley 1991).

There is some evidence that the HCFA (1991) report continued to identify too many high-mortality outlier hospitals. Green, Passman, and Wintfeld (1991) reported that the number of outlier hospitals declined by half (to 101) if the following four proxy measures for case severity were added to the regression analysis: share of patients age 85 or over, percentages of patients with pneumonia and with urinary-tract infections, and discharges to a nursing home (as opposed to HCFA's less accurate variable "transfers from a nursing home"). The HCFA (1991) report was superior to earlier federal lists because mortality was shown for 30, 90, and 180 days after admission (rather than only for 30 days after admission). The 1991 HCFA list also adjusted the rates for new subdiagnoses not used in previous reports.

On April 17, 1985, the Health Care Financing Administration (HCFA 1985), controlling almost $100 billion in medical expenditures, announced that the 54 local professional review organizations (PROs) would be required to release data on hospital quality by DRG and department to the public. Confidentiality would be maintained as to the identity of specific doctors and patients. PROs and hospitals could provide their own interpretations concerning the quality of care. From a political perspective this is a unique issue, in which strange bedfellows like Ralph Nader and Milton Friedman (1965) are in agreement that consumers must be provided with information as a basis for shopping for health care. For both liberals and conservatives, if the data are collected with public funds, they must be made available to consumers, employers, and insurance companies. Consumer information is the fuel that fosters cost-decreasing competition, quality enhancement, and innovation in the marketplace. Improving quality and productivity through improved information to the multiple buyers, especially in a local service market (e.g., health care), puts into practice the economic theory concerning the benefits of a better buyer's knowledge of the supplier (Stigler 1961). For consumerists, the battle cry is "Select your providers on facts, not just hopes."

Provider concern for quality is not new (Sahney 1991). However, the type of systematic inquiry that characterizes the contemporary quality-assurance field has evolved within the health-services research community over the past two decades. Donabedian (1967) and Roemer, Moustafa, and Hopkins (1968) laid the groundwork for quality-measurement and quality-control activities. Donabedian outlined three basic approaches to quality assessment: structure (credentials, accreditation, licensure, certification), process (what is done for patients, checklists, or criteria-mapping protocol, including the coordination and sequence of the activities), and outcomes (fatality, infection, and other adverse events or positive results, assessed from medical records or interviews). As a number of Rand Corporation researchers in the quality arena attest, measures of care by outcome are the best yardstick because they reflect net changes that occur in the patient's health status (Brook and Lohr 1985). Milton Roemer, as a strong advocate of both outcome measures and consumerism, proposed in 1968 a hospital quality index based on fatality rates crudely adjusted for case severity. A more refined version of that index by hospital product lines may soon be published on a regular basis in local community newspapers (Eastaugh 1986).

INJECTING QUALITY INTO THE COST-CONTAINMENT EQUATION

Are consumers smart enough to interpret quality statistics? The most basic answer to that question is yes, if we make the summary statistics comprehensible to the nontechnical reader. Just as buyers weigh a multitude of attributes in complex purchases, from televisions to cars, so payers and patients can shop for providers with better information at their fingertips. Many hospital visits cost as much as luxury cars, and some outpatient visits cost as much as televisions. Sensitivity to quality is even more acute in the case of health care. Consequently, buyer awareness is high, and the resources invested are not trivial.

A comprehensive review of the entire range of quality-measurement techniques is beyond the scope of this chapter. We shall briefly review methodological issues first and then examine the federal role in information data collection and dissemination. The danger if employers utilize Medicare PRO quality measures is that they may represent inappropriate tracers for overall facility quality. Employer groups may privately contract with the PROs to gather information on younger patient populations. The Commission on Professional and Hospital Activities (CPHA) offers normative quality data on 29 million nonelderly patients.

The prevalence of empty beds across the board has destroyed a low cost (easy to get) signal of quality—the degree of empty beds in a facility. Many hospitals, of good and bad quality, currently have low occupancy rates much of the year. Consumers may close inferior quality hospitals and reward quality facilities. A high level of unnecessary and inappropriate care has contributed to the litigious atmosphere in our medical care system. Redoubling our efforts in the area of quality control is not only consumerist but assists in reducing the headaches and prestige-deterioration implicit in a high malpractice volume. During their September 1986 meeting, the Joint Commission on Accreditation of Healthcare Organizations (JCAHO) voted to evaluate clinical outcomes as part of its ongoing accreditation process. JCAHO and HCFA must come to the realization that to recognize true hospital quality (the signal) one must be able to adjust for differences in case-mix (bias) and account for random variation (random noise). Although adjustment for case mix differences has been discussed extensively in the literature, the effect of random variation has not been adequately addressed. Predictive error rates with respect to "quality" for both "outlier" and "non-outlier" hospitals show that death rates are not yet a good indicator of underlying quality. HCFA and the PROs must continue to improve the predictive error rates of their quality measures. Large hospitals with large sample sizes that are high fatality rate outliers for several years in a row may be, with high probability, hospitals with low quality of care. However, it is likely that only a small number of hospitals would be identified this way. As the number of patients served by the hospital increases, because more years of data are included in the analysis, classification may grow more reliable. JCAHO and regulators will have difficulty in their efforts to find and recognize low-quality hospitals by looking at (case-mix adjusted) mortality rates because random variation appears to swamp the quality signal. Mortality rates will not be our only measure of quality. Des-Harnais, McMahon and Wroblewski (1991) report that some hospitals that rank well when compared with mortality rates do not do as well on quality measures such as readmission rates or complication rates.

QUALITY STATISTICS: LARGE STATISTICAL PROBLEMS

Quality measures that are inaccurate either because the case is one of a hundred conditions that require a severity adjustment in the analysis or because the sample is too small, can yield an unjustified slur against, or recommendation for, a given hospital (Daley and Kellie 1991). For example, the March 1986 DHHS Health Standards and Quality Bureau report on 269 "atypical" hospitals nationwide (Krakauer 1986) identified providers with abnormal fatality rates. The *New York Times* coverage of this story focused on two cases: (1) inferior hospital A, having a mortality rate of 6.0 percent when the predicted DRG-adjusted national average rate should have been 2.7 percent, and (2) good hospital B, having a 4.4 percent mortality rate, compared to the national standard rate of 6.2 percent (if the average hospital treated the same mix of DRGs) (Sullivan 1986). However, these statistical estimates were based on a 5 percent sample of Medicare patients. The lower limit of the 95 percent confidence interval for hospital A was a 1.9 percent fatality rate, and the upper limit for hospital B was a 7.3 percent fatality rate. In other words, hospital A may not have been worse than the national average, hospital B may not have been better than average, and there was a small chance that hospital A might be better than hospital B. For instance, two very severely ill heart-attack or gastrointestinal-hemorrhage cases could have made hospital A look bad. In summary, one should not be quick to generalize from 5 to 20 percent samples; analysts and consumer groups need the full data tape. Moreover, the performance of small hospitals may have to be analyzed with two to three years of compiled data to make statistically significant statements about the 10 to 20 most popular DRGs.

HCFA has tried to improve the predictive ability of the statistical model used in the 1991 release of "Medicare Hospital Mortality Information." This latest model included information on patient characteristics such as: principal diagnosis (grouped into 17 analytical risk categories), age, sex, previous hospital admissions within the prior six months, admission source (e.g., physician reference, skilled nursing facility reference), admission type (e.g., elective or emergency), and the presence of up to four comorbid conditions—cancer, chronic cardiovascular disease, chronic renal disease, and chronic liver disease. Two additional adjustments for patient risks were also carried out. First, account was taken of the effect of the specific reason for admission—the principal diagnosis within each analytic category—on the probability of patient death. Second, additional information was carried by the grouping of patients into clinically informative categories. This last adjustment proved particularly important in the case of the surgical categories. The early 1986 HCFA reports gave high grades to the hospitals that were efficient at discharge planning (minimizing terminal cases). For example, in the March 1986 report, the predicted death rate for Georgetown Hospital Medicare patients was, if equal to national average performance, 5.4 percent (Krakauer, 1986). The actual death rate was 1.9 percent, making this facility one of the fifty hospitals rated best. However, these ratings only considered case fatality rates, DRGs, and patient demographics. In reality, hospitals would have differing scores and severity ratings across departments and from year to year. The challenge for researchers is to make the rankings meaningful both statistically and for consumers trying to choose a hospital.

We have surveyed a number of severity systems in chapter 8, including the Horn et al. (1985) severity-of-illness (SOI) index and her computerized severity index (CSI), Brewster et al.'s (1985) key clinical findings (KCFs), Gonnella's (1984) disease staging, and Young's (1984) patient-management categories. The KCF system (MedisGroups) has the widest application, being used by over 600 hospitals (Iezzoni 1991). A fifth severity measure, the APACHE index (acute physiology and chronic health evaluation), done by Knaus et al. (1986), has been validated on intensive-care patients (Zimmerman 1989). This APACHE index is the only severity-of-illness measure that has been validated using clinical outcomes such as mortality and morbidity (Keeler et al. 1990). The streamlined second version of APACHE requires only 12 routine physiologic measurements, patient age, and chronic health status. The Knaus et al. (1986) study contained 10 teaching and 3 nonteaching hospitals. The best hospital had 41 percent fewer deaths among ICU patients than predicted utilizing the physiologic severity index. This particular teaching hospital had 69 predicted fatalities, but only 41 observed deaths, statistically significant at the 0.0001 level. In contrast, the worst-rated teaching hospital in the sample had 27 percent more deaths than expected (predicted 44, observed 56). The worst nonteaching hospital in the sample had 58 percent more deaths than expected (predicted 33, observed 52). There is much room for improvement in refining severity systems (Stearns 1991) and in refining the DRGs (MacKenzie, Steinwachs, and Ramzy 1991).

Pine et al. (1990) explored the limited effectiveness of quality-assurance screening using large but imperfect data bases. A number of studies have suggested that the federal approach at HCFA still has imperfections (HCFA 1991; Hartz et al. 1989). State government officials have been equally cautious in drawing conclusions. For example, the New York State Cardiac Surgery Reporting System labeled only 4 of 28 hospitals as having significantly low-quality mortality rates (Hannan et al. 1990). While there is no evidence in the October 1990 Rand Corporation study that Medicare quality of care has been harmed by the DRG system of payment (Kahn et al. 1990), more states need to fund Medicaid quality-assurance programs.

A Harvard University evaluation team (Leape et al. 1991) identified 27,179 adverse events involving negligence in New York hospitals during one year. Some adverse events may result from limited medical knowledge, and a large percentage result from simple management errors that are preventable. The Deming (1986) or Juran (1964) approaches to statistical quality control are two approaches to identifying causes and developing systems to prevent error or reduce its harmful impact on the patient. Quality-assurance (QA) programs are slowly improving in this direction (Casanova 1990; Kuperman et al. 1991; Kritchevsky and Simmons 1991).

SEVERITY MUST BE BALANCED WITH APPROPRIATENESS REVIEW

Quality scorecards without severity measures may lead to needless apprehension among patients for the one-third of DRGs that are severity sensitive. Brook et al. (1990) reported that being treated by a surgeon who performed a high volume of carotid endarterectomies decreased the likelihood of an appropriate operation by 35 percent. This type of severity-adjusted appropriateness review can attempt to document the additional increments of severity caused by bad-quality medicine or poor medical judgment (e.g., doing an elective operation on a terminal cancer case). For example, one teaching hospital defended its high fatality rates on the HCFA outlier list (Krakauer 1986) as being the result of seven unfortunate (fatal) operations on six terminal cancer cases and one total hip replacement operation on a wheelchair-bound patient with above-knee amputations. The fact that these cases were more severe explains why the fatality rates were high, but why were the operations done at all? Was the hernia operation going to cure the cancer? Was the hip operation going to make the patient walk? All concerned agreed that the answer to these questions was no. However, provider motivation to do inappropriate care had two aspects: senior attending physicians desired the additional income, and residents desired the extra patient volume since the teaching hospital occupancy rate had declined rapidly. The determinants of fatality rates (Alhaider and Wan 1991) are as difficult to model as predicting hospital choice (Adams et al. 1991).

Such ethical problems, producing needless pain and suffering, can be addressed with more aggressive appropriateness review. The more basic question is whether we run our medical care system for doctors or for patients. The question is raised not so much to nettle as to alert teaching hospitals that attempt to misuse severity as a defense for their high fatality rates. Such hospitals will discover that the defense that their patients are more severely ill may get the hospital into more hot water if the public discovers that the elderly were overtreated.

Each year, according to the Centers for Disease Control (1991), 20,000 Americans die because of nosocomial infections. One-third of the hospital-acquired infections could easily be prevented with better quality-control techniques, saving society an estimated $2 billion in direct hospital care costs (not counting the billions of dollars of other costs, forgone earnings, and pain and suffering). The very nature of Medicare PPS payments has fueled renewed interest in investing in quality control (Keeler et al. 1990). Fewer hospital-caused complications translate into a shorter patient stay at lower cost, more in line with the prospective payment price for the case. Consider one simple example, the common "catheter fever" nosocomial infection. One should take a catheterized patient's urine specimen out of the plastic bag with a syringe, rather than unhooking the bag and draining the urine into a specimen cup. This example also highlights the fact that quality is a function of both medical-staff and hospital employee behavior (Eastaugh 1986).

The Federal Role

Federally financed PROs are surveying a wide array of quality measures, including (1) department fatality rates for cases with length of stay in excess of one day (given that some hospitals receive a disproportionate share of critically ill patients who cannot be immediately stabilized); (2) abnormally high rates of inpatient admission following outpatient surgery; (3) abnormally high readmission rates 30 to 60 days following discharge; (4) abnormally high rates of transfer for medical complications after the hospital treated the patient for more than two days; and (5) excessively high rates of adverse patient occurrences (APO morbidity events, i.e., an infection not present on admission, unexpected cardiac or respiratory arrest, unexpected deterioration leading to transfer into a critical-care unit, unplanned return to the operating room, or pathology tissue diagnosis not matching the patient diagnosis). If all these alternative measures of quality agree, then they provide independent confirmation of the validity of labeling a hospital good or bad.

Consumers also have their foibles. Just as individual doctors have a practice-style pattern or "clinician signature," so certain consumers have a consumption pattern or "demander signature" (e.g., to get the inappropriate drug prescribed or procedure done). Increased consumer education is warranted. If the federal government cannot afford it, employers may have to finance the effort (Eastaugh 1986; McClure 1985). If consumers are to reap the benefits of information disclosure on quality, they could assist the effort through personal word-of-mouth advertising and alert value shopping for the best providers to meet their needs.

Shifting Concerns in Consumer Behavior

Health care consumers are beginning to learn that ''what you don't know can hurt you.'' Current questioning of the traditional model of the physician acting as the patient's agent, called agency theory, offers a number of challenges to the medical profession. If doctors do not send their patients to the best hospitals, but in fact make decisions for reasons of income maximization or travel minimization, as suggested by a number of studies (Luft et al. 1990b; Flood, Scott, and Ewy 1984), one should bury the idea that ''doctor knows best.'' Hospital quality does vary widely, and the public would benefit from reading a valid summary scorecard on quality, disaggregated by logical groupings of similar elective conditions (high, moderate, or low risk; probable surgical versus non-surgical). Information on nonelective conditions would be less valuable for shopping considerations, especially for trauma cases. Consumers are increasingly coming to realize that it would be desirable to have the facts before choosing a hospital and, in turn, a doctor. This is a reversal of past tendencies to select the doctor first and let the doctor make the subsequent decisions. Surveys by the American Hospital Association suggest that physicians made only 39 percent of all nonemergency hospital selection in 1983 (Professional Research Consultants 1984). Consumers have become even more involved in selecting the hospital where they are to be treated over the last four years. Consequently, this figure now may be well below 25 percent. Consumers often make the de facto selection of a hospital by selecting certain HMOs or managed-care options.

Consumers select providers on the basis of imperfect information, and the extent of their rational (and semirational) search behavior suggests an ongoing process in which they seek their own balance between technical quality (e.g., outcome statistics), personal care-giving quality, and out-of-pocket price. If their perceptions of these three attributes become, on balance, sufficiently unattractive, they will search for new providers (Bolton and Drew 1991; MacStravic 1991). Shock waves would resonate through the provider community if only 10 to 20 percent of patients comparison shopped. The health care delivery system has always been controlled by the element in short supply: previously the doctors, currently the patients. A lack of response from the majority of consumers can be predicted if two basic conditions occur: (1) information overload from too many conflicting and divergent sources, and (2) information ''underload'' because the informational content of the data is low. Information disclosure will be most effective when the data are packaged in nontechnical simplified ratings and reported for a list of possible local providers. The data presentation could be popularized in a convincing manner with a five-star rating system for a number of inpatient service lines. Five stars imply excellent quality; one star implies poor quality.

MORTALITY RATES: ONE MEASURE OF SERVICE QUALITY

In December 1989 an article by Hartz et al. (1989) confirmed the conventional wisdom of a link between hospital mortality rates and the quality of care. The

Table 9.1
Confidence Intervals of 90 Percent for Binomial Distributions of 1991 Death Counts and Severity-adjusted Mortality at Hospital Z

DRG	Number of Patients	Severity-adjusted Expected Dead	Actual Dead at Z	Upper 90 Percent Confidence Interval
127	986	92.39	151*a	127
14	571	74.84	82	97
89	549	63.92	90*	83
82	173	40.53	59*	53
87	168	38.20	55*	50
416	140	31.89	32	41
79	104	24.15	31	31
296	393	19.85	18	26
299	368	19.70	25	26
110	152	17.68	24*	23
239	156	13.29	20*	18
138	393	11.92	14	17
130	195	11.48	19*	16
403	99	10.96	15	16
132	150	9.03	11	14
182	853	8.87	13	14
209	348	6.99	6	10
15	349	3.65	4	6
243	396	3.64	7*	6

[a]The asterisk denotes mortality rates in excess of the 90 percent confidence interval.

Hartz study linked an outcome measure (mortality, severity adjusted to some degree) with peer review judgments of quality of care in PRO panels. These results may apply only to inpatient elderly Medicare cases, but other researchers are studying data bases for all ages (Lohr 1990).

External users of quality-control information utilize the 10 and 90 percentile confidence interval in a different way. The regulatory emphasis is on tagging bad performers annually, rather than plotting performance at one facility over a number of days or weeks and trying to improve it. Consumers should try to vote with their feet to avoid the hospital in table 9.1, where actual death rates fall at the high end of the predicted range for half the most prevalent DRGs. The opposite situation applies in table 9.2, where the hospital is better than 9 in 10 hospitals for two-thirds of the DRGs listed. The risk-adjusted mortality rates

Table 9.2
Confidence Intervals of 90 Percent for Binomial Distributions of 1991 Death Counts and Severity-adjusted Mortality at Hospital A

DRG	Number of Patients	Severity-adjusted Expected Dead	Actual Dead at A	Lower 90 Percent Confidence Interval
127	2,071	205.41	126*a	137
14	1,319	186.72	109*	125
89	1,235	155.96	101*	104
82	414	104.84	72	70
87	369	89.38	51*	60
416	266	64.72	39*	43
79	211	50.31	29	34
296	917	48.63	39	33
299	718	40.58	22*	27
110	280	35.18	29	24
239	359	31.89	18*	21
138	882	28.25	11*	19
130	394	23.72	14*	16
403	181	20.95	10*	13
132	266	16.93	12	10
182	1,442	15.07	8*	9
209	678	14.21	11	8
15	802	8.51	1*	3
243	733	6.94	3	2

aThe asterisk denotes mortality rates better (lower) than the 90 percent confidence interval.

presented in these tables employ different statistical techniques depending on the frequency of mortality. For most DRGs, representing 84 percent of patient admission, a contingency-table model must be employed because the mortality rate is less than 5.0 percent (DesHarnais 1990). Low-mortality DRGs are not reported in the tables. However, a more detailed logistic model can be employed for the 65 DRGs, representing 74 percent of deaths and 16 percent of discharges, where the mortality rate is 5.0 percent or higher. These logistic regressions should include items like patient-severity comorbid conditions (Medical Technology and Practice Patterns Institute [MTPPI] 1991). Earlier work with smaller sample sizes (e.g., Greenfield et al. 1988) revealed wide variations among hospitals in patient age, severity, and the burden of comorbid conditions. The teaching hospitals with high crude-mortality rates may also have the highest comorbidity burden, and this must be corrected for in any valid risk-adjusted mortality index (RAMI). The hospital listed in table 9.2 was a below-average performer in mortality-rate terms in the federal HCFA statistics, but the results from the RAMI demonstrate that the facility is in fact better (fewer deaths) than 90 percent of hospitals when patient severity is factored into the analysis.

All great hospitals are not equally great across all departments. Moreover, effectiveness for certain services like ambulatory care cannot be measured by mortality rates or morbidity rates (Taulbee 1991). A certain teaching hospital may be in the 99th percentile for mortality rates, morbidity rates, or consumer satisfaction in some departments and rated between the 40th and 80th percentiles in other departments. In some cases the best hospitals in certain service product lines may be small or moderate-sized facilities. Consumers should inquire about quality ratings of specific departments where possible.

PATIENT-CENTERED SELF-REPORTING OF QUALITY?

The basic data sources for quality and access studies are presented in table 9.3. A consumers' utility function in weighing the multiattribute dimension they label as "quality care" may vary widely according to education of the rater, experience, and the clinical disease in question (Lehr and Strosberg 1991). Technological sophistication may be highly important to the educated cardiology consumer, but less relevant in selecting a rheumatology provider. Participation in clinical trials may be a positive attribute for cancer and AIDS patients, but irrelevant to the average consumer seeking neurology, ear, or eye care. The quality of nursing services may be highly important for AIDS care or rehabilitation, but less important for ophthalmology care (SHS 1991). The crude RN-to-patient staffing ratio is a poor predictor of nursing quality; for example, San Francisco General Hospital with 0.8 RNs per patient can give better-rated nursing care than facilities with 50 percent more RNs and very few nurse extender technicians.

The 1990 Institute of Medicine study, *A Strategy for Quality Assurance*, was groundbreaking for a National Academy of Sciences study team because it went beyond using the model of expert/professional dominance to suggest that consumers have a right to assess quality. The Institute of Medicine study team suggested that perhaps in a restructured PRO program some patient-centered perspectives on quality might be studied. The report cited the Picker/Commonwealth patient-centered project of Dr. Thomas Delbanco at Beth Israel Hospital in Boston. He will publish in 1992 a book on patient-centered care, patient education, and patient satisfaction, based on surveys of 6,500 patients at 62 hospitals. With patient satisfaction come better patient compliance and higher-quality long-run clinical outcomes. Medicine and surgery have to become more patient focused if the quality of our health care system is to improve. This viewpoint is also endorsed by DHHS Secretary Dr. Louis Sullivan, who often states that consumers and physicians must work together to enhance quality and

Table 9.3
Three Data Sources for Obtaining Information on Quality, Utilization, and Access to Health Care

	Patient Report	Administrative Data	Medical Record
1. Outcomes of care	Richest source of data on patient function.	Useful for assessing mortality and other selected outcomes likely to be recorded on claims.	Useful for some outcomes, but data on many outcomes are frequently missing, and functional status is missing.
2. Technical aspects of care	Patients may be good reporters, but recall of past visits is untested.	Not useful.	Data may be available only on most important processes.
3. Diagnostic tests	Patients recall testing in general terms but may not know details.	If available, may be best source of data, although test results will not be available	Good source, particularly for abnormal test results, but hospital records may miss data on outpatient tests.
4. Medications	Fair source of information on current medications.	If available, may be good source for certain types of medications.	Good source for important drugs; other drugs may not be recorded.
5. Symptoms	May be best source of information.	Not useful.	Limited data, generally on most important symptoms.
6. Access to care	May be best source of information.	Data on frequency of visits only.	Data on frequency of visits only.

Sources: Eastaugh 1986; Siu et al. 1991.

solve the corrosive problems that cloud our future as a leading nation and as a strong, yet compassionate people.

ORGANIZED MEDICINE AND REGULATORY PHILOSOPHY

In practice, hospitals will trim low-quality, low-volume departments before they consider closing the entire hospital. For these low-volume, poor-quality, high-cost departments, the best solution may well be competition through information disclosure. Patients can break the habit of going to such a facility, whereas professional groups often try to hide the problem. For lack of competition and information, low-quality operators have been able to avoid bankruptcy; cost reimbursement underwrote their unit costs, no matter how high. If one in six hospitals goes out of business, how will this affect the careers of physicians?

Organized medicine has offered a festoon of arguments for not releasing report cards on provider quality. Analysts are correct in pointing out that without a severity adjustment per patient, one may not be able to discriminate between a 38th percentile two-star hospital and a 62d percentile four-star hospital. In such cases where the measurable differences in quality may be small and may fluctuate up and down from year to year, the differences in cost may be more relevant to the purchaser of care. Consequently, one could advise employees and employers to utilize economic criteria, access, and other criteria to differentiate two- to four-star hospitals. Users of the ratings should be confident that a one-star hospital is in fact a below-average hospital. Likewise, a five-star hospital is in fact an above-average hospital. What will happen if we do not tout the good news about five-star hospitals? Patient flow to such hospitals may decline in a price-competitive marketplace. One business executive of a large Fortune 500 company had a chilling rejoinder: "I don't care if 900 to 1,000 hospitals close over the coming five years, just as long as 100 of those Council of Teaching Hospitals members close. They are too expensive in the states we do business." Valid quality report cards, and not economics, may well be the trump card for survival among the expensive five-star hospitals.

WANTED: QUALITY ENHANCEMENT

Five-star hospitals might gain more patients than they can, or wish to, accommodate. However, higher volume will allow the hospital departments to, in the jargon of economics, slide down their average cost curves and take advantage of economies of scale (Eastaugh and Eastaugh 1986). Because consumers are constrained by travel costs, time costs, and out-of-pocket care costs, the problem of too many patients going to good hospitals seems a minor problem in the current low-occupancy marketplace. On the other end of the scale, perhaps the low-quality hospitals will be "disciplined" by the marketplace to go out of business. Those patients who shop deserve and receive better value for their money. Conservatives would suggest that those who remain with their inferior-quality providers deserve whatever they receive. Regulators would argue that the government should close some low-quality hospitals. If the medical profession gets more serious about its own independent investigations and fullfills the paradigm of the self-policing professional, licensing groups will give out more sanctions, expulsions, punishments, and mandatory exams.

If the medical profession does not police itself, and protect the public from low quality providers, government review programs will expand. Market philosophy views technical quality as being simply another attribute, taken together with price, place (access), bedside manner, and hospital religious orientation, on which customers may or may not choose. Government's role is limited to breaking the information asymmetry between providers and consumers by providing PRO statistics and data for private reanalysis on care quality.

One of the difficult problems for researchers is that it will be hard to discriminate between a hospital that has two or three unethical senior attending physicians and a facility where the majority of physicians and nurses could benefit from a substantial upgrade in performance quality. A retrospective data base may never by capable of pinpointing whether quality is a problem with 3 or 40 people in the organization. Researchers may have to expose the quality shortfalls and leave it up to the hospital to develop an effective remedial quality-control program. The hospital can then decide whether it desires to be ranked poor or excellent in the eyes of its public, in which case many hospitals may finally get tough with providers of inappropriate care who in the past produced appropriate revenue for the hospital and infrequent reprimand.

One could ask, especially if we have a doctor surplus, how many doctors should be disciplined by the marketplace and whether the discipline should end careers. Some substantial fraction of physicians suffer from problems that significantly impair their functioning at some point in their careers. The number so impaired at any one time may remain small, perhaps under 5 percent. Who do we have to monitor competence? As one "60 Minutes" television segment documented in November 1985, the state of Massachusetts had two medical licensure investigators, in contrast to eight hairdresser investigators. In comparison to the hairdressing profession, health-service consumer awareness is higher, and the dollar amounts are more significant. Physicians tend to be dedicated, hardworking individuals, subject to human foibles and fearful that quality disclosure will further erode the patient-physician relationship.

One could ask if there is a way to obtain consumer attention without resorting to overstatement. Politicians often sensationalize issues such as "premature discharges" and hospital deception concerning "what day your Medicare benefits run out under DRGs." Senator John Heinz (R., Pa.), chairman of the Senate Special Committee on Aging, claimed frequently during 1985–86 that "seriously ill Medicare patients are catapulted out of hospital doors prematurely." However, in the vast majority of these "documented abuse cases," physicians kept their patients in the "facility" until it seemed safe to discharge them (Ray, Griffin, and Baugh 1990).

The definition of what is included in the "facility" has substantially changed as hospitals diversify, initiate less expensive and more appropriate settings for patient care, and "unbundle" the patient episode. For example, hospitals increasingly transfer patients to "swing beds" (lower-cost nursing beds; Shaughnessy 1992), thus maintaining the elderly patient within a more appropriate setting, yet preserving continuity of care across the hospital/campus. When appropriate, providers often discharge the patient with follow-up home health care services (often owned and marketed by the hospital). In the marketing literature this situation is often summarized by the rather unattractive word "demarketing"—that is, directing the patient to more appropriate channels of cost-effective service distribution. If the measures of quality for the individual patient do not erode under this demarketing/diversification strategy, then no harm is done. Customers would be left to decide whether a differential advantage, or shortfall, in comparing providers is substantial enough to change their behavior. For some Americans a small differential on fatality or infection rates may be substantial, but to other customers this difference is insignificant, even if it is statistically significant at the 5 percent level.

DIRECT REGULATION OR BUYER BEWARE

The chief failing of the proregulatory school is in defining a "significant" national or local cutoff point beyond which the quality of care is judged so substandard as to justify closing the provider. The issues are more complex in medical care because the quality measures are more complex and subject to future refinements than in truck safety or meat safety. In the 1986 case of naval heart surgeon Donal Billig, a fatality rate 1.24 times the national average was judged "terrible." If 18 fatal cases among 240 is terrible because the national average performance is 5.9 percent (or 14 cases in 240), should the regulatory protectors of the quality of care be charged with finding those four bad results? Billig was tried on five cases (five of 65 died) and convicted on three. In some sense a 7.3 percent fatality rate was surprising, considering that Billig was legally blind with vision of 20/400, certainly a handicap for a member of the surgical profession.

Reactionary providers lobbying against consumer disclosure argue that patients should be interested in two attributes: access and continuity of service. They refuse to even call patients "consumers." In other words, consumers should know as much about the quality of health providers as they know about the quality of electricity. One might recall the ad copy "All you need to know about electricity is that it is there when you need it." Considering the highly personal and potentially final (critical, life-threatening) nature of health care, most of the population would desire more comprehensive information concerning provider quality. Everyone likes competitive information about what we buy, not about what we sell or provide.

Ultimately it is a question of regulatory philosophy as to whether one makes normative or absolute judgments about quality of care. The liberal proregulatory school of thought suggests that the national PRO should make absolute judgments as to what a minimum standard of care is and should close those 5 to 20 percent of hospitals that do not meet this standard. However, any imposed national standard is by definition arbitrary; for example, should we set it such that it closes 8 or 16 percent of hospitals? On the other side, the conservative market-oriented school would suggest that we simply publish the information, promote consumer awareness, and let the customers vote with their feet to close poor-quality hospitals. Customers would be left to decide whether a differential advantage or shortfall in comparing providers is substantial enough to change their behavior. For some Americans a small differential on fatality or infection rates may be substantial, but to other customers this difference may be insignificant, even if it is statistically significant at the 5 percent level.

Advocates of more regulation ask whether market mechanisms and the courts will close providers fast enough. Regulators, while having problems defining minimum standards or "fast enough," do have a point. Low-quality providers will be harmed by consumer disclosure in two ways (business volume and further quality erosion), but will not close if enough patients continue to visit. With more information, low-quality providers will lose even the patient volume necessary to maintain their substandard level of performance and will decline further in quality rating (if they can stay in business). At this point Peterson et al.'s (1956) "out-of-practice" (negative impact on quality) effects come into play, and it may be in the best interest of society to close the provider. However, most economists would counterargue that the press and the provider's financial state could close the business quicker than the courts.

CONSUMERISM AND RATIONING

Are hospitals to be more like restaurants, in which the public servant assures us against food poisoning, and the PRO critic provides a zero- to five-star rating of the quality before the discriminating consumer decides to trust the kitchen? Or do we leave the decision totally up to government regulators, as with taxicabs, to save us from making personal calculations on car safety and cost before consuming the service? Considering this mixed metaphor, physicians and hospital managers should weigh which hassle they dislike less: (1) answering the critics and improving the kitchen or (2) being rationed like taxicabs and burdened with substantially more paperwork. The facts seem to suggest that medical care providers are more like restaurants than taxicabs: The variability in quality is substantial, and taste is highly personalized. Sorting single-handedly through a barrage of restaurant or hospital ad copy is an onerous task. But having a five-star hospital guide available seems prudent. The guide would have a brief summary section for 6 to 12 basic hospital case types, followed by what would be a seldom-used lengthy appendix listing actual numerical quality scores on a number of measures by hospital department for popular DRGs.

People spend more time shopping for restaurants than selecting health care providers. Good information concerning quality has heretofore not attracted much attention. Customs will change over time. As the population listens to friends who summarize or share information from *Consumer Reports* on health care provider quality, behavior will change. To utilize the very frank term, "excess deaths" will decline. If providers attempt to falsely discredit *Consumer Reports* on quality, they will experience the lament of deregulated bankers and airline executives: Information talks, people walk (to those with the better numbers). Doctors can either steer patients to the best-quality hospitals for which they have admitting privileges or try to gain privileges at better hospitals.

The cash flow now channeled to low-quality hospitals and doctors is destined to decline because of better consumer information. If society lets the low-quality providers fail, closing out their fixed costs, the average quality-of-care level improves. This method would cost less than any regulatory method of rationing through price controls done by Medicare DRGs or alternative delivery systems. If we trust consumers with an array of quality ratings, the public will have the ability to directly insist on better-quality care. The surviving providers would function in a better-equipped and less tightly reimbursed environment. Resources dedicated to health care would certainly be better spent, which is good economics and good medicine (Epstein 1990).

Specialization can yield better service quality (Couch 1992). However, specialization of product-lines does not always occur, especially in two-hospital towns with equal financial strength and with equally matched medical staffs. For example, no product-lines have been dropped in the two-hospital city of Kalamazoo, Michigan. The 462 bed Catholic hospital Borgess Medical Center is in a medical arms race with the 478 bed Bronson Methodist Hospital. Each tries to maintain a prenatal center and cardiovascular team; while the local newspaper editor argues for consolidation of the duplicated $5.1 million helicopter service and specialization of certain product-lines. One hospital is better in prenatal care, while the second hospital is better in cardiovascular surgery. Dysfunctional competition prevents cost control and quality enhancement. Consequently, C. Everett Koop is correct in his 1991 public television assertion that two-hospital towns have 30 percent higher cost than one-hospital towns.

CONCLUSIONS

Relman (1988) labeled the rising outcomes/quality-measurement movement as the "third great revolution in medical care." If this dream is to come true, more research should be financed in the area of national practice standards. Perhaps Robert Brook was correct in stating that national practice standards will make better doctors, because a good cook always starts with a cookbook. The Brook generalization is also true in long-term care (Davis 1991).

Aggressive use of information on quality and cost has always been the principal advantage of any competitive industry (Dunlop 1980; Stigler 1961). Valid quality measures that provide easily understandable rankings for public consumption will prove eye-opening for patients, payers, and physicians (Fleming 1991). Hospitals and physicians will have to exist in a world of more aggressive comparison shoppers, including individuals, employers, and insurance companies. The major weakness that researchers perceive in the current vision of scorecards and directories is a failure to adjust for patient severity of illness within DRGs. Consumer power, from the provider viewpoint (more irritating, but better informed), will force institutions to invest more in quality-enhancing efforts.

In a quality-competitive marketplace, it becomes even more important for clinicians to ally themselves with good-quality hospitals and more strongly support the Deming approach (1986, 1982). Until recently a simple doctrine existed that said that competition would not work in health care, patients would not shop, and all "credentialed" doctors and hospitals offered approximately the same quality of care. The simple doctrine has died. Consider the popular joke among medical school students concerning what they should call the lowest-quality graduate in their class. Answer: doctor. A quality physician is as unhappy as anybody else about incompetent clinicians who give physicians a bad name. Future research should consider how accurately performance in residency programs and medical school predict postgraduate quality of care in practice.

REFERENCES

Adams, E., Houchens, R., Wright, G., and Robbins, J. (1991). "Predicting Hospital Choice: Role of Severity of Illness." *Health Services Research* 26:5 (December), 566–584.

Alhaider, A., and Wan, T. (1991). "Modeling Organizational Determinants of Hospital Mortality." *Health Services Research* 26:3 (August), 303–24.

American Hospital Association. (1992). *Quality Measurement and Management*. Chicago: HRET Report, AHA.

Anderson, J., Bush, J., and Berry, C. (1986). "Classifying Function for Health Outcome and Quality of Life Evaluation." *Medical Care* 24:5 (May), 454–470.

Benson, D., and Townes, P. (1991). *Excellence in Ambulatory Care*. San Francisco: Jossey-Bass.

Berwick, D. (1989). "Continuous Improvement as an Ideal in Health Care." *New England Journal of Medicine* 320:1 (January 5), 53–56.

Bodendorf, F., and Mackey, F. (1986). "Evaluating a Hospital's IQ: Indicators of Quality." *Medical Benefits* 3:9 (May 15), 1–3.

Bolton, R., and Drew, J. (1991). "Multistage Model of Customers' Assessments of Service, Quality and Value," *Journal of Consumer Research* 17:4 (March). 375–384.

Brewster, A., et al. (1985). "MEDISGRPS: A Clinically Based Approach to Classifying Hospital Patients at Admission." *Inquiry* 22:4 (Winter), 377–387.

Brewster, J. (1986). "Prevalence of Alcohol and Other Drug Problems among Physicians." *Journal of the American Medical Association* 225:14 (April 11), 1913–1920.

Brook, R., and Lohr, K. (1985). "Efficacy, Effectiveness Variations, and Quality: Boundary-Crossing Research." *Medical Care* 23:5 (May), 710–722.

Brook, R., Park, R., Chassin, M., and Solomon, D. (1990). "Predicting Appropriate Use of Carotid Endarterectomy, Upper Gastrointestinal Endoscopy, and Coronary Angiography." *New England Journal of Medicine* 323:17 (October 25), 1173–1177.

Caldwell, C., McEachern, J., and Davis, V. (1990). "Measurement Tools Eliminate Guesswork." *Healthcare Forum Journal* 11:4 (July/August), 23–28.

Casalou, R. (1991). "Total Quality Management in Health Care." *Hospital and Health Services Administration* 36:1 (Spring), 134–146.

Casanova, J. (1990). "Status of Quality Assurance Programs in American Hospitals." *Medical Care* 28:11 (November) 1104–1109.

Centers for Disease Control. (1991). *Study on the Efficacy of Nosocomial Infection Control.* Washington, D. C.: DHHS.

Couch, J. (1992). *Health Care Quality Management for the 21st Century.* Tampa: American College of Physician Executives.

Cunningham, L. (1991). *The Quality Connection in Health Care.* San Francisco: Jossey-Bass.

Daley, J., and Kellie, S. (1991). *Guidebook on Uses of Mortality Data: Applications in Hospital Quality Assurance Activities.* Chicago: American Medical Association.

Dans, P., Weiner, J., and Otter, S. (1985). "Peer Review Organizations: Promises and Potential Pitfalls." *New England Journal of Medicine* 313:18 (October 31), 1131–1137.

Davis, M. (1991). "Nursing Home Quality: A Review and Analysis." *Medical Care Review* 48:2 (Summer), 129–165.

Deming, W. (1986). *Out of the Crisis.* Cambridge, Mass.: Massachusetts Institute of Technology Press, Center for Advanced Engineering.

Deming, W. (1982). *Quality, Productivity, and Competitive Position.* Cambridge, Mass.: Massachusetts Institute of Technology Press.

DesHarnais, S. (1990). "Current Uses of Large Data Sets to Assess the Quality of Providers: Construction of Risk-adjusted Indexes of Hospital Performance." *International Journal of Technology Assessment in Health Care* 6:2 (Spring) 229–238.

DesHarnais, S., McMahon, L., and Wroblewski, R. (1991). "Measuring Outcomes of Hospital Care Using Risk-adjusted Indexes." *Health Services Research* 26:4 (October), 425–446.

Donabedian, A. (1968). "Promoting Quality through Evaluating Patient Care." *Medical Care* 6:1 (January), 181–202.

Dubois, R. (1990). "Inherent Limitations of Hospital Death Rates to Assess Quality." *International Journal of Technology Assessment in Health Care* 6:2 (Spring) 220–227.

Dunlop, J. (1980). *Business and Public Policy.* Cambridge, Mass.: Harvard University Press.

Eastaugh, S. (1986). "Hospital Quality Scorecards: The Role of the Informed Consumer." *Hospital and Health Services Administration* 31:6 (November/December), 85–102.

———. (1983). "Placing a Value on Life and Limb: The Role of the Informed Consumer." *Health Matrix* 1:1 (Winter), 5–21.

Eastaugh, S., and Eastaugh, J. (1986). "Prospective Payment Systems: Further Steps to Enhance Quality, Efficiency, and Regionalization." *Health Care Management Review* 11:4 (Fall), 37–52.

Epstein, A. (1990). "The Outcomes Movement—Will It Get Us Where We Want to Go?" *New England Journal of Medicine* 323:4 (July 26), 266–270.

Fleming, S. (1991). "The Relationship between Quality and Cost: Pure and Simple." *Inquiry* 28:1 (Spring) 29–38.

Fleming, S., McMahon, L., and DesHarnais, S. (1991). "The Measurement of Mortality: Risk-adjusted Variable Time Window Approach." *Medical Care* 29:9 (September), 815–828.

Flood, A., Scott, W., and Ewy, W. (1984). "Does Practice Make Perfect?" *Medical Care* 22:2 (February), 98–125.

Friedman, M. (1965). *Capitalism and Freedom*. Chicago: University of Chicago Press.

Gonnella, J., Hornbrook, M., and Louis, D. (1984). "Staging of Disease: A Case-Mix Measurement." *Journal of the American Medical Association* 251:5 (February 3), 637–644.

Green, J., Passman, L., and Wintfeld, N. (1991). "Analyzing Hospital Mortality: The Consequences of Diversity in Patient Mix." *Journal of the American Medical Association* 265:14 (April 10), 1849–1853.

Greenfield, S., Aronow, H., Elashoff, R., and Watanabe, D. (1988). "Flaws in Mortality Data: The Hazards of Ignoring Comorbid Disease." *Journal of the American Medical Association* 260:15 (October 21), 2253–2255.

Greenfield, S., Nelson, E., and Zubkoff, M. (1992). "Variations in Resource Utilization among Medical Specialties." *JAMA* 267:12 (March 25), 1624–1630.

Guaspari, J. (1989). *I Know It When I See It: A Modern Fable about Quality*. New York: AMACOM.

Hall, J., Epstein, A., and McNeil, B. (1989). "Multidimensionality of Health Status in an Elderly Population." *Medical Care* 27:3 (March), 168S–177S.

Hannan, E., Kilburn, H., O'Donnell, J., Lukacik, G., and Shields, E. (1990). "Adult Open Heart Surgery in New York State: Analysis of Risk Factors and Hospital Mortality Rates." *Journal of the American Medical Association* 264:21 (December 5), 2768–2774.

Hartz, A., Krakauer, H., Kuhn, E., Young, M., and Jacobsen, S. (1989). "Hospital Characteristics and Mortality Rates." *New England Journal of Medicine* 321:25 (December 21), 1720–1725.

Hass, D., and Savoca, E. (1990). "Quality and Provider Choice: A Multinomial Logit-Least-Squares Model with Selectivity." *Health Services Research* 24:6 (February), 791–809.

Health Care Financing Administration (HCFA). (1991). *Medicare Hospital Mortality Information: Summary Information and Methodology*. Washington, D.C.: HCFA, DHHS.

———. (1985). *Federal Register* 50:12 (April 17), 312–322.

Herrmann, J. (1990). "Buying Health Services from a List of the Highest Quality: The Cleveland Initiative." *Federation of American Health Systems Review* 23:6 (November–December), 26–31.

Horn, S., and Horn, R. (1986). "The Computerized Severity Index: A New Tool for Case-Mix Management." *Journal of Medical Systems* 10:1, 73–79.

Horn, S., et al. (1985). "Interhospital Differences in Severity of Illness: Problems for

Prospective Payment Based on DRGs.'' *New England Journal of Medicine* 313:1 (July 4), 20–24.

Iezzoni, L., Ash, A., and Coffman, G. (1991). "Admission and Mid-Stay MEDISGRPS Scores as Predictors of Death.'' *American Journal of Public Health* 81:1 (January), 74–78.

Institute of Medicine. (1990). *A Strategy for Quality Assurance*. Washington, D.C.: National Academy of Sciences Press.

Ishikawa, K. (1989). *Guide to Quality Control*. Tokyo: Asian Productivity Organization.

Joint Commission on Accreditation of Healthcare Organizations (JCAHO). (1991). *Report of the Joint Commissions Survey*. Chicago: Joint Commission on Accreditation of Healthcare Organizations.

Juran, J. (1964). *Managerial Breakthrough*. New York: McGraw-Hill.

Kahn, K., Rubenstein, L., Draper, D., Kosecoff, J., Keeler, E., and Brook, R. (1990). "Effects of the DRG-based PPS on Quality of Care for Hospitalized Medicare Patients.'' *Journal of the American Medical Association* 264:15 (October 17), 1953–1961.

Keeler, E., Kahn, K., Draper, D., and Sherwood, M. (1990). "Changes in Sickness at Admission Following the Introduction of PPS.'' *Journal of the American Medical Association* 264:15 (October 17), 1962–1968.

Kisner, K. (1992). "Partnership Takes Gamble to Measure Quality.'' *Business and Health* 11:3 (March), 20–27.

Knaus, W., Wagner, D., and Joanne, L. (1991). "Short-term Hospital Prediction for Critically Ill Hospital Patients.'' *Science* 254:18 (October 18), 389–394.

Knaus, W., Draper, E., Wagner, D., and Zimmerman, J. (1986). "An Evaluation of Outcome from Intensive Care in Major Medical Centers.'' *Annals of Internal Medicine* 104:3 (March), 410–418.

Krakauer, H. (1986). "The Prediction of Statistical Outliers Based on Medicare Fatality Rates, Report (March), Office of Medical Care Review.'' Health Standards and Quality Bureau, Health Care Financing Administration, DHHS.

Kritchevsky, S., and Simmons, B. (1991). "Continuous Quality Improvement.'' *Journal of the American Medical Association* 266:13 (October 2), 1817–1823.

Kuperman, G., James, B., Jacobsen, J., and Gardner, R. (1991). "Continuous Quality Improvement Applied to Medical Care.'' *Medical Decision Making* 11:4 (October–December), S60–S64.

Leape, L., Brennan, T., Laird, N., Lawthers, A., Newhouse, J., Weiler, P., and Hiatt, H. (1991). "The Nature of Adverse Events in Hospitalized Patients.'' *New England Journal of Medicine* 324:6 (February 7), 377–384.

Lehr, H, and Strosberg, M. (1991). "Quality Improvement in Health Care: Is the Patient Still Left Out?'' *Quality Review Bulletin* 17:10 (October), 326–330.

Lohr, K. (1990). "Use of Insurance Claims Data in Measuring Quality of Care.'' *International Journal of Technology Assessment in Health Care*. 6:2 (Spring), 263–270.

Luft, H., Garnick, D., and Mark, D. (1990). "Does Quality Influence Choice of Hospital?'' *Journal of the American Medical Association* 263:21 (June 6), 2899–2906.

Luft, H., Garnick, D., Mark, D., and McPhee, S. (1990). *Hospital Volume, Physician Volume, and Patient Outcome: Assessing the Evidence*. Ann Arbor, Mich.: Health Administration Press.

Luft, H., and Hunt, S. (1986). "Evaluating Individual Hospital Quality through Outcome

Statistics.'' *Journal of the American Medical Association* 255:20 (May 30), 2780–2784.

Lynn, M., and Osborn, D. (1991). "Deming's Quality Principles: A Health Care Application.'' *Hospital and Health Services Administration* 36:1 (Spring), 111–119.

MacKenzie, E., Steinwachs, D., and Ramzy, A. (1991). "Trauma Case-Mix and Hospital Payment: Refining DRGs.'' *Health Services Research* 26:1 (April), 3–22.

MacStravic, R. (1991). *Beyond Patient Satisfaction: Building Patient Loyalty*, Ann Arbor, Mich.: Health Administration Press.

McClure, W. (1985). "Buying Right: The Consequences of Glut.'' *Business and Health* 2:9 (September), 43–46.

Manheim, L., Feinglass, J., and Hughes, R. (1992). "Regional Variation in Medicare Mortality Rate.'' *Inquiry* 29:1 (Spring), 55–65.

Medical Technology and Practice Patterns Institute (MTPPI). (1991). "Report on Medicare Hospital Mortality Statistics: A Detailed Analysis of the Mortality Profile.'' Medical Technology and Practice Patterns Institute, Washington, D.C.

Milakovich, M. (1991). "Creating a Total Quality Environment.'' *Health Care Management Review* 16:2 (Spring), 9–20.

Morley, J. (1991). "Cleveland Health Quality Choice Program.'' *Federation of American Health Systems Review* 24:1 (January–February), 40.

Murray, J., Greenfield, S., and Yano, E. (1992). " Ambulatory Testing for Capitation and Fee-for-service Patients: Relationship to Outcomes.'' *Medical Care* 30:3 (March), 252–261.

Neuhauser, D. (1988). "The Quality of Medical Care and the 14 Points of Edwards Deming.'' *Health Matrix* 6:2 (Summer), 7–10.

O'Leary, D. (1986). "JCAH New Series of Quality Indicators Based on Outcome, Clinical Standards.'' *Federation of American Health Systems* 19:3 (May/June), 26–27.

Peters, G. (1991). "Fixing the Quick Fixes to Physician Relations.'' *Healthcare Financial Management* 45:11 (November), 36–50.

Peterson, O., et al. (1956). "An Analytic Study of North Carolina Medical Practice, 1953–54.'' *Journal of Medical Education* 31:12 (December), 1–165.

Pine, M., Rogers, D., Morgan, D., and Beller, R. (1990). "Potential Effectiveness of Quality Assurance Screening Using Large But Imperfect Databases.'' *Medical Decision Making* 10:2 (April–June), 126–134.

Poses, R., Bekes, C., Copare, F., and Scott, W. (1990). "What Difference Do Two Days Make? Inertia of Physicians' Sequential Prognostic Judgements.'' *Medical Decision Making* 10:1 (January–March), 6–14.

Professional Research Consultants, Inc. (1984). "Marketing Surge Tied to Consumers.'' *Hospitals* 58:12 (June 16), 33–35.

Ray, W., Griffin, M., and Baugh, D. (1990). "Mortality Following Hip Fracture before and after Implementation of the Prospective Payment System.'' *Archives of Internal Medicine* 150:10 (October), 2109–2114.

Re, R., and Krousel-Wood, M. (1990). "How to Use Continuous Quality Improvement Theory and Statistical Quality Control Tools in a Multispecialty Clinic.'' *Quality Review Bulletin* 16:11 (November), 391–397.

Relman, A. (1988). "Assessment and Accountability: The Third Revolution in Medical Care.'' *New England Journal of Medicine* 319:23 (December), 1220–1222.

Roemer, M., Moustafa, A., and Hopkins, C. (1968). "A Proposed Hospital Quality

Index: Hospital Death Rates Adjusted for Case Severity.'' *Health Services Research* 3:2 (Summer), 96–118.

Sahney, V. (1991). ''Quest for Quality and Productivity in Health Services.'' *Frontiers of Health Services Management* 7:4 (Summer), 3–22.

Sahney, V., Dutkewych, J., and Schramm, W. (1989). ''Quality Improvement Process: Foundation for Excellence in Health Care.'' *Journal of the Society for Health Systems* 1:1, 17–30.

Shaughnessy, P. (1992). *Shaping Policy for Long-term Care: Learning from the Effectiveness of Hospital Swing Beds*, Ann Arbor, Michigan: Health Administration Press.

Siu, A., McGlynn, E., Morgenstern, H., and Brook, R. (1991). ''A Fair Approach to the Quality of Care.'' *Health Affairs* 10:1 (Spring), 62–75.

Sloan, F., Perrin, J., and Valvona, J. (1986). ''In-Hospital Mortality of Surgical Patients: Is There an Empirical Basis for Standard-Setting?'' *Surgery* 99:4 (April), 446–454.

Sloan, F., Valvona, J., Perrin, J., and Adamache, K. (1986). ''Diffusion of Surgical Technology: An Exploratory Study.'' *Journal of Health Economics* 5:1 (March), 31–62.

Society for Health Systems (SHS). (1991). *Proceedings of the Quest for Quality Conference*, Norcross, Georgia: Industrial Engineering & Management Press.

Stearns, S. (1991). ''Hospital Discharge Decisions, Outcomes, and the Use of Unobserved Information on Case-Mix Severity.'' *Health Services Research* 26:1 (April), 27–51.

Stigler, G. (1961). ''The Economics of Information.'' *Journal of Political Economy* 69:3 (May), 213–225.

Stoskopf, C., and Horn, S. (1992). ''Predicting Length of Stay.'' *Health Services Research* 26:6, 749–765.

Sullivan, R. (1986). ''Leading Hospital Accused of Poor Care.'' *New York Times*, March 4, B–3.

Tarlov, A., Ware, J., Greenfield, S., Nelson, E., Perrin, E., and Zubkoff, M. (1989). ''The Medical Outcomes Study: Application of Methods for Monitoring the Results of Medical Care.'' *Journal of the American Medical Association* 262:6 (August 18), 925–930.

Taulbee, P. (1991). ''Outcomes Management: Buying Value and Cutting Costs.'' *Business and Health* 9:3 (March), 28–39.

U.S. Congress. (1986). Health Care Quality Improvement Act, Title IV of Public Law, 99–660.

Veney, J., and Kaluzny, A. (1991). *Evaluation and Decision Making for Health Services*, 2d ed. Ann Arbor, Mich.: Health Administration Press.

Walton, M. (1990). *Deming Management at Work*. New York: G. P. Putnam's, 99.

Ware, J., and Berwick, D. (1990). ''Patient Judgements of Hospital Quality: Report of a Pilot Study.'' *Medical Care* 28:9 (September), S39–S48.

Webber, A. (1986). ''Status of the PRO Program.'' *Federation of American Health Systems Review* 19:3 (May/June), 28–29.

Williamson, J. (1988). ''Future Policy Directions for Quality Assurance: Lessons from Health Accounting Experience.'' *Inquiry* 25:1 (Spring), 67–77.

———. (1978). *Assessing and Improving Outcomes in Health Care: The Theory and Practice of Health Accounting*. Cambridge, Mass.: Ballinger.

Wolfe, S. (1986). "Consumer Information on Hospital Quality." *Public Citizen Health Letter* 2:4 (September/October), 1.
Young, W. (1984). "Incorporating Severity and Comorbidity in Case-Mix Measurement." *Health Care Financing Review* 5:4 (Supp.), 23–32.
Zimmerman, J. (1989). "APACHE III Study Design: Selected Articles." *Critical Care Medicine* 17:12 (December Supplement), S169–S221.

10 Health Manpower Policies, Physician Extenders, and Nursing Education

The study of costs for nursing education, in a decade which forecasts curtailing enrollments in general and further economic retrenchment, cannot be overemphasized.

—Elsa L. Brown

Hospitals have shifted an increasingly costly nurse training program onto the public sector.... with a decline in subsidy many programs will have to close. To the extent that the earnings of an RN plus the nonmonetary benefits of nursing provide a "surplus" above the most attractive alternative occupation, a student will be willing to pay for part or all of their training. As one moves from the truly dedicated nurse to those whose attachment to the profession is more marginal, the amount they are willing to invest declines.

—Stuart H. Altman

The health economy is the nation's second-largest employer. In the period 1989–91 the health sector gained nearly 1 million jobs, bringing total industry employment to 8.8 million. During the 1990–91 recession, when manufacturing lost 550,000 jobs and construction lost 420,000 jobs, the health care business was expanding. After years of policy studies concerning low wages in the nursing sector (e.g., Aiken 1990), nurses' wages improved markedly. Annual inflation in the starting wage for registered nurses (RNs) increased from 3.8 percent in the period 1983–87 to 5.4 percent in the period 1988–91. The wage improvement was even more pronounced for annual inflation in the maximum wage rate for RNs: 4.5 percent in the period 1983–87, more than doubling to 9.7 percent in the period 1988–91. The labor market has worked more effectively in recent years, as senior RNs in short supply get better wage hikes (Roberts et al. 1989). However, a number of noneconomic problems exist in the nursing profession that go beyond the creation of better career ladders for nurses (Stein, Watts, and

Howell 1990; Hepner 1990). Nurses are changing roles and placing their profession in the center of the cost/quality/access debate (Zander 1990).

In the period 1970–91 the number of nurses working in the nation increased from 751,000 to 1.66 million. Hospitals that employed 0.48 nurses per patient in 1970 now employ 1.15 nurses per patient on average. Nurses are also branching into specialty midlevel provider areas like nurse anesthetists or geriatric nurse practitioners. Some optimistic health care professionals claim that health workers will continue to grow in the 1990s as the need for RNs expands by 42 percent, the need for home health aides and occupational therapists expands by 53 percent, the need for physical therapists expands by 64 percent, and the need for medical records personnel expands by 75 percent (Department of Health and Human Services [DHHS] 1991; Ginzberg 1990). As a number of sage labor economists have pointed out, such projections are biased upward (e.g., who really thinks that government will continue to expand medical records workload at the record-setting pace of the 1983–88 era?). Consequently, we will not get 75 percent more medical records employees in the 1991–2000 era; but the larger policy point is whether we need and can produce 42 percent more RNs in this period. Nursing schools are closing, and the federal government should assess how effective its subsidy programs were in the past two decades before launching any major expansion in federal supports in the mid–1990s. The role of the nurse is changing in society (Begun and Feldman 1990; Fralic, Kowalski, and Llewellyn 1991).

In this chapter we discuss the impact of federal policy on the market for nursing education. Whether the marginal price paid per additional nurse trained is a "good buy" as a federal program is discussed in the context of other current nurse labor-market issues. The second half of the chapter surveys trends in nurse practitioner and physician assistant markets. Due in large part to a lack of physician acceptance, the physician extender market is faced with what many consider a paradox. The nation faces a shortage of primary-care, low-cost providers in certain locations, yet many physician extender programs that emphasize such a social mission have had to close (U.S. Congress, Office of Technology Assessment [OTA] 1989).

Since 1965 the federal government has been providing financial assistance for the training of registered nurses. Federal support began in 1964 with the passage of the Nurse Training Act (NTA); subsequent legislation has extended and expanded this initial commitment to nursing education. Government assistance for nurse training began as an attempt to increase the supply of RNs because health care institutions demanded more RNs on their staffs to meet the increased utilization of health services by the population. The provisions of the Nurse Training Act were specifically designed to increase the number of nurse graduates by subsidizing operating costs for nurse training programs and lowering tuition levels for nursing students. Support is awarded to training programs and students who meet certain criteria based on enrollment levels and financial need (Department of Health, Education, and Welfare [DHEW] 1974). In addition, special project grants were available to (1) increase the quantity and quality of nurse training programs, (2) increase enrollment levels of disadvantaged students, (3) increase the supply of nurses in underserved areas, and (4) upgrade the skills of existing nurses.

LONG-STANDING SHORTAGES: FACT OR FICTION?

In the 1980s the willingness of federal and state governments to support nurse education declined for two basic reasons. First, governments did not have the financial resources to underwrite the promises of the past. Second, the prevailing belief in the need for government subsidies for the previous two decades dissipated as conventional wisdom concerning the nurse "shortage" eroded. Indeed, a 1983 Institute of Medicine study (IOM 1983) concluded that the national nurse shortage was over. From 1962 to 1983 the number of nurses per capita grew 100 percent. The IOM report recommended continued, but increasingly targeted, funding of the Nurse Training Act. Direct funding for student aid was considered especially crucial, given that most students come from families with moderate incomes and that further federal support reductions could cause a future shortage of RNs.

Some analysts may argue that there has been no nursing shortage since 1969. For example, the principal stimulus for passing the NTA program was a 1963 surgeon general's report that provided manpower targets. The report recommended (1) increasing the nursing supply to 675,000 (a figure actually achieved five years ahead of schedule in 1969) and (2) improving the quality of nursing education by expanding bachelor of science in nursing (BSN) programs. McNally (1981) estimated a "shortage of 1.3 RNs per hospital, hardly a situation which might be described as a crisis." However, for some health professionals, if the "correct number of nurses" does not exist on each and every shift to staff a unit at 85 percent target occupancy, even if actual patient occupancy is 20 to 30 percent less, a "crisis" shortage of nurses exists. Professional guesstimates of the need for nurses have ranged from 110,000 in 1945 to 70,000 in 1955, 150,000 in 1969, 100,000 in 1980, and, most recently, 160,000 forecast for 1995. Estimates have not been developed by type of nursing program.

There are three basic educational training programs for the training of registered nurses. Each program is administered in a different educational setting and varies in length of time from start to completion. The two-year associate degree (AD) is earned at a community or junior college; the three-year diploma certificate is earned at a hospital-sponsored school of nursing; and the four-year baccalaureate degree (BSN) is earned at a college or university.

In 1988, BSN programs constituted 34 percent of all nursing programs and 41 percent of all graduates. The three-year diploma programs conducted in hospitals emphasize on-the-job training within the facility. In 1988 diploma programs constituted 17 percent of all nursing programs and 15 percent of all graduates. Total federal NTA subsidies per BSN student per year were twice as high as support for AD and diploma students over the first 20 years of federal funding. If the federal donors for nurse education had been interested only in maximizing the quantity of RNs, the government would have directed its expenditures to AD and diploma programs. The costs of educating a nurse in either AD or diploma schools is substantially less than the cost of a BSN degree in terms of money (as well as the opportunity costs of forgone labor). A measure of the cost of the quality objective was obtained by Edgren (1976) by comparing the cost of the subsidy program with what it would have cost to support diploma and AD programs exclusively. Edgren estimated that approximately 17,000 additional active RNs would have graduated from 1966 to 1972 if the decision to emphasize quality as well as quantity had not been made. Undoubtedly there have been some positive shifts in educational and service quality, but some undetermined amount of these quality improvements might have occurred without NTA federal donations.

CHANGES IN THE NURSING PROFESSION AND THE SCHOOLS

There have been three empirical estimates of the effectiveness of the NTA program in expanding the supply and type of nurses. In 1976 Edgren estimated that 7 percent of the total supply of RNs, or an additional 13,535 licensed RNs, could be attributed to the federal program from 1966 to 1972. Using an econometric simulation model initially developed by Deane (1971), Edgren calculated a second estimate of the number of newly trained RNs produced by the federal program. In Deane's model the number of entrants to nursing schools was a function of the wages of RNs, the wages of other professional women, and the number of female high-school graduates. Using this equation, Edgren calculated the total change in graduations from schools of nursing between 1966 and 1972. Comparing the cumulative net change in graduates with predicted change, Edgren found approximately 6,813, or 3.5 percent, more graduates than expected because of the federal program. A third estimate, provided by Yett (1975), suggested that approximately 1,330 additional trained RNs graduated per year between 1968 and 1970 as a result of the NTA program. If these three estimates can be used as a range, anywhere between 1,300 and 3,000 extra RNs per year can be attributed to the NTA program during its initial seven years.

Edgren estimated that over the first decade, the costs of an NTA-subsidized education were roughly six times greater than his hypothetical alternative (a direct wage-subsidy program). Thus the cost of increasing the nurse labor force by one additional nurse was approximately $50,000 because of the federal policy. If a wage subsidy had been used, however, the cost of each additional RN would have been only $7,936 in 1969 dollars. This $7,936 estimate assumed that the wage elasticity of RNs with respect to nurse participation in the labor market was 1.0 (i.e., a 1 percent increase in wages produced a 1 percent increase in employment).

Various attempts to measure the accomplishments of the Nurse Training Act have concluded pessimistically that the increase in the supply of RNs resulting from the federal program does not appear to justify the cost. Health providers and nursing groups still contend, however, that federal support for nursing schools and students is necessary. Further research is required in view of the most recent substantial reductions in federal support. This chapter provides an empirical test of the enrollment behavior of nurse training programs. A viable policy for government support of nurse education must be based on reliable measurements of the sensitivity of nursing school enrollments to tuition, government subsidies, and educational costs. These measurements will permit estimates of the effects that future changes in subsidy levels will have on enrollment behavior and, ultimately, on the supply of registered nurses.

THE DONOR MODEL OF SCHOOL BEHAVIOR

How have nursing schools responded to the NTA program and other subsidies? Nursing schools could have attempted to utilize subsidies to train more students, train the same number of students more intensively, engage in more community services, raise faculty salaries, or even purchase better office equipment. Without an economic model of the nursing school, we cannot test predictions of how schools respond to donations (including loans) from the government or the private sector. We shall adopt the donor model of medical school behavior developed by Hall and Lindsay (1980) to the nursing school context.

The single most important demanders of nursing education are the donors, including public agencies, that provide one-third to one-half of school revenues. The support for educational institutions is most frequently predicated on the distribution of "in-kind" dividends to the gift givers (i.e., the donors) in the form of increased supply and quality of nursing manpower and thus improved access to quality of health-services delivery for the donors and society (Eastaugh 1985). In the Hall and Lindsay (1980) model, the public donors care about the quantity of school output, whereas the private donors are concerned with the quality of output. In the nursing education context, most of the donors are public sources, but they care about both the quantity and the quality of output as stated in the Nurse Training Act. One might hypothesize that nursing schools have more internal control because they have a less diverse stakeholder (donor) group.

Let us consider how nursing schools have reacted to the rise and fall of donor support. Because nursing schools have received few large private donations in the past, one might predict a reversal of this trend in the near future. In fact, there is evidence that this is already occurring. Alumni are also becoming a more important donor group. However, the "giving power" of the typical middle-aged nurse is substantially less than the giving power of the "old-boy" medical school alumnus. Physician and nurse markets are very different, and the theories applicable to one may not be transferable to the other. It is the basic contention of the empirical portion of this chapter that the donor model is applicable to nursing education, even if donors' contributions to schools of nursing represent a smaller fraction of total school revenues (one-fourth to one-third; by comparison, one-half to two-thirds of medical school revenues come from government and private donors). In fact, a donor model of nursing school behavior might be as effective as the Hall and Lindsay medical school model for predicting behavior, for six basic reasons:

1. Nurses are less mobile and thus more likely to practice in the state in which they were trained and subsidized (a critical point for state government donors who want to donate for long-term increases in the state's supply of nurses).
2. Nurses exist in a more competitive job market with less control of their wages and demand functions.
3. Potential students face narrower variation in tuition across nursing schools; thus the existence of a subsidy may determine whether a student goes into nursing. In contrast, potential medical students face a tenfold variation in tuition that allows a student to shop for a school with a lower price, ceteris paribus.
4. Once training is completed, nurses face fewer barriers to practice entry (e.g., licensure exams are easier and less frequent than those for physicians).
5. Given the differences between medical and nursing students in socioeconomic backgrounds and given the perceived opportunity costs of forgoing short-term employment at $600 a month to go to schools, a net $3,000 subsidy to a potential nurse may be more of a "lure" to that field than a much larger subsidy for a medical student with dreams of $80,000 in annual income. In other words, the absolute levels of subsidy per student may be lower in nursing education, but the dollars may be more critical to an 18- to 22-year-old individual facing the decision of whether to enter or forgo a career in nursing.
6. The number of nursing schools is much larger for hypothesis testing (Hall and Lindsay studied 16 of 128 medical schools; we shall consider data from 639 nursing schools in this analysis).

Nursing schools have good reasons to exercise discretion over matriculants (and their faculty). Analogously, baseball ticket buyers donate only one-fourth of the revenues to support the game, these "donors" largely determine the number and quality of the players. Donors may not be as important in the nursing education industry as they are in medical education, but their dollars do help determine the quantity and educational quality of our nursing labor force. If nursing schools competitively produce trained licensed nurses for donors and their health programs, one can model the donors' demand for first-year students. Figure 10.1 graphically shows the three critical variables of the model: H is the demand curve of all hopeful applicants for first-year admission, D is the demand curve by that fraction of applicants judged qualified and allowed to matriculate, and M is the marginal cost of education per student per year. A nursing school will select a class size of A_1 if it can collect T, R, A_1, and O dollars of tuition after budgeting for T, R, O, and M dollars of donations. If the dollars of donations expand to $T_2 R_2 O_2 M$, as happened during the period 1965–71, nursing schools

Figure 10.1

Demand Schedule for Nursing Education as a Function of Tuition Supports (MT₁, MT₂) in Periods T₁ and T₂

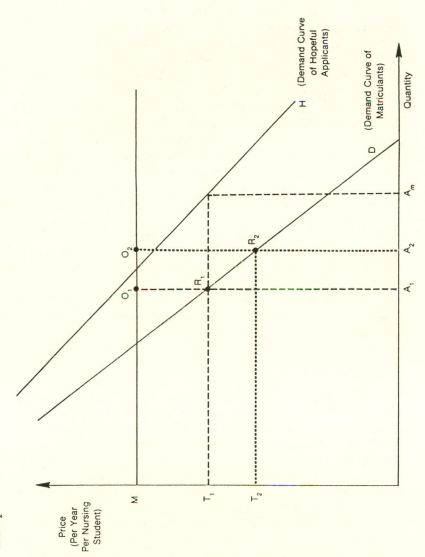

can lower tuition (in real dollar terms) and expand enrollment (price T_2, class size A_2). Large numbers of potential nursing students are still rationed on a nonprice basis, but fewer qualified applicants are "available" than under equilibrium T_2.

One could hypothesize that during the period 1971–74 we reached a new equilibrium (figure 10.2) with donations at their maximum in real dollar terms $(T_3R_3O_3M)$, tuition falling to T_3, and enrollment expanding to A_3. The demand for nursing services and thus for nursing education shifted outward from D to D_3 thanks to increased medical technology and the demand-pull medical-expenditure inflation fueled by expansion in Medicaid and Medicare coverage. Some would argue that during this "golden era," a large number of poorly qualified "marginal" nursing students were admitted, nearly one-third of whom did not graduate. Perhaps the correct equilibrium to balance quality and quantity is point A_u. However, a steady retrenchment of donations occurred from 1974 to 1980 back to T_2, and a more drastic retrenchment during 1981 to 1984 back to T_1. Consequently, nursing school administrators have been pressured to raise tuition, which somewhat curtails class size (closer to A_u). Finally, nursing school faculty have become more highly trained and costly, driving up the marginal cost curve M. Increases in training costs created pressures to raise tuition and downsize enrollment. This simple model assumes that it is equally costly to train each of the class levels (years 1, 2, 3, and 4) within a given nursing program.

We shall next test the validity of the donor model for the nurse training equilibrium market where the supply and demand for medical training is determined by the level of donations (mostly government subsidies). In fact, the equilibrium price and quantity of training actually faced by prospective students and schools depends to a great degree on donor subsidies.

Data Analysis

Data were collected for 639 U.S. nursing schools for each of the academic years from 1974–75 through 1983–84. A fixed-effects analysis of covariance was used to pool the time-series, cross-sectional data. The dependent variables were tuition and first-year enrollments. The models involved simple linear approximations of the reduced-form equations for nursing school tuition and enrollments. Annual subsidies, marginal training costs, and annual applications were the primary independent variables. The reduced-form equations were estimated using two different model specifications, two functional forms (linear and semilog), and two estimation procedures (ordinary least squares and instrumental variables).

We shall measure equilibrium enrollment (A) and tuition (T) as linear functions of donor subsidies (G), marginal training costs (C), and actual applications (H). In contrast to Hall and Lindsay (1980), we have the advantage of having data for applications by school annually. Hall and Lindsay utilized aggregate applicants to all schools annually in combination with superior physician wage data

Figure 10.2
Demand Schedule for Nursing Education as Tuition Supports Increase (to MT₃) and the Demand for Nurses and Consequent Demand for Nursing Education Increases

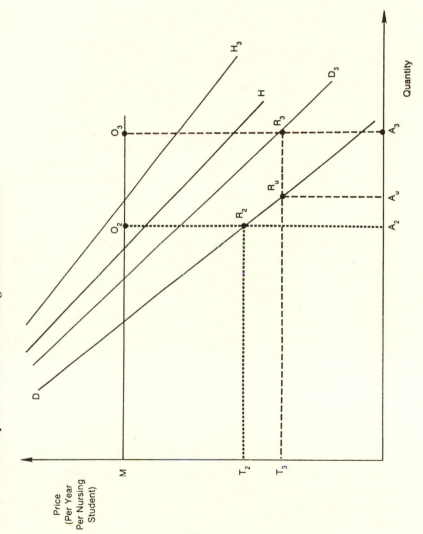

(Average Number of Nursing Students Per Year Per Class)

to impute optimal physician stock. The nurse wage data from the Bureau of Labor Statistics are too spotty (they are irregular and do not include all of the school catchment regions), and the sample sizes are too small (50 to 100 respondents per area, rather than over 1,000 physicians per standard metropolitan statistical area [SMSA]) to properly regress an optimal nursing labor stock. The number of applicants per school acts herein as the device to meter demand shifts directly.

In simplest form, the initial regression specifications can be written as

$$A = \beta_0 + \beta_1 H + \beta_2 C + \beta_3 G + e \qquad (10.1)$$

$$T = \alpha_0 + \alpha_1 H + \alpha_2 C + \alpha_3 G + u \qquad (10.2)$$

The model leads one to expect that regressions (10.1) and (10.2) will yield positive signs for β_1, β_3, α_1, and α_2 and negative signs for β_2 and α_3. The estimated coefficients from these equations allow one to test whether the derivatives of the true reduced-form equations for tuition and enrollment are nonzero and of the correct sign. One should point out that our reliance on actual observations of enrollment (A) and tuition (T) to measure equilibrium levels assumes that changes in exogenous conditions are correctly anticipated and that adjustments to such changes are made fully within each academic year. Nothing in the nursing literature suggests consideration of a more complex distributed-lag model (Eastaugh 1985). The only variable in the analysis we shall lag is subsidies (G), which are assumed to affect school behavior the following year (year $n + 1$).

Next we shall estimate the structural equations for the demand for nursing education (A) as a linear function of estimated tuition values ($\hat{T}$) from equation (10.2), as well as a function of applications (H). The regression specification for demand may be written as

$$A = \delta_0 + \delta_1 \hat{T} + \delta_2 H + v \qquad (10.3)$$

Coefficients obtained from this equation will be used to calculate the elasticity of enrollment with respect to tuition and to achieve closer approximations to the partial derivatives of the true reduced-form equation for enrollment.

Equation (10.1) can be estimated from data for each of the ten academic years, 1974 to 1983. The tuition data, however, are very poor prior to 1978; therefore, equations (10.2) and (10.3) are estimated over the six academic years 1978 to 1983. Two final caveats are in order. First, implicit in our definition of H is the assumption that the proportion of multiple applications to nursing schools remains relatively constant over the study period. Second, faculty salaries are used as a proxy for the marginal training cost (C) variable, for two reasons. First, as an

Institute of Medicine (1974) study suggested, faculty salaries are 50 percent of total costs per student for a wide range of nursing schools, plus or minus 5 percent. Faculty salaries are clearly a consistent underestimate of marginal cost and average cost, but a procedure for estimating error in variables is used to minimize this problem. Faculty are clearly the most elastic component of a nursing school's cost function. Alternatively, one could also argue that salaries are a proxy for average cost, which is itself a proxy for marginal costs. Economists often use average cost as a proxy for marginal cost, under the assumption that returns to scale in the proportion of students are constant.

The total number of nursing programs increased only 3 percent during the study period 1974–83. The mix of program types, however, changed significantly over this time period. The 50 percent decline in diploma programs was offset by increases in both associate and baccalaureate degree programs (up 55 and 45 percent, respectively). Our sample represented 639 of the 650 largest nursing programs in 1974. These 639 schools matriculated 79 percent of the first-year RN enrollments in 1974 and 81 percent in 1983. Our sample included 68 private BSN schools, 74 public BSN schools, 250 public AD schools, 28 private AD schools, 196 private diploma schools, and 23 public diploma schools. The sample represented the larger, more stable nursing schools that were more likely to report financial data to the National League for Nursing (NLN). The NLN survey is annually administered to all state-approved schools of nursing each October. Because of its consistency during the period 1974–1983, it was used as the basis for developing the sample of nursing schools used in this chapter.

The data for the federal component of the variable G were taken directly from the *Annual Directory of Grants, Awards, and Loans to Schools of Health Professions* of the U.S. Department of Health, Education, and Welfare, Bureau of Health Manpower. These data reflect all award actions administered by the Bureau of Health Manpower in each fiscal year. Only those appropriations made specifically for the purpose of training nursing students, however, were included in the measurement of G. The data for the state, local, and private donation terms of G were obtained from the annual *Financial Statistics of Institutions of Higher Education Survey* of the National Center for Education Statistics. Due to the long lead time necessary for government funds actually to go into effect, the data for the public component of G were lagged by one year.

Model Specification

The reduced-form model that specifies individual school effects can be written as

$$y = X_{it}\beta + Z\alpha + u_{it},$$
(10.4)

where y = a vector of observations on the dependent variable (i.e., annual tuition or first-year enrollment),

X = observations on the regressors (i.e., applications H, marginal training costs C, and annual subsidies G),

u = a random error term, and

Z = a design matrix for school effects.

Let $i = 1, 2, \ldots, 639$ cross-sectional units (schools), $t = 1, 2, \ldots, 10$ years for enrollment, and $t = 1, 2, \ldots, 6$ years for tuition. The total number of observations is 6,390 for enrollment and 3,834 for tuition. Assuming that only cross-sectional effects are important and that X includes an intercept term, Z contains 628 dummy variables where each column is 1 for the respective ith school and 0 otherwise. Thus Z is $6,390 \times 638$ for the enrollment equation and $3,834 \times 638$ for tuition, and α is 638×1 for both equations.

To estimate equation (10.4), one usually specifies dummy variables for each school in the sample. However, because N is large, an alternative approach was followed. The mean of each variable was computed for each school from the unpooled observations. Performing ordinary least squares (OLS) regression on observations that have been modified in this way yields the same slope coefficients as those obtained by incorporating individual dummy variables into the model. Given results obtained from equation (10.4), the second reduced-form model specification examined categories of effects, which permitted study of the variability of slope coefficients across financial control (public and private).

The expected signs of the coefficients of the three focus variables (G, C, H) vary across the tuition and enrollment equations. The subsidy variable (G) is expected to have a negative effect on tuition (less is charged if there is more subsidization) and a positive effect on enrollment (more subsidy, more students). The expected sign of the marginal-costs (C) coefficient is positive for tuition (more costly faculty, higher tuition) and negative for enrollment (expensive faculty, less student demand because of inability of students to pay their way). Finally, the applications (H) coefficient is expected to be positive for both equations (more applications, greater capability to raise tuition and enrollment). The structural equation for demand contains two focus variables. The expected sign of the estimated tuition variable (T) is negative, and the applications variable (H) is expected to be positive.

Empirical Results

The tuition equation results for public and private schools are presented in tables 10.1 and 10.2, respectively. The signs of the coefficients are as expected for the three focus variables: G, C, and H. The one exception is the negative but statistically insignificant sign for applications in the diploma school equation in table 10.1. With only 23 schools and 114 degrees of freedom, however, this result is hardly disturbing. The relatively small t ratios corresponding to the coefficients of H in the five equations indicate the lack of importance of applications in explaining tuition levels in public schools. One possible explanation for this is that public schools have much less internal control in pricing because of their more diverse stakeholder or donor group. Consequently, interaction between student demand for application and tuition prices is less pronounced than in private schools.

One can place some confidence in the model, given the expected signs of the coefficients in table 10.1. Although some variation is expected, no clear meaning can be given, for example, to the 3.5-fold variation in the slope coefficients of the subsidy variable across program type. These coefficients indicate that the effects of subsidies on tuition levels are approximately 250 percent higher for diploma programs than for associate programs. Interpreted in terms of the dependent variable, the coefficient of G in the aggregate equation indicates that annual tuition levels for public nursing programs would decrease by $1.10 to $1.23 if per school subsidy levels increased by $1,000 annually. The coefficient of C in this equation indicates that a $100 increase in marginal training cost will increase annual tuition levels by $12.31, ceteris paribus. However, this estimate may be low, and thus we shall reduce the effect of measurement error in C by reestimating the equation (table 10.1, line 3) using the instrumental variables (IV) technique (Durbin's IV method; Eastaugh 1985). These results, as reported in Table 10.1, show that the IV estimator increased the magnitudes of the coefficients of G and C and improved their corresponding t ratios compared to the OLS estimation of the same equation. The coefficient of C in this best equation for public schools indicates that a $100 increase in the marginal training cost will increase annual tuition levels by $19.82.

The tuition equations in tables 10.1 and 10.2 are impressive in that they explain more than two-thirds of the variance. All coefficients are of the expected signs in table 10.2. Private schools appear to be twice as responsive to subsidies and applications as public schools. The relatively small t ratios and coefficients of H in table 10.2, however, indicate that subsidies (G) are more important in explaining tuition levels in private schools. The tuition levels for private nursing schools would be expected to decrease $2.69 for every $1,000 increase in subsidy per school per year. Each $100 of increase in marginal cost per student will, ceteris paribus, increase annual tuition per student by $47.40. Private schools appear to be more responsive to market signals, such as declines in government subsidies or increases in educational costs. Before placing too much confidence in such a conclusion, however, one should consider potential sources of reporting bias between the two types of financial control. For example, private-school tuition might more accurately reflect the actual costs of training a student.

The enrollment equation results for public and private schools are presented in tables 10.3 and 10.4, respectively. The signs are in the expected directions, and the t ratios are more impressive than those of the tuition equations. The

Table 10.1
Regression of Tuition Equations, Public Schools (t Ratios in Parentheses)

Equation	Number of Schools	(G) Subsidies[a]	(C) Marginal Training Cost	(H) Applications	BSN Dummy	Diploma[b] Dummy	Intercept	R^2	d.f.
1. Disaggregate									
Associate	250	-.476 (-2.8)	9.25 (3.6)	.326 (1.7)			6.5	.798	(55,1444)
Baccalaureate	74	-1.274 (-4.1)	7.09 (3.9)	.156 (1.3)			28.7	.739	(49,394)
Diploma	23	-1.682 (-3.7)	20.36 (4.2)	-.064 (-.3)			34.8	.694	(23,114)
2. Aggregate	347	-1.195 (-4.0)	12.31 (4.1)	.298 (1.2)	163.4 (9.3)	207.7 (10.4)	15.2	.715	(59,2016)
3. Aggregate: IV estimation[c]	347	-1.231 (-4.5)	19.82 (4.8)	.340 (1.7)	159.7 (8.9)	198.7 (9.6)	9.9	—	(59,2016)

[a] Coefficients of subsidy and marginal training cost have been multiplied by 1,000 and 100, respectively.
[b] All equations include state and time dummy variables not reported in this table.
[c] All coefficients are significant at the .05 level except coefficient H (significant at .06).

Table 10.2
Regression of Tuition Equations, Private Schools (*t* Ratios in Parentheses)

Equation	Number of Schools	(G) Subsidies[a]	(C) Marginal Training Cost	(H) Applications	BSN Dummy	Diploma[b] Dummy	Intercept	R^2	d.f.
1. Disaggregate Associate	28	-2.261 (-2.0)	18.28 (1.8)	.285 (1.1)			456.5	.721	(26,141)
Baccalaureate	68	-2.135 (-4.3)	38.79 (2.7)	.472 (1.9)			399.0	.596	(35,372)
Diploma	196	-4.974 (-5.1)	25.91 (1.6)	.398 (2.0)			368.2	.640	(41,1134)
2. Aggregate	292	-2.508 (-4.9)	36.72 (4.5)	.550 (2.1)	302.7 (4.5)	302.7 (-6.2)	343.1	.686	(47,1710)
3. Aggregate: IV estimation[c]	292	-2.693 (-6.0)	47.40 (7.1)	.619 (2.4)	295.1 (4.2)	-438.3 (-6.3)	327.4	—	(47,1710)

[a]Coefficients of subsidy and marginal training cost have been multiplied by 1,000 and 100, respectively.
[b]All equations include state and time dummy variables not reported in this table.
[c]All five coefficients are significant at the .05 level.

269

Table 10.3
Regressions of Enrollment Equations, Dependent Variable A, First-Year Enrollment, for Public Schools
(*t* Ratios in Parentheses)

Equation	Number of Schools	(G) Subsidies[a]	(C) Marginal Training Cost	(H) Applications	BSN Dummy	Diploma[b] Dummy	Intercept	R^2	d.f.
1. Disaggregate Associate	250	.106 (36.7)	-2.88 (-9.9)	.276 (18.3)			39.3	.82	(59,2440)
Baccalaureate	74	.049 (19.2)	-1.79 (-7.4)	.141 (7.6)			62.4	.84	(53,686)
Diploma	23	.117 (31.3)	-1.52 (-4.9)	.310 (10.9)			21.9	.91	(27,202)
2. Aggregate	347	.048 (22.5)	-2.52 (-7.5)	.207 (10.3)	19.2 (11.6)	5.2 (2.3)	45.9	.687	(63,3394)
3. Aggregate: IV estimation[c]	347	.051 (22.8)	-3.06 (-9.1)	.238 (10.3)	21.9 (10.8)	7.8 (3.0)	54.6	—	(63,3394)

aCoefficients of subsidy and marginal training cost have been multiplied by 1,000 and 100, respectively.
bAll equations include state and time dummy variables not reported in this table.
cAll five coefficients are significant at the .05 level.

Table 10.4

Regressions of Enrollment Equations, Dependent Variable A, First-Year Enrollment, for Private Schools
(t Ratios in Parentheses)

Equation	Number of Schools	(G) Subsidies[a]	(C) Marginal Training Cost	(H) Applications	BSN Dummy	Diploma Dummy[b]	Intercept	R^2	d.f.
1. Disaggregate									
Associate	28	.184 (17.0)	-1.57 (-2.4)	.329 (17.6)			1.7	.90	(30,249)
Baccalaureate	68	.058 (6.6)	-1.14 (-5.9)	.126 (14.8)			48.4	.81	(39,640)
Diploma	196	.115 (13.5)	-2.39 (-6.5)	.317 (22.9)			31.1	.762	(45,1914)
2. Aggregate	292	.060 (12.9)	-2.47 (-6.5)	.294 (23.5)	-17.9 (-8.6)	-15.7 (-8.2)	53.2	.739	(51,2880)
3. Aggregate: IV estimation[c]	292	.062 (14.0)	-3.19 (-9.2)	.301 (23.4)	-17.1 (-7.9)	-13.2 (-6.3)	57.8	–	(51,2880)

[a]Coefficients of subsidy and marginal training cost have been multiplied by 1,000 and 100, respectively.
[b]All equations include state and time dummy variables not reported in this table.
[c]All five coefficients are significant at the .01 level.

instrumental-variable estimation procedure again improves the magnitude of the coefficient and t ratios, especially for the intended target (C). The coefficient of C under IV estimation suggests that first-year public-school enrollment would be expected to increase by one student if annual subsidies increased by approximately $19,600 per school. This benefit-to-cost ratio represents an improvement on the $50,000 estimate (1969 dollars) reported by Edgren (1976).

Applications appear to be more significant in determining the enrollment equation than in affecting the tuition equation. The estimates in table 10.3 suggest that first-year enrollment per school would increase by one student if applications at the margin increased by 4.2 per public school. However, BSN public nursing schools appear to be more selective—that is, less driven by applications. The coefficients for H indicate that, ceteris paribus, the enrollment per public BSN program would increase by one student if applications increased by 7.1 per school per annum.

The results for the private-school enrollment estimates are shown in table 10.4. Private schools are even more sensitive to subsidies. The estimates suggest that first-year enrollment would be expected to increase by one student per $16,100 of subsidies added per school per year. The effectiveness ratio of subsidy programs is more dramatic if one factors inflation into the equation. If Edgren's estimates are revalued in 1983 dollars, one nurse was added to the labor supply per $123,200 of NTA subsidies invested in the period 1966–72. Expressed in 1983 dollars, one nurse was added to the first year of private nursing school programs for each $25,400 invested in NTA and other subsidies, and one graduated nurse was added to the nursing labor pool for each $35,800 of subsidies (1974–83). In 1983 dollars, one nurse was added to the first year of public nursing school programs for each $30,485 invested into NTA and other subsidies (state, local, and so on), and one graduated nurse entered the labor supply for each $43,550 of subsidies (1974–83). Although there are differences between the design of the present study and that of Edgren's study, nursing schools appear to have become three to four times more efficient in producing nurses from donations during the period 1974–83 than during the years 1966–72.

Two final points should be made regarding table 10.4. The coefficient for C suggests that first-year enrollment should, other factors being equal, decline by 3.19 students per school if marginal costs increase by $100. This suggests that private and public nursing schools are equally responsive to shifts in marginal costs. Second, the coefficient of H suggests that first-year enrollment would increase by 3.1 students per school. However, the coefficient of H for BSN schools is substantially lower (i.e., they are more selective). First-year BSN enrollment would increase by one student if applications at the margin increased by 7.94 students per school per year.

Enrollments for private schools appear to be 22 percent more sensitive to subsidy levels than public schools. One possible interpretation may be that a large portion of government subsidies are in the form of loans and scholarships that go directly to students. If this source of funding is cut back, rather than pick up the full (higher) tuition bill of a private nursing education, students would probably enroll in public nursing programs. Private schools could retain enrollment levels by cutting back on their marginal costs, but private schools appear to be no more successful at further improving educational productivity than public nursing schools. Annual private-school expenditures on faculty salaries are, on average, $53 less per student per year in diploma programs, $151 less per student per year in associate programs, and $548 less per student per year in BSN programs than public-school expenditures. Dramatic reductions in marginal costs may have to be made in the diploma programs, the dominant type of private schools, if they are to survive in the 1990s. Many will not survive because of downward pressure on hospital payment rates. The typical private diploma program in our sample has 10 students per faculty member, in contrast to 15 for BSN programs and 18 for the few private associate programs. Thus reducing faculty is the most obvious way in which a nursing school could cut its costs.

Finally, the results for the equation estimating the demand for education (first-year enrollment) as a function of price (tuition), applications, and type of program are presented in table 10.5. Private-school demand appears to be more sensitive to price. From the coefficients of T in table 10.5, private-school enrollments would increase by one student for each $7.75 decline in tuition, and public-school enrollments would increase by one student per $10.65 decline in tuition. Also, public-school enrollment is less sensitive to applications (H) than private-school enrollment. Public-school applications would have to increase by 4.4 per school to yield an increase in enrollment of one student. However, the coefficient for private schools (correcting for type of program) suggests that applications need only increase by 2.9 to yield one more student per year. Because variable H may be a proxy for such effects as RN wage levels, marriage status, and so forth, this result could reflect a difference in the socioeconomic backgrounds of the students who attend private and public nursing schools. More research is needed to determine why students select nursing careers and how they select nursing schools (Hafer and Ambrose 1983; Record, McCally, and Schweitzer 1989; Mechanic and Aiken 1983).

A more complete examination of nursing school behavior should include factors that affect demand for education, such as expected future wages. How do prospective nurses acquire information on this issue? For example, one recent issue of *RN* magazine reported that (1) general-duty nurses in Kansas City earned 21.1 percent less per hour than grocery cashiers and 28.4 percent less than head grocery clerks, (2) Boston nurses earned 28.6 percent less than head grocery clerks, and (3) Atlanta nurses earned 13.8 percent less than grocery cashiers and 29.8 percent less than head grocery clerks. The nursing profession seems insensitive to the two potential negative ramifications of such articles. First, young people pondering investment of time and money in nursing school might think twice after reading such information. Second, the nursing profession seems insistent that it operates independently of all other labor markets. While the health-services sector is a ''special'' industry, one is nonetheless struck by the

Table 10.5
Regressions of Demand Equations (*t* Ratios in Parentheses)

Equation[a]	Dependent Variable	(*T*) Tuition[b]	(*H*) Applications	Dummy	Diploma Dummy	Intercept	d.f.
Private schools	First-year enrollment	-.129 (-14.6)	.343 (31.2)	23.06 (8.0)	-27.95 (-10.3)	150.78	(46,1711)
Public schools	First-year enrollment	-.094 (-7.0)	.229 (25.1)	49.52 (10.7)	38.66 (11.5)	37.20	(58,2017)

[a]All equations include state and time dummy variables not reported in this table.
[b]All variables are significant at the .01 level.

apparent difficulty of the nursing profession to respond proactively to the coming cuts in hospital-based nursing positions and wages. If the Medicare prospective payment system is going to withdraw $19 to $22 billion of reimbursement out of the hospital sector from 1987 to 1993, the principal losers will be nurses, not physicians or administrators. If the "nursing shortage" was the issue in the past, more bed closures and forced unemployment may become the nurse labor-market issues for the mid–1990s.

In summary, the best statistical results for all four equations were obtained from the aggregate model, which allows the slope coefficients to vary across financial control and includes dummy variables for time, state, and program-type effects. A significant trend in our analysis of state effects is that California has the third-highest tuition levels for private nursing schools but the second-lowest tuition levels for public schools. The southern states, by contrast, appear to have relatively high public-school tuitions. Concerning time effects, increases in private-school tuitions exceeded those in public schools from 1978 to 1981. Furthermore, first-year enrollments have been declining since 1980 for both BSN and associate degree schools. The decline in enrollments for the 196 private diploma schools began in 1978. The moderate variability of the slope coefficients across program type for the disaggregated model suggests that the results reported in this section should be considered good approximations.

NURSING SCHOOLS AND THE FUTURE

Two central measurement problems exist in this study. First, we did not have a good measure of marginal cost, but IV estimation procedures (Intriligator 1978) minimized this problem. Second, we did not have wage data for the 300 nursing markets in which the 639 schools operate. Applications served as a proxy for demand factors, especially wage levels. Given that nursing education is an input to the market for RNs, an examination of school behavior should include factors that affect demand for education, such as expected future wages. Prospective payment for hospital services may prove to have a downward impact on nurse wages and employment.

Despite the limitations of the regression, the equations strongly indicate that nursing schools respond to market signals from government and other donors, applicants, and faculty costs. These responses differed over the 10-year period for all three types of private and public schools. Schools appear to have improved their efficiency in producing nurses as a function of donations and loans since the Edgren study. Our estimates of a NTA effectiveness of $35,800 to $43,550 per additional nurse graduated can be interpreted as the marginal price to the federal government of additional nurses produced. Whether this is too high a price to pay, even if nursing schools more than doubled their efficiency in the 1970s, is a political decision. Most nursing educators hope that the federal government will continue to be the final guarantor of financial access to nursing school for students otherwise qualified.

Increasing subsidies in the 1960s and 1970s slightly increased class size and lowered tuition (below what tuition would have been), just as declining subsidies are now decreasing class size and raising tuition. The Bush administration questioned the validity of subsidizing nursing education in the absence of a nursing shortage during an era when many inefficient hospital beds might have to close. Nursing subsidies can be criticized for continuing the operation of inefficient and obsolete schools and promoting the training of "marginal" nursing students. In contrast to medical education, however, nursing schools do not have a large pool of excess applicants; indeed, there are excess schools. Nursing educators might refute the various arguments for discontinuing NTA subsidies by pointing to the fact that qualified students could not afford the investment in a nursing education without government subsidy. Political support for the nursing loan program appears to be dissipating in the face of vexing and persistent problems in collecting on the loans. Nursing loan defaults became a major issue when the DHHS announced that if nurses merely paid the amounts they were delinquent (not their total debt), another 24,000 nursing students could receive loans.

In attracting donors to substitute for declining federal support, nursing school deans will have to address the issue of attrition and educational standards to win the support of private donors. Deans of medical schools have a somewhat easier task because the donors are financially better off and may face less uncertainty in the medical education business. A medical student admitted is a practicing doctor down the educational pipeline, with very few dropouts and little voluntary inactivity from work. The nursing pipeline can be much more leaky, with an average 30 percent dropout rate in nursing school and up to one-third of licensed nurses not working. There never has been an aggregate shortage of trained nurses, just a presumed shortage of working nurses. Job satisfaction and wages are critically important in retaining practicing nurses. Levels of dissatisfaction may increase, however, if education and training continue to far exceed practical needs and duties. The progressive educator will lobby for providing nurses with more interesting and challenging duties and responsibilities.

HOSPITAL NURSING: VACANCY RATES AND WAGES

The official DHHS policy under the past four administrations since 1975 has been that the aggregate supply of nurses is adequate. The American Nursing Association (ANA) acknowledged the American Hospital Association's (AHA) and state hospital associations' estimates of a nurse shortage of 130,000 in 1991. However, the ANA characterizes the market as geographically maldistributed, "crying out" for the specialized nurses with BSN training. Both the AHA and the ANA characterized the nurse shortage as a "crisis" since 1983. The AHA reported that 88 percent of the nation's hospitals could not fill their nursing vacancies. The long-standing "crisis" is most critical in certain states. In 1991 a number of state hospital associations reported especially high nurse vacancy rates: 16 percent in Illinois, 17 percent in Texas and Maryland, and 18 percent in California. However, one should suspect the validity of such "evidence." What are the social costs of not filling 20 percent of the maximum possible "full-staffing" nursing slots, given that 42 percent of the beds in California are empty on average? Statistics on budgeted vacancies are poor evidence of a shortage but could be indicative of a geographic or specialty-skill maldistribution in the market.

In pondering the "budgeted vacancy" issue, a number of points might be made regarding the major employer of trained nurses. Hospitals employ two-thirds of active nurses. Hospitals are monopsony buyers of nurse labor, and each hospital faces an upward-sloping labor supply curve (in contrast to a horizontal curve under perfect competition); thus hospitals are wary of raising nurse wages. For hospitals, the short-run supply of nurses is inelastic; that is, increases in wages will yield only small increases in nurse labor availability. Raising wages increases the entire nurse-staff budget while yielding minuscule returns in terms of reentry by inactive nurses. Therefore, the rational hospital will purposefully control nurse wages at low levels (but not so low as to lose too many nurses to neighboring providers), and the hospital's state association can complain about a "crisis in budgeted vacancies."

State hospital associations might better spend their resources considering incentives to make more nurses careerists, such as increasing the differentials between beginning and top-level salaries. Managers should trade off the costs of providing incentives to induce nurses to pursue a hospital-based career versus the continuous high costs of retraining new nurses who turn over every three to four years. In the process of professional development, nurses have questioned the dated "doctor-knows-best" rules and replaced self-doubt with self-esteem. In the 1970s an assertive prospective nurse might have asked, "How can I fit into this hospital's goals?" Increasingly, nurses can ask, "How will the hospital fit into my goals?" "How will it impact on my life-style?" "Will the work be interesting?" "Will I grow in my field of expertise?" Flexible employment opportunities, improved automated scheduling systems, and elimination of non-nursing tasks from the daily routine can be optimal for both nurses and employers. Nurses can stay in nursing and overcome conflicts between home and career, and management can reduce nursing costs.

Over the last 15 years federal appropriations under the NTA have amounted to almost $5.2 billion in 1991 dollars. Table 10.6 lists the amounts of federal support appropriated to each provision of the Nurse Training Act over the last 23 years, representing 7 to 13 percent of the total expenditures for nursing education in any given year. According to the American Nursing Association's inventory of registered nurses, the supply of nurses per 100,000 citizens increased from 280 in 1960 to 356 in 1970, 506 in 1980, and an estimated 564 in 1991 (ANA 1991). This doubling over 31 years in the fraction of the labor force working as nurses has brought with it a trend to specialize. Specialization in nursing has often focused more on high-technology inpatient care rather than on long-term care or primary care. However, the demand for hospital nurses has

Table 10.6
Nurse Training Act and Research Program Appropriations and Other Special-Purpose Projects, 1969–1991 (in Millions of Dollars)

	Student Support (1-3)			4	5	6	7	8	Research (9-10)		11	12
	1 Scholar-ships	2 Trainee-ships	3 Loans[a]	Special Projects	Formula and Capi-tation	Advanced Nurse Training	Nurse Practi-tioner	Construc-tion	9 Fellow-ships	10 Grants	Other	Total
1969	6.5	10.5	9.6	4.0	3.0			8.0	1.4	2.6		45.5
1970	7.2	10.5	16.4	8.4				8.0	1.4	2.6		54.4
1971	17.0	10.5	17.1	11.5				9.5	1.4	2.6		69.4
1972	19.5	11.5	21.0	19.0	31.5			19.7	1.4	2.5	12.0	138.0
1973	21.5	12.5	24.0	25.0	38.5			21.0	1.7	2.5	14.0	160.6
1974	19.5	13.0	24.4	19.0	34.3			20.0	1.4	2.5	5.4	139.5
1975	6.0	13.0	24.4	19.0	34.3			20.0		1.2	4.8	122.7
1976	6.0	13.0	23.5	15.0	44.0	2.0	3.0	1.0				107.5
1977	6.5	13.0	25.5	15.0	40.0	9.0	9.0		1.0	5.0		124.0
1978	9.0	13.0	24.0	15.0	30.0	12.0	13.0	3.5	1.0	5.0		125.5
1979	9.0	13.0	14.3	15.0	24.0	12.0	13.0		1.0	5.0		106.3
1980	9.0	13.0	14.3	15.0	24.0	12.0	13.0		1.0	5.0		106.3
1981		13.0	14.3	12.0	10.0	12.0	13.0		1.0	5.0		80.3
1982		9.6	7.66	6.18		11.5	11.5		.96	3.4		50.8
1983		9.6	1.61	6.33		13.2	11.8		.96	5.0		48.5
1984		9.6	1.56	6.9		13.8	12.0		.96	5.0		50.0
1985		11.4	1.0	9.5		16.4	12.0		.65	5.0		56.0
1986		10.9		9.0		15.8	11.5		.53	4.8		52.7
1987		11.8		11.2		16.8	12.0		.77	2.1		54.5
1988		12.4		11.7		16.8	11.5		.91	1.8		55.0
1989		12.8		12.0		17.2	11.8		1.8	2.0		56.9
1990		13.5		12.9		12.8	13.4			5.0		57.6
1991		13.7		10.5		12.5	14.6			1.5		52.8

Source: Congressional Budget Office.
Note: Some lines do not add due to rounding.
[a]Includes loan repayments.

declined since 1983 and may continue to decline in the future. Nursing schools that adapt best to the emergence of growth markets, such as long-term care (discussed in chapter 5), will be in the best position to place their students after graduation.

One final word of caution is in order concerning hospital managers setting nurse wages. Many hospital executives anxious to reduce labor costs incorrectly envision a long-run, large supply of unemployed nurses. This attitude may be true in the short run, but nurses are already shifting in large numbers to other care settings and may be less interested in a return to hospital nursing. Managers must work to enhance nurse productivity by using nurse extenders (Eastaugh and Regan 1990) and to improve job satisfaction (Friss 1990). Nurses will face a variety of sources of job stress in the 1990s (Eastaugh 1991; Aiken 1990), and the task of enhancing employee retention will not be easy. However, the surviving nursing schools have improved both their marketing (new matriculants increased 18 percent) and their graduation efficiency (the fraction of matriculants actually graduating, up 16 percent over the period 1989–91).

NEW PROFESSIONALS: PHYSICIAN EXTENDERS

If the market for nurses and nursing education is in a turbulent state in 1986, the market for physician extenders is in far worse shape by comparison. Projections of 25,000 physician extenders in practice by 1985 (Eastaugh 1981) were not realized until 1989. The supply of physician extenders has become a captive of high-technology medicine and not a substantial source of primary care in underserved areas. Physician extender programs over the years from 1981 to 1991 have closed or adapted to the "funding realities." While limited funding support exists for primary-care extenders, most dollars are offered in high-technology areas—for example, the federal budget contained funds for nurse anesthetists and surgical assistants.

In theory, a set of new professionals was to emerge in order to provide care in a fashion that would be more conducive to serving consumer needs than traditional solo physician practice. Since 1971 federal support of physician extender (PE) training programs has been the primary federal response to the perceived shortage and maldistribution of providers of primary care. The term physician extender includes both nurse practitioners (NPs) and physician assistants (PAs) with formal training that has equipped them for functions beyond the scope of the traditional nurse. The rapid growth in PE training programs in the 1970s was a by-product of the unmet consumer demand for primary care and the perceived neglect of the human side of medicine. PEs frequently take the family approach to health education and contact the spouse or relative of the patient in an attempt to improve patient compliance with treatment and to convince the individual that a healthier life-style is attainable. With the growth in concern for the caring function, prevention, health promotion, and care of the chronically ill came a fivefold increase in the supply of PEs from 1970 to 1980.

However, the PE supply rose only two-fold 1981 to 1991. In the current era of governmental retrenchment, concern over the nation's medical bill should not a priori lead to a freeze at the current annual level of the number of PEs trained. Physician fears of competition should not change the fact that many underserved patients increasingly demand nonphysician personnel to act as counselors, educators, and ombudsmen.

The promise of PEs is best described in terms of improved access to care, health education counseling, comprehensive planning in patient-care management, and potential gains in productivity. PEs can meet a previously unmet need in two basic senses: if they are not hospital based, they are more likely than physicians to reside in medically underserved areas, and they specialize in often-neglected areas of medical practice. Physician resistance to employing more PEs has called into question the service-delivery rationale for federal funding of training programs. The intent of the following sections is to suggest that PEs can increasingly become a medically and economically popular solution to the problem of providing health care in underserved rural and inner-city areas. However, PE expansion into these markets did not occur from 1980 through 1991.

For nearly two decades the terms ''doctor shortage'' and ''primary-care shortage'' have been bandied about. The ''crisis'' was defined in the 1970s as one of both geographic and specialty maldistribution. One of the most vexing questions asked by labor economists is whether, and to what extent, PEs act to improve productivity and decrease average costs by performing delegable tasks (DHHS 1991; Zeckhauser and Eliastam 1974), or whether they free physician time to perform less necessary and more costly complex tertiary medical care. In the parlance of economics, to what extent do PEs act as substitutes and/or complements for physician time? Another, less tangible, unanswered question is to what extent PE training programs have had a positive spin-off effect on physician education—that is, making physicians more aware of primary care and the need for the caring function and preventive counseling. Any benefit-cost framework for assessing the projected expansion in the supply of PEs should not underestimate the tangible benefits to society of health promotion, self-care, and prevention activities (Eastaugh 1991).

CURRENT LEVELS OF MANPOWER SUPPLY AND TRAINING SUPPORT

In January 1980 there were an estimated 11,000 physician assistants, including 1,000 certified PAs who did not graduate from a formal training program. The PA class size declined from 1,600 graduates in 1981 to only 700 graduates in 1986. An estimated 70 percent of certified PAs are presumed active. Most PA programs are university based and require two years of training. Between 1972 and 1980 approximately 7,200 PA students received $66 million in direct and indirect federal support (Eastaugh 1981). However, the level of federal support per annum has been frozen at approximately $8 to $11 million for the past 13 years.

Certificate and master's NP training programs vary in emphasis over a range of disciplines: family medicine, pediatrics, maternity care, midwifery, and psychiatric care. In 1991 an estimated 29,000 NPs had graduated from formal training programs. An estimated 80 percent are presumed to be active. (Data were provided by the Bureau of Health Manpower, Division of Nursing, Public Health Service, DHHS.) The American College of Nurse-Midwives estimates that 3,000 of the NPs are actively engaged in midwifery. Between 1972 and 1981 approximately 12,000 NP students and about half of the NP programs received $88 million from the Nurse Training Acts of 1971 and 1975. The level of federal support from the 1975 Nurse Training Act has been frozen at $49 to $56 million for the past ten years. Since 1978 the traineeships have been awarded to individuals who were willing to perform postgraduate service in areas designated as underserved by the federal government.

One seldom-mentioned benefit resulting from the emergence of PE training programs was the public questioning of the resistance of organized medicine to task delegation. Since 1847 the American Medical Association has committed itself to the trade-union objective of promulgating restrictions on nurses or would-be doctors (Kessel 1958). According to the report of the Macy Foundation (1976), the continued success of PEs will not only have a positive impact on the quality of health care, but will also encourage the development of other nonphysician competitors to physician subspecialist and solo practitioners. If consumers prefer high accessibility to care and cost containment, then training PEs seems a better bargain than training physicians at five times the cost (Ginzberg 1990; Sturmann, Ehrenberg, and Salzberg 1990).

PHYSICIAN SUPPLY AND REIMBURSEMENT ISSUES

An Institute of Medicine (1978) study questioned the need to train additional PEs if the anticipated supply of physicians in 1990 would be at least adequate and if the projected specialization trend is a return to family practice and primary care. While the need for a comprehensive strategy that coordinates the supply and distribution of PEs and physicians is clear, it seems a shortsighted policy to presume that physicians in oversupplied areas will suddenly decide to serve the poor and less profitable locations. There is limited statistical evidence, however, that doctors have increasingly moved to rural underserved areas, thus alleviating some of the original impetus for many PE training programs. Physicians began to disperse to relatively underserved locations in response to competitive pressures as early as 1979 (Newhouse et al. 1982). In 1990 Congress resolved to reimburse physicians on the basis of a relative-value system rather than on the basis of prevailing charges, and the financial disincentives to work in a region of low physician density were diminished. A mass exodus of physicians from the suburbs under this new reimbursement climate would seem highly unlikely. Despite the fact that personal life-style preferences dominate the physician's location decision, it seems poor public policy to pay more in areas where doctors are needed less and to pay less in areas where they are needed most.

Medicaid regulations typically permit reimbursement for PE services that are performed under "general" physician supervision. Some states are more liberal on this point—for example, the South Dakota legislature required health insurers to cover all PE services starting in 1980. Since 1976 the state of Nevada has directly reimbursed PAs at 100 percent of physician rates and NPs at 55 percent of physician rates. To liberalize the reimbursement climate among insurance payers in areas of physician shortage, Congress passed the 1977 Rural Health Clinic Services Act (Pub. L. 95–210), which provided Medicare and Medicaid reimbursement for PE services rendered without direct physician supervision in certified clinics. Congress changed the law in FY 1987, but the volume of PA billing was still very small in 1991 (DHHS 1991).

Although one-fifth of PEs are employed in HMOs and clinics, the majority of PEs were employed by physicians in private practice until 1983. A number of outside surveys have suggested that physicians' reluctance to hire PEs might be accounted for by conflicting perceptions about the PE role (Prescott and Driscoll 1979). Five rationales have been suggested to explain why physicians may hire PEs. First, they may wish to improve the quality of care by creating a less crowded and more comprehensive schedule. Second, they may want to increase the quantity (minutes) of care delivered per visit. Third, they may indulge in the purely economic desire to expand practice profits. Fourth, physicians may desire more leisure time and a shorter workweek. Last, employment of a PE may result in lower malpractice premiums in the long run, if improved patient rapport diminishes the incidence of nuisance suits.

PRODUCTIVITY AND COST CONSIDERATIONS

Many early comparative cost studies tried to portray PEs either as a financial windfall or as a liability. Some of the earliest pro-PE studies came from HMOs in which nonphysician personnel provided care in a majority of the visits. Other studies were flawed because they loaded a large amount of overhead unnecessarily onto PE practices only (Nelson et al. 1975). The Systems Sciences (1978) study avoided such methodological pitfalls. The productivity component of its analysis focused on an economic efficiency measure, the number of ambulatory visits per $1,000 of cost. When the study considered group practices, it found no differential in economic efficiency between PE and non-PE comparison practices; both kinds of group practice produced 66 visits per $1,000 of cost. However, the Systems Science study found that solo physician practices produced 81 visits per $1,000 of reimbursable cost (cost to society) when a PE was part of the team, compared to 57 visits per $1,000 of cost in solo physician practices without a PE. Three other major conclusions of the study were that (1) the average charge per visit was lower in PE practices, (2) physician job satisfaction increased in PE practices as the perceived workload decreased, and (3) process measures of quality of care were better on average in the PE practices.

The demand for PEs is a function of the consumer demand for medical services, physician supply, physician reimbursement policy, PE reimbursement policy, and the willingness of physicians to hire PEs. For example, legal constraints, such as requirements for direct supervision of PEs by physicians, are cited by physicians as a rationale for not employing PEs. Another rationale for not employing PEs is the American physician's distaste for staff management (Scott and Harrison 1990). In estimating that physicians could profitably employ one to five PEs, Reinhardt (1972) suggested that physicians react with rather high psychic costs to employing a larger staff—that is, they hate to manage people. It is difficult to generalize these study results over time, but if we update the figures to 1991 dollars, Reinhardt estimated the marginal disutility of each additional PE employed to be between $520 and $680 per week. If the economic conditions of the 1990s erode a physicians' ability to maintain a high living standard, the medical community may increasingly discount the marginal disutility of employing additional extenders and hire more PEs. However, the anticipated productivity gains may be overstated. For example, a study by Hershey and Kropp (1979) suggested that the productivity gain from employing a PA may be as small as 20 percent and the increase in net income may be negligible. The authors' optimization-simulation model did not consider the possibility that shifts in the patient mix following addition of a PA might cause the measured productivity improvement to be understated. However, if income gain was negligible for the doctor in a period when office visits were increasing, the incentive to employ a PE is nonexistent in a market where visits per annum declined and the physicians often have empty appointment calendars. The declines in dental visits have been even larger.

TOUGH TIMES FOR SOME SCHOOLS

Enrollment in nursing schools declined by 40 percent in the period 1984–90. However, the declines in nursing students stabilized at the start of the 1990s. Other professions have experienced a decline in enrollment, for example, a 21 percent decline in dental students since 1984. Including the closure of Georgetown Dental School in 1991, the number of dental schools declined from 60 to 53 in the period 1988–91. PE and PA schools have experienced a lower rate of closure in recent years (American Academy of Physician Assistants [AAPA] 1991).

Nurse practitioners have subspecialized to remain viable in the market. Pediatric nurse practitioners have proven valuable in rural areas and in urban medical centers. They can provide a wide range of functions vital to a multispecialty setting (Cruikshank, Clow, and Seals 1986). The normative ideals for pediatric NPs, as developed at three HMOs, were consistently higher than their actual job roles (Weiner, Steinwachs, and Williamson 1986). Nurse practitioners maintain their linkage to nursing by performing nursing functions—for example, patient advocacy, health education, and patient support (McNamara and Smith 1984). Rather than acting as "junior house staff" to supplement inpatient care, NPs and PAs might find greater growth potential in caring for the elderly (chapter 5). The federal government invested $220 million in NP and PA training programs to provide primary care, not to produce a cheap source of labor for teaching hospitals. Geriatric medicine is one specialty area where the physician community may cede increasing independence to these physician extenders. Expansion of the physician extender work force has been retarded by inadequate marketing, lack of community understanding, and lack of acceptance by community physicians (Kelly 1985). If specialists are increasingly successful in attracting PEs away from hospital practice, the total demand for PEs could increase.

The federal government might better serve the public interest by concentrating a higher proportion of PE funds into traineeships with a service obligation. As an added inducement to increase retention of PEs after completion of the service payback requirement, DHHS might subsidize the malpractice premiums and office equipment costs of individuals remaining in medically underserved regions. The DHHS could further target direct grants and contracts to programs that offer curricula that track students into primary care. Finally, the federal government should have an increased concern for research in the area of primary-care manpower. For example, we need to ascertain the volume or critical mass of population necessary to allow an independent PE practice to attain financial self-sufficiency after three to five years of growth in an isolated rural area (Moscovice and Rosenblatt 1979). Specifically, PAs have a proven ability to decrease per visit costs by up to 20 percent in large urban practices (Greenfield et al., 1978), but the introduction of PAs into smaller practices has not led to an equal reduction in unit cost or increase in patient volume (Frame, Wetterav, and Parey 1978).

Another potential area for further research is the difference in productivity between PAs and NPs. A study of 455 matched paired comparison practices suggested that PAs are 6 to 36 percent more productive than NPs, depending on practice arrangement (Mendenhall, Repicky, and Neville 1980). The NPs in this study were employed in larger practices—practices with an average of 9.5 physicians, compared to 4.7 in the average PA practice situation. However, the cause of the productivity differential was not explained by practice size.

The wisdom of increasing support for PE programs depends on judgments about future reimbursement incentives, PE responsiveness to required service location, PE retention in underserved areas following completion of the service requirement, and assumptions about competition in health care markets. In the short run, if PEs merely add to the aggregate level of demand, they will, acting as an add-on, produce a net inflationary impact on medical costs. Although there are many reasons for the very slow emergence of PEs as a profession, a dominant one is the concern for efficiency. Why must a $40 per hour physician spend 30 minutes with the anxious patient, when a $10 per hour PE can do an equally good or even better job in one hour at half the cost? Rather than spend a few rushed minutes with the physician, that patient can spend more time with a PE who can take the time to emphasize the caring function, yielding greater patient self-respect and improved rates of compliance. Managed-care systems may well discover that PEs offer good value for their wage rate. Managed-care systems, consumerism, and the emerging public desire for a low-cost health care adviser could promote a renaissance of interest in primary-care PEs.

REFERENCES

Aiken, L. (1990). "Increasing the Supply of Health Personnel: What Has Been Gained?" *Frontiers of Health Services Management* 7:2 (Winter), 23–27.

Altman, S. (1970). "The Structure of Nursing Education and Its Impact on Supply." In H. Klarman (ed.), *Empirical Studies in Health Economics*. Baltimore: Johns Hopkins University Press, 343.

American Academy of Physician Assistants (AAPA). (1991). *General Census Data on Physician Assistants*. Alexandria, Virginia.

American Nurses' Association. (1991). *Facts about Nursing*. Kansas City, Mo.: American Nurses' Association (ANA).

Baldwin, L., Hutchinson, H., and Rosenblatt, R. (1992). "Professional Relationships between Midwives and Physicians: Collaboration or Conflict?" *American Journal of Public Health* 82:2 (February), 262–264.

Begun, J., and Feldman, R. (1990). "Policy and Research on Health Manpower Regulation: Never Too Late to Deregulate?" In *Advances in Health Economics and Health Services Research*, edited by R. Scheffler. Greenwich, Conn.: JAI Press, 79–109.

Brown, A. (1985). "The Uncertain Future of the Nurse Practitioner." *Health Matrix* 3:2 (Summer), 49–54.

Brown, E. (1982). *Analyzing the Cost of Baccalaureate Nursing Education*. National League of Nursing Publication 15–1880. New York: National League of Nursing, 13–25.

California State Division of Health Professions Development. (1991). *Annual Report to the Legislature, State of California Healing Arts Licensing Board*, Sacramento.

Cruikshank, B., Clow, T., and Seals, B. (1986). "Pediatric Nurse Practitioner Functions in the Outpatient Clinics of a Tertiary Care Center." *Medical* Care 24:4 (April), 340–349.

Deane, R. (1971). "Simulating an Econometric Model of the Market for Nurses." Ph.D. diss., Department of Economics, University of California at Los Angeles.

Department of Health and Human Services (DHHS). (1991). *Eighth Report to the President and Congress on the Status of Health Personnel in the United States*. HRSA, Bureau of Health Professions. Washington, D.C.: U.S. Government Printing Office.

Department of Health, Education and Welfare. (1974). *Report to the Congress: Nurse Training*. Publication (HRA) 75–41. Washington, D.C.: U.S. Government Printing Office.

Eastaugh, S. (1991). "Valuation of the Benefits of Risk-free Blood: Willingness to Pay for Hemoglobin Solutions.'' *International Journal of Technology Assessment in Health Care* 7:1 (Winter), 51–59.

————. (1990). ''Health Insurance Reform in the 1990s.'' *Journal of the American Academy of Physician Assistants* 3:5 (July/August), 384–395.

————. (1985). ''Impact of the Nurse Training Act on the Supply of Nurses, 1974–1983.'' *Inquiry* 22:4 (Winter), 404–417.

————. (1981). ''Physician Extenders: Potential for Improved Productivity.'' *Hospital Progress* 62:2 (February), 32–45.

Eastaugh, S., and Regan, M. (1990). ''Nurse Extenders Offer a Way to Trim Staff Expenses.'' *Healthcare Financial Management* 44:4 (April), 58–62.

Edgren, J. (1976). ''The Nursing Shortage and the NTA: Should the Federal Government Be Paying for the Education of Nurses?'' Health Manpower Studies Group Working Paper A–12 (September). Ann Arbor, Mich.: School of Public Health, University of Michigan.

Elbeck, M. (1992). ''Patient Contribution to the Design and Meaning of Satisfaction.'' *Health Care Management Review* 17:1 (Spring), 91–95.

Fralic, M., Kowalski, P., and Llewellyn, F. (1991) ''The Staff Nurse as a Quality Monitor.'' *American Journal of Nursing* 91:4 (April), 40–43.

Frame, P., Wetterav, N., and Parey, B. (1978). ''A Model for the Use of Physician Assistants in Primary Care.'' *Journal of Family Practice* 7:12 (December), 1195–1204.

Feldstein, P. (1979). *Health Care Economics*. New York: John Wiley, 375.

Friss, L. (1990). *Strategic Management of Nurses: A Policy-oriented Approach*. Baltimore: National Health Publishing.

Ginzberg, E. (1990). ''Health Personnel: The Challenges Ahead.'' *Frontiers of Health Services Management* 7:2 (Winter), 3–19.

Greenfield, S., Kamaroff, A., Pass, T., Anderson, H., and Nessim, S. (1978). ''Efficiency and the Cost of Primary Care by Nurses and Physician Assistants.'' *New England Journal of Medicine* 288:6 (February 9), 305–309.

Hafer, J., and Ambrose, D. (1983). ''Psychographic Analysis of Nursing Students: Implications for the Marketing and Development of the Nursing Profession.'' *Health Care Management Review* 8:3 (Summer), 69–76.

Hall, T., and Lindsay, C. (1980). ''Medical Schools: Producers of What? Sellers to Whom?'' *Journal of Law and Economics* 23:2 (April), 55–80.

Hepner, J. (1990). ''What Else Is New for Health Professionals?'' *Frontiers of Health Services Management* 7:2 (Winter), 33–36.

Hershey, J., and Kropp, D. (1979). ''A Re-appraisal of the Productivity Potential and Economic Benefits of Physician's Assistants.'' *Medical Care* 17:6 (June), 592–606.

Iglehart, J. (1992). ''American Health Care.'' *NEJM* 326:14 (April 2), 962–968.

Institute of Medicine. (1989). *Allied Health Services: Avoiding Crises*. Washington, D.C.: National Academy of Sciences.

————. (1983). *Study of Nursing and Nursing Education*. Washington, D.C.: National Academy of Sciences.

————. (1978). *A Manpower Policy for Primary Health Care*. Washington, D.C.: National Academy of Sciences.

————. (1974). *Costs of Education in the Health Professions*. Washington, D.C.: National Academy of Sciences.

Intriligator, M. (1978). *Econometric Models, Techniques, and Applications*. Englewood Cliffs, N.J.: Prentice-Hall.

Kelly, K. (1985). "Nurse Practitioner Challenges to the Orthodox Structure of Health Care Delivery: Regulation and Restraint on Trade." *American Journal of Law and Medicine* 11:2 (December), 195–225.

Kessel, R. (1958). "Price Discrimination in Medicine." *Journal of Law and Economics* 1:1 (October), 20–53.

Kruijthof, C. (1992). "Career Perspectives of Women and Men Medical Students." *Medical Education* 26:1 (January), 21–26.

Lamb, G., and Napodano, R. (1984). "Physician-Nurse Practitioner Interaction Patterns in Primary Care Practices." *American Journal of Public Health* 74:1 (January), 26–29.

Macy Foundation. (1976). *Physicians for the Future: Report of the Josiah Macy Commission*. New York, 27.

McNally, J. (1981). "Nursing Shortage: Fact or Fiction." *Hospital Financial Management* 11:5 (May), 16–25.

McNamara, J., and Smith, R. (1984). "Management Issues in an Ambulatory Care Consortium." *Journal of Ambulatory Management* 2:1 (January), 1–11.

Mechanic, D., and Aiken, L. (1983). "A Cooperative Agenda for Medicine and Nursing." *New England Journal of Medicine* 307:12 (September 16), 747–750.

Mendenhall, R., Repicky, P., and Neville, R. (1980). "Assessing the Utilization and Productivity of Nurse Practitioners and Physician's Assistants: Methodology and Findings on Productivity." *Medical Care* 18:6 (June), 609–623.

Mennemeyer, S., and Gaumer, G. (1983). "Nursing Wages and the Value of Education Credentials." *Journal of Human Resources* 18:4 (Winter), 32–48.

Moscovice, I., and Rosenblatt, R. (1979). "The Viability of Mid-Level Practitioners in Isolated Rural Communities." *American Journal of Public Health* 69:5 (May), 503–505.

National League of Nursing (1991). *NLN Nursing Data Book*. New York: National League of Nursing.

Nelson, E., Jacobs, A., Cordner, B., and Johnson, K. (1975). "Financial Impact of Physician Assistants on Medical Practice." *New England Journal of Medicine* 293:11 (September 11), 527–530.

Newhouse, J., et al. (1982). "Where Have All the Doctors Gone?" *Journal of the American Medical Association* 247:17 (May 7), 2392–2396.

Perry, H. (1976). "Physician Assistants: An Empirical Analysis." Ph.D. diss., Department of Social Relations, Johns Hopkins University.

Petersdorf, R. (1992). "Primary Care Applicants." *New England Journal of Medicine* 326:6 (February 6), 408–409.

Pope, G., Butrica, B., and Pitcher, J. (1991). "CRNA Manpower Forecasts: 1990–2010." *Medical Care* 29:7 (July), 628–644.

Prescott, P., and Driscoll, L. (1979). "Nurse Practitioner Effectiveness." *Evaluation and the Health Professions* 2:4 (December), 387–418.

Record, J., Blomquist, R., Berger, B., and O'Bannon, J. (1977). "Quality of PA Performance at a HMO." In A. Bliss and E. Cohen (eds.), *The New Health Professionals*, chap. 12. Germantown, Md.: Aspen Systems.

Record, J., McCally, M., and Schweitzer, S. (1989). "New Health Professions after a

Decade and a Half: Delegation, Productivity, and Costs in Primary Care." *Journal of Health Policy, Politics, and Law* 5:3 (Fall), 470–497.

Reinhardt, U. (1975). *Physician Productivity and the Demand for Health Manpower.* Cambridge, Mass.: Ballinger.

————. (1972). "A Production Function for Physician Service." *Review of Economics and Statistics* 54:1 (February), 55–66.

Roberts, M., Minnick, A., Ginzberg, E., and Curran, C. (1989). *A Commonwealth Fund Study: What to Do about the Nursing Shortage.* New York: Commonwealth Fund.

Rosenblatt, R. (1992). "Specialists or Generalists: On Whom Should We Base the American Health Care System?" *JAMA* 367:12 (March 25) 1665–1666.

Scott, C., and Harrison, A. (1990). "Direct Reimbursement of Nurse Practitioners in Health Insurance Plans of Research Universities." *Journal of Professional Nursing* 6:1 (January–February), 21–25.

Simms, L., Dalston, J., and Roberts, P. (1984). "Collaborative Practice: Myth or Reality?" *Hospital and Health Services Administration* 29:6 (November/December), 36–48.

Sorkin, A. (1979). *Health Economics.* Lexington, Mass.: D. C. Heath.

Stein, L., Watts, D., and Howell, T. (1990). "The Doctor-Nurse Game Revisited." *New England Journal of Medicine* 322:8 (February 22), 546–549.

Sturmann, K., Ehrenberg, K., and Salzberg, M. (1990). "Physician Assistants in Emergency Medicine." *Annals of Emergency Medicine* 19:3 (March), 304–308.

Systems Sciences, Inc. (1978). *Survey and Evaluation of the Physician Extender Reimbursement Experiment.* Contract No. 55A–600–76–0167, Social Security Administration, Washington, D.C.

Thorpe, K., Hendricks, A., and Newhouse, J. (1992). "Reducing the Number of Uninsured by Subsidizing Employment-based Insurance." *Journal of the American Medical Association* 267:7 (February 19), 945–948.

U.S. Congress, Office of Technology Assessment (OTA). (1989). *Nurse Practitioners, Physician Assistants, and Certified Nurse-Midwives: A Policy Analysis.* Washington, D.C.: U.S. Government Printing Office.

Wallen, J. (1980). "Considerations in the Use of Nonphysician Health Care Providers in Physician-Shortage Areas." Unpublished report, Division of Intramural Research, National Center for Health Services Research, DHEW.

Weiner, J., Steinwachs, D., and Williamson, J. (1986). "Nurse Practitioner and Physician Assistant Practices in Three HMOs: Implications for Future U.S. Health Manpower Needs." *American Journal of Public Health* 76:5 (May), 507–511.

Weston, J. (1984). "Ambiguities Limit the Role of Nurse Practitioners and Physician Assistants." *American Journal of Public Health* 74:1 (January), 6–7.

Yett, A. (1975). *An Economic Analysis of the Nursing Shortage.* Lexington, Mass.: D. C. Heath.

Zander, K. (1990). "The 1990's: Core Values, Core Change." *Frontiers of Health Services Management* 7:2 (Winter), 28–32.

Zeckhauser, R., and Eliastam, M. (1974). "The Productivity of the Physician Assistant." *Journal of Human Resources* 9:1 (Winter), 95–116.

VI EFFICIENCY, EFFECTIVENESS, AND COST-BENEFIT ANALYSIS

11 Cost-Effectiveness and Cost-Benefit Analysis

It is better to put a fence at the top of the cliff than an ambulance at the bottom.

—James Mason

The highest quality providers are also the most cost-effective because they make fewer mistakes and know how to treat conditions properly, avoiding traumatic expensive procedures when there are less intensive but equally effective alternatives.

—Charles Jacobs

Cost management means the delivery of all the care that is medically needed, for as long as it is needed, but not for a day or a dollar more.

—Robert Shelton

Cost-effectiveness and cost-benefit analysis have been applied in many preventive, diagnostic, and treatment contexts. Over the past decade methods have improved for prospectively collecting better data sets and incorporating intangible quality-of-life valuations into the calculus for weighing benefits against costs. Further cooperation between clinicians, economists, and epidemiologists is a healthy trend. Political scientists are prone to argue over valuation in dollars, reflecting a basic misunderstanding of the trade-off concept and a need to combine and compare benefits and costs in comparable units. The purpose of this chapter is to review the state of the art of cost-effectiveness and cost-benefit analysis in evaluation of medical technologies. Economic evaluation of new or expensive technologies has become a central issue in the public debate about rising medical care costs (Sisk 1990). Historically, the growth in technology has stimulated a concomitant increase in the numbers and salaries of health care employees. Warner and Luce (1989) and Fuchs (1986) characterized the new health technologies prior to 1955 as being cost-saving (physician time-saving and usually quality-enhancing), whereas the technologies introduced since 1955 have tended to be cost-increasing. Physicians and economists frequently express their hope that these expensive and/or physician-using technologies are partially justified by their quality-enhancing properties. Sometimes expensive new technologies can be cost-saving. The price of a kidney transplant in 1980 was about $26,000, equivalent to about $63,000 in 1991. In 1991 the actual price of a kidney transplant was $41,000, including the expensive anti-rejection drug cyclosporine, unavailable in 1980. A kidney transplant costs $63,000 the first year, then you have an immunosuppression cost of $4,600 a year. The alternative, dialysis costs $33,000–37,000 each year.

BASIC CONCEPTS

The objective of cost-benefit analysis is to maximize net benefits (benefits minus costs, appropriately discounted over time). The objective of cost-effectivness analysis is to rank order the preferred alternatives for achieving a single goal or specified basket of benefits. Cost-effectiveness analysis is not any easier to perform than cost-benefit analysis if multiple varieties of benefit are specified (person-years, work-loss days, reduced angina), except that in doing cost-benefit analysis one must value the intangible benefits in commensurate dollar terms. Operationally, ethical questions can be raised if the benefits and costs accrue to different social groups. For example, a clinic scheduling system that minimizes wasted time for the physician through multiple overlapping appointments may be a net benefit of a few hundred dollars per doctor at the expense of many more dollars of patient time.

In economic sectors where competitive markets fail to exist, such as the health care or water resource sectors, cost-benefit analysis aims to do what supply and demand forces accomplish in competitive markets. The price system will not equalize marginal benefits and marginal costs if market failure exists—that is, price disequilibrium occurs in highly insured consumer markets (Fuchs 1986). Another criterion of choice is to maximize the ratio of benefits to costs, discounting the numerator and denominator to present-value dollars. Alternative programs (or procedures or services) are then ranked by benefit-cost ratios, and the programs with the highest payoff ratios are selected until resources are exhausted or until the ratio equals one. This approach is equivalent to maximizing net present value within a budget constraint. A third, outmoded decision criterion is to support a project if the internal rate of return exceeds the predetermined discount rate. The internal rate-of-return criterion can lead to different resource decisions from the net-present-value criteria if programs are of different sizes or have varying time horizons.

If a technology is found to be the most cost-effective alternative, then the next question is whether it is cost-beneficial. For example, Acton (1973) first evaluated which of five program alternatives was most efficacious and which was most cost-effective in reducing deaths from heart attacks, which he followed by a valuation of life and intangible benefits to assess whether the benefits made the program worth the costs for society. One obvious advantage of cost-benefit analysis is that it leads to a positive (go) or negative (no-go) net present value for the procedure being evaluated and does not require a cost-effectiveness cutoff level to decide whether a project can be done within the resource constraints. However, many more complete cost-effectiveness analyses are performed than cost-benefit analyses, because intangible benefits pose difficulties with valuation, and the choice of a discount rate is simpler in cost-effectiveness evaluations (Eastaugh 1983).

If a technology is found to be cost-beneficial, the only question left is whether the risk is socially acceptable for public financing of the service. Society may have some preference for the social classes that are to face an unacceptable risk, even if it is known in advance that the total risk is insufficient to make the benefit-to-cost ratio less than one. Safety, as measured by risk analysis, is a relative concept. No test or therapy that provides any benefit has ever been completely safe. Physicians, like all professionals, have learned to live comfortably with the reasonable notion that we must forgo some safety to achieve any net benefit (Shortliffe 1991).

THE MERITS OF PREVENTION AND EXPERIMENTATION

One may consider the efficiency of medical care in a broader context by taking output as the overall health of the nation rather than simply as days of care. Victor Fuchs (1986) stated that ''when the state of medical science and other health-determining variables are held constant, the marginal contribution of medical care to health is very small in modern nations.'' In other words, one cannot simply add more doctors and hospitals and expect an equivalent improvement in health. Fuchs gives several reasons for this low marginal contribution. First, patients and physicians use more discretion when physicians are scarce—that is, patients seek medical care less often when it is difficult to obtain, and physicians tend to concentrate on those patients who need care most. Second, many highly effective treatments such as vaccinations do not require the huge amounts of resources required by many generally less effective treatments such as heart transplants. Third, as medical care proliferates, iatrogenic disease becomes a problem, exemplified by highly risky surgical interventions. Fourth, it is difficult to measure the output of medical care in terms of health, in that many factors other than medical care contribute to health—for example, nutrition and environment (Fuchs 1986).

It is certainly not necessary to conduct economic analysis and randomized clinical trials on every new technology, and certainly not on most existing ones. However, the uncontrollable economic pressures for efficiency are apt to result in more careful economic analysis. Some of these studies will severely disrupt the conventional wisdom. For example, Russell (1985) studied a number of preventive programs, from immunization to exercise programs, and concluded that society's total health care costs increased (i.e., prevention was a cost add-on, not a cost-saving investment). Investments that cost very little on a per person basis become very expensive when applied on a national basis. Russell cited the example of a blood pressure check, which is very inexpensive on an individual basis, but becomes very costly when applied to 20 to 30 million people. A well targeted work-site blood pressure control program can result in $1.72 to $2.72 in reduced health care claims per dollar spent operating the program (Foote and Erfurt 1991). Harvard professor Tom Schelling (1986) suggested that smoking cessation programs may not be cost-beneficial for society. However, Ershoff, Mullen, and Quinn (1989) performed a randomized trial to test the effectiveness of a prenatal self-help smoking cessation program, and 20 percent of the women in the program quit smoking, versus 8.8 percent of the control group.

Two basic truths seem apparent. First, society should not be oversold on prevention and health promotion as a strategy to slow (or reverse) the rise in national health expenditures. If health officials oversell their programs as a cost-saving vehicle, the inevitable disillusionment will cause excessive additional cuts in public health programs (i.e., a backlash against such programs). Second, prevention may not save money, but such programs can often be justified in terms of a worthwhile investment in improved quality of life. Keeping people happy is expensive, but quality of life is something worth paying for in the minds of most citizens. Analogously, while many medical technologies may be cost-increasing, they are strongly supported by the public. Schwartz and Aaron (1984) summarized this issue best with the following example: Hip replacements are much more expensive than providing an elderly person with aspirin and a walker, but wouldn't most people want the quality-of-life mobility of a new hip?

Newcomer (1990) suggested that the reason prevention is not covered by insurance companies is that it may not be effective, or, if effective, it may not be cost-saving. While this attitude toward exclusions seems purely economic, some decisions by private insurance companies to include experimental therapy (e.g., bone marrow transplants for certain cancers) have more to do with public relations. A March 1991 public poll listed lack of insurance coverage for experimental therapy as the number two health problem (cost control was the number one problem). There is an irony in this listing, because the number two problem was a reaction by private insurance companies designed to combat the number one problem (excessive costs). Medical costs are excessive for the population, but not for identified individuals. Medical costs are too high, but if the money is to be spent on an identified person—you, a family member, or a nice person on the television set—then many political leaders (and followers) say, "Spend the money, even if the therapy is untested and seldom successful." We shall return to the topic of "identified individuals" and our willingness to pay in chapter 13. Redelmeier and Tversky (1990) have outlined the basic difference between the individual perspective and the group perspective in making health policy. An individual with a medical condition spins the wheel of chance for treatment once or a few times, but a policy maker must play the leadership role of spinning the wheel for millions of unseen individuals and aggregate the costs, risks, and benefits (a difficult task that will frame our discussion in chapter 12). Individual providers at the bedside take patients in groups of one and have a bias for action and treatment in America, an instinct dubbed the rule of rescue by Jonsen (1988).

Why are proven preventive services underinsured? Even in the event that preventive services are cost-saving, the gains may be so far in the future or the elasticity of supply in the industry may be so high that insurance companies are unable to reap any benefits (Cohen 1989; Robinson 1990). One of the problems with preventive screening examinations is that the cost of treating false-positive results, along with adverse psychological effects, may outweigh the benefits of detecting a disease in its early stages (Leaf 1989). In the same vein, Fuchs (1986) suggested that if expensive cancer-treatment programs did not exist, people might be more likely to follow their own prevention programs. In this case it might be more important to encourage a change in behavioral patterns rather than to support research into expensive cancer treatments. The critical need for better technology-assessment studies was highlighted in the 1986 federal government decision to pay for heart transplants on a limited basis. If heart transplants were performed on all patients who could marginally benefit from them, the cost per year would be an estimated $8 billion; that estimate compares to an annual expense of $950 million for liver transplants.

Some 133,000 Medicare beneficiaries will have coronary bypass surgery at a cost of $3.1 billion in 1992. To trim this expense, HCFA is trying a PPO approach to regionalized heart surgery at four hospitals: St. Joseph Mercy Hospital in Ann Arbor, University Hospital in Boston, St. Joseph's Hospital in Atlanta, and Ohio State University Hospital in Columbus. HCFA will pay one combined fixed fee for all expenses (surgeon fees and hospital costs). HCFA will receive a 9 to 20 percent discount for this PPO "package rate" in FY 1992, and the patients will receive lower copayments and quality service in a highly specialized teaching hospital. As patients are encouraged to go to designated Medicare PPO specialty centers in the mid–1990s, fatality rates should decline and costs should be controlled. The only loser under PPO/Medicare is the hospitals that have no specialty designation and are experiencing declining patient revenues.

The traditional basis of clinical medicine suggests that the physician should make every effort to provide all possible avenues of care to the patient. The idea of scarcity of resources has no role in this code of ethics, except during wartime (Hiatt 1990). The medical ethic is increasingly being criticized relative to the public health ethic, which suggests that every clinician has an obligation to inquire about underserved potential patients and forgone person-years of life for conditions that go untreated because physicians serve a technological imperative and a profit imperative (that is, they serve the patients who are technically interesting or profitable, then attend to the other cases; Callahan 1991). Decision making is increasingly affected by computer monitoring, surveillance of the quality of care, and appropriateness review (Evans, Larsen, and Burke 1986; Kanouse, Winkler, and Kosecoff 1989; Chassin, Kosecoff, and Park 1990).

METHODS OF ANALYSIS

There has been a high degree of public and political disenchantment with model builders who provide narrow definitions of direct benefits and ignore the limitations of their very crude data bases. The typical accounting costs of billed charges or incurred expenses are too narrow a definition of cost for the economic analyst. Confusion frequently exists when members of the medical profession attempt to do a cost analysis. For example, the cost to society of not having airbags must not exclude accident victims who are DOAs (dead on arrival). In the arena of cost-effectiveness analysis between medical treatment versus surgery, surgeons frequently omit DOTs (dead on table) from the analysis in order to make surgery look better relative to medical treatment. The tendency is to go far afield in counting benefits and to neglect some costs, such as the pain of surgery or the overhead costs of the operating room. Cash expenditures are too limited a definition of cost. True cost to society can only be measured in opportunity-cost terms. In the parlance of economics, the cost of any item or service is the forgone benefit that you sacrificed in order to obtain it.

Estimating the economic burden of a disease involves the measurement of prevalence, the assessment of impact on the individual's health status and other people's well-being, and the eventual quantification of direct and indirect costs associated with these impacts. For example, Berry and Boland (1977) estimated the cost of alcohol abuse at $31.4 billion in 1971. Half of the alcohol abuse burden on the economy resulted from lost economic production ($14.9 billion), $8.3 billion was generated in direct health care service costs, and the residual $8.2 billion resulted from motor vehicle accidents, fires, crime, and other less tangible impacts.

Pauly and Held (1990) suggested a number of sources of uncertainty in making economic decisions. The first source of analytical uncertainty results from incomplete mastery of available knowledge in medicine coupled with the fact that medicine is in a constant state of flux and revision. A second source results from limitations in current medical knowledge. HIV-1, HIV-2, Lyme disease, Legionnaires' disease, and eosinophilia-myalgia syndrome were only characterized in the 1980s, and new disease entities are being discovered every year. The third source of uncertainty, derived from the first two, is the difficulty in distinguishing between ignorance and the limitations of current medical knowledge: the fear of the untaught versus the fear of the unknown. Acquired immune deficiency syndrome (AIDS) is a major social issue, and we shall consider a risk-analysis assessment in chapter 13. Hardy et al. (1986) estimated that the first 10,000 AIDS cases in the United States required 1.6 million hospital days at a direct cost of $1.4 billion and $4.8 billion in lost (forgone) wages from 8,387 lost years of work from disability and premature death. In most cases indirect costs can be the largest component of the analysis. Klarman (1965) estimated the present value of eradicating syphilis at $3.1 billion, with 42 percent of this total benefit accounted for by erasure of the "stigma" associated with the discovery of the disease. The study assumed that people were willing to forgo 1.5 percent of their earnings to avoid the stigma associated with the disease.

MEASUREMENT OF INDIRECT BENEFITS

Direct benefits of health services or public health programs are measured by the forgone medical care costs. Often the direct benefits of eliminating a disease are a fraction of the indirect benefits. For example, in 1979 the Department of Health, Education, and Welfare (DHEW) estimated the direct benefits of eliminating medical expenditures on smokers at $5 billion annually, and the indirect benefits were estimated at $12 billion in terms of forgone worker productivity. Mushkin (1962) separated indirect benefits of health programs into three categories: reducing premature death, avoiding lost working time (morbidity), and avoiding lost capacity to be productive after returning to work (debility). The first and second measures, mortality and morbidity, have been well researched. However, our ability to quantify debility remains a topic for future research. Expected earnings replaced income as the relevant measure of indirect benefits in the 1960s (Rice 1966). Cooper and Rice (1976) produced annual tabulations of the present value of lost earnings due to mortality under alternative discount rates and annual estimates of the forgone earnings due to disability. In some cases potential morbidity reduction represents 90 percent of indirect benefits (skin diseases), and in other cases potential mortality reduction represents 90 percent of indirect benefits (neoplasms). Rice, Hodgson, and Kopstein (1985) estimated the cost of illness at $455 billion: $211 billion for direct costs, $176 billion for mortality, and $68 billion for morbidity. Diseases of the circulatory system and injuries were the most costly conditions.

The value of housewives' services has also recently entered the benefit picture, although their services are still omitted from the gross national product. Klarman (1967) measured housewives' services by the wages they could earn (using alternative wages they could earn as an opportunity-cost measure), while Weisbrod (1968) measured their replacement value by the cost of employing a housekeeper. The only strength of the Weisbrod approach is that it estimates housewives' worth as an increasing function of family size: A housewife is more expensive to replace in larger families. The opportunity-cost concept is more persuasive, since housewife value is a function of education attainment and occupation. Forgone earnings as an estimate of indirect benefits are relatively easy to estimate, although some radical economists might question the assumption that earnings are a suitable measure of social benefit. The resultant biases implicit in measuring benefits in terms of earnings reflect imperfections in the labor market such as racism and sexism.

Most economists became disenchanted during the 1970s with the gross-output approach of valuing a person's life as discounted expected future earnings. For example, the conclusion that visits to a rheumatology clinic were cost-beneficial only for males merely reflects an artifact of the sex bias in earnings data: Women earn less (Glass 1973). A variant of this approach—subtracting out consumption to yield net output—was considered ill advised, because killing elderly or handicapped individuals would be "valued" as an act that confers a net benefit to society. Fromm (1965) suggested a third approach, valuing life on the basis of the life insurance premiums one is willing to pay. However, the life insurance approach only measures a person's willingness to compensate others following death rather than the value set on one's own life.

The most prevalent assessment approach in the 1970s was the "willingness-to-pay" approach suggested by Schelling (1968) and measured initially by Acton (1973). Both authors realized that quantity multiplied by price was at best equal to a minimum benefit of health services to the society, since it does not account for the many consumers who would be willing to pay more than the price.

A consumer's surplus of benefit involves estimating a measurable proxy, the area under the entire demand curve. Figure 11.1 illustrates the concept of measuring benefit by the amount of money that each person is willing to pay rather than go without the service. For a hypothetical example of selling bone marrow transplants to people with aplastic anemia, figure 11.1 shows some 48 individuals willing to pay $100,000 to receive the treatment.

Not all individuals are willing to pay the same amount under hypothetical conditions of equal wealth across all individuals. Individuals face different risks; for example, the treatment is painful and often causes potentially fatal side effects under which the new transplanted marrow cells attack the liver, skin, and other organs. The ABC shaded area above the price line AB is the sum of money equal to the consumer's surplus. The surplus represents a dollar measure of the excess of satisfaction over consumer dissatisfaction. Individuals 1 to 6 are willing to pay an extra $100,000 above the price ($100,000), individuals 7 to 11 are willing to pay an extra $80,000 each, individuals 12 to 15 are willing to pay an extra $60,000, individuals 16 to 25 are willing to pay an extra $40,000, and individuals 26 to 40 are willing to pay an additional $20,000 each. Consequently, the net benefits are $4,800,000 (price times quantity) plus $1,940,000 consumer's surplus.

This analysis assumes that the consumer is well informed and that the social value of transplants for anemia patients is the sum of the individual values. One might argue for adding on a psychic benefit for expressing the value that all members of society place on the assurance that if they have this rare type of anemia, the bone marrow transplant will be available.

Whether the bone marrow transplant makes economic sense depends on the expected survival rate and the probability of complications beyond the standard (average) case. An aggregate figure for cost per year of life saved may be $62,500, as in Welch and Larsen (1989). However, the cost with complications

Figure 11.1
Hypothetical Demand Curve for Bone Marrow Transplant Therapy (Aplastic Anemia Patients)

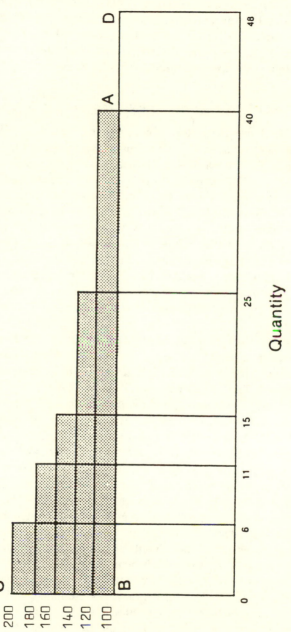

The shaded regions represent the consumer's surplus.

has a wide coefficient of variation (Viens-Bitker, Fery, and Blum, 1989), and the averages vary widely: $43,000 for allogenic bone marrow transplant in adult acute myelogenous leukemia, $50,000 for chronic granulocytic leukemia, $108,000 for severe combined immunodeficiency, and $180,000 for severe aplastic anemia. One of the technical problems with the Oregon Medicaid approach to health care resource allocation (using cost-benefit ratios) is the wide variety of clinical subdivisions within each of the program's 1,800 listed conditions.

The Oregon Approach to Rationing by Cost-Benefit Estimation

The choice for society is not rationing: yes or no? We ration services now based on a number of factors (money, time, and all the other factors covered in chapter 3). The question is whether rationing should be implicit or explicit. The public has little explicit knowledge of the process, but we ration now at the bedside based on do-not-resuscitate orders (Hackler and Hiller 1990; Tomlinson and Brody 1990). In addition to this implicit micro form of rationing, Americans also ration at the macro level every time they make a capital-asset decision (not to build that public hospital in Illinois or Louisiana). Oregon is the first state to try to make rationing explicit, scientific, and also consumerist (by asking people for their opinion). The difficulty Oregon Medicaid officials will have defending their list of unreimbursed conditions with an insufficient (low) cost-benefit ratio reflects the social difficulties of withholding any useful technology (Mechanic 1989).

A brief background of the evolution of the Oregon approach is necessary. The physician leader of the Oregon senate (mentioned in chapter 7) viewed rationing medical progress as the way to affordable health care and expanding access to the poor. This would help 119,000 poor people, and the federal government would pay 63 percent of the $149 million expense. The idea (beginning in 1988) was to use Medicaid funds to expand basic health services to all Oregonians below the poverty line. In most states less than half of the poor citizens are eligible for Medicaid. To provide expanded primary care and universal access to all poor citizens, Oregon officials enlisted consumers and physicians to construct a priority-based list of over 1,800 conditions. The state payments will extend as far down the list as available funds allow. The approach to developing the list was ad hoc, based on opinions of social value and clinical effectiveness (Kitzhaber 1990). The 1990 draft list of services was not based on cost-benefit analysis, but rather was a political compromise imputing values to qualitative estimates of cost, risk, and benefit. The Oregon Health Services Commission public meetings attracted only 260 nonphysician consumers and 330 providers during 1989–90. Some of the listings were indefensible, like ranking cosmetic breast surgery higher than treatment for an open thigh fracture, and the list makers were sent back to work to develop a 1992 list for pilot testing.

More defensible lists could be developed if they involved a wider cross-sectional survey of the general public (Eastaugh 1991). Alternatively, economists could impute values to national statistics and make explicit decisions based on expert opinion. Both approaches to list making have been tried in Canada (Linton and Naylor 1990) and the United Kingdom (Klein 1991). Political reaction to the Oregon approach has ranged from positive to negative: Joseph Califano thinks that government should not play King Solomon and decide who benefits from new technology, and the poor are not the place to look for funds to benefit the poor. National Institutes of Health (NIH) physicians and private firms in the biomedical area think that list making by cost-benefit will narrow our horizons, inhibit vision, slow the progress of researchers, and trap America within the limitations of today's technology.

Arnold Relman (1990) argued that we should expand basic care for all (regardless of ability to pay) by redistributing funds to primary care and away from high-tech firms and high-cost, low-effectiveness transplants. To make significant progress toward reducing the rapidly increasing financial strains on the health care system, a complete "realignment" of expectations is needed. Two of the most vocal and articulate proponents of this shift in values are Daniel Callahan of the Hastings Center and Richard D. Lamm (1990), director of the Center for Public Policy and Contemporary Issues at the University of Colorado.

Three of the steps toward rationing that were suggested by Callahan (1990) are the following:

1. Stringent assessments of technology before dissemination
2. Social and economic standards for the assessment that are biased toward restrictiveness
3. An understanding that beneficial applications may have to be passed over on grounds of cost and other, more pressing social priorities

He argued that any change must encompass both a strict cost-containment movement and a shift in fundamental values. Both Callahan and Lamm pointed to Oregon's health care rationing program as a step in the right direction. The Oregon experiment will be interesting to watch. Schwartz and Aaron (1990) suggested that Oregon Medicaid assign priorities to specific medical interventions on the basis of cost-benefit considerations but take into account individual circumstances.

The next two chapters survey a number of normative economic models. The techniques, such as cost-benefit analysis and cost-effectiveness analysis, are decision-making models designed to guide resource decisions, from building a facility to deciding what technique should be the standard operating procedure. The truth is, of course, that normative techniques are typically used to help provide better-informed decisions at the margin, rather than dictate cookbook decision making. In our pluralistic society, the decision makers are wise to keep the experts on tap, rather than on top (Eastaugh 1983). A number of willingness-to-pay techniques are presented in chapter 13. The willingness-to-pay approach is an improvement relative to the economic theory of human capital developed by Becker (1964) and others. In contrast to the human-capital approach for measuring forgone expected earnings, the willingness-to-pay approach provides a consumer measure of the sum total of indirect benefits and intangible benefits.

Economics and Patients

The critical point to convey to the reader is that cost-effectiveness analysis and cost-benefit analysis are increasingly taking their appropriate position in the evaluation (prediffusion) stage prior to the marketing decision. The rationale of this emerging public policy is that the costs (in lives and in dollars) of forgoing economic and efficacy evaluation may often be much greater than the costs of a well-designed evaluation. One "consumerist" benefit of increasing reliance on economic evaluation is that it must force those in power to be explicit about (1) valuation-of-life biases (across social class) in cost-benefit calculations and (2) the resource cutoff level utilized in cost-effectiveness analysis.

As the public increasingly understands the degree to which medicine involves decision making under uncertainty, the doctor-god model must give way to a more realistic paradigm. Consumers might better think of their doctor as a "senior partner" (SP) in health care. This abrupt relabeling of the professional title, from M.D. to SP, highlights the rising popularity of health promotion and education and the declining perception of infallibility in medicine. Moreover, outcome measures of quality and patient satisfaction and compliance are inseparable. Patient compliance is critical to improving health status (Eastaugh and Hatcher 1982). SPs enhance patient compliance and provide a better level of informed consent; omniscient practitioners claim that their "hands are touched by the god." Gods give out proclamations; SPs give probability estimates and explain them. For some patients, the explanation of odds and conditional probabilities may be so complex as to best be labeled "overinformed consent." The sensitive SP knows when to stop with the detail, whereas a god would never become schooled in such detail or provide it to a patient. The SP will wait for the junior partner (patient) to say either "Enough detail, go for XYZ" or "What shall we do, doctor?"

MEASUREMENT OF INTANGIBLE BENEFITS

Valuation is not a consideration in competitive markets, because marginal benefit is assumed to be equal to price. However, when prices fail to exist (water resources) or price is deemed a defective measure of value (health services), an attempt is made to impute value or "shadow price." Shadow-price values can be imputed by asking individuals what they would be willing to pay for relief from pain, grief, discomfort, and disfigurement. For example, if a year of life is valued by a willingness-to-pay measure of $28,000, and a woman would sacrifice a year of life to avoid losing her breast(s) (Abt 1977), this suggests a shadow price of $28,000 for a mastectomy. In this situation, Abt suggested that the additional costs for a few more drugs and drinks would bring the annual average shadow price of grief and worry to about $3,000. Often the analyst can only identify the need to shadow-price an intangible benefit. For example, one intangible that is difficult to shadow-price is the benefit of restored fertility capacity that follows a successful kidney transplant.

The shadow-price concept can also be applied to arrive at quality weights for adjusting the value of additional years of existence. Klarman (1965) utilized an analogous-disease approach to measure the willingness-to-pay value of escape from early manifestations of syphilis by the proxy disease psoriasis and from the late manifestations of syphilis by the proxy of terminal cancer cases. Direct data acquisition for "unstigmatized" medical conditions like cancer and psoriasis was more easily accomplished than working directly with syphilis victims. Economists must work with physicians to develop proxies and weighting schemes for capturing the multiplicity of dimensions of health care outputs. Inappropriate priorities might be set if survival probabilities are not integrated with quality-of-life factors.

A growing number of physician surveys have focused on diagnostic decisions. Two suggested approaches present evidence as to just how advanced and complex medical risk assessment became in the 1980s. Spiegelhalter and Knill-Jones (1984) favored computing diagnostic probabilities by forming a control group that is a combination of all the other diagnostic categories. This conceptual approach deals with the real-world problem in which patients may possess several diagnoses simultaneously. Alternatively, Begg and McNeil (1985) suggested a decomposition in which each diagnostic group is separately treated with a baseline (normal) category as more appropriate in the absence of complex, equally critical, multiple-condition cases. Both approaches are equally valid, but the second approach may be more generalizable (and easier to explain to clinicians).

Individual physicians will not see a large number of instances of any specific rare condition in their practice, but individual subjective opinion is useful. As Kahneman, Slovic, and Tversky (1982) pointed out, most predictions contain an irreducible intuitive component. The intuitive threshold estimates of good clinicians contain useful information, even if they are biased in a predictable manner. Doctors often have more specific observations about the patient than can be evaluated by long-run statistical analysis. As Neuhauser (1991) indicated, subjective probabilities are not just the stuff we do before the statistician arrives.

Consumer surveys are prevalent in the area of decisions (Eastaugh 1983). The consumer utility literature has benefited from the development of more sophisticated scales for measuring preference functions and indifference curves. Stewart, Ware, and Johnston (1975) and Grogono and Woodgate (1971) developed refined, but unvalidated, scales for measuring physical, social, psychiatric, and mobility limitations. The psychometric approach provided only marginal improvements over the 1948 Visick scales. Multiattribute utility theory has been applied to evaluate the benefits of treating sore throats (Giaque and Peebles 1976) and cleft lips in children (Krischer 1976). Indifference-curve analysis has been suggested as another approach to quantifying benefits. Fuchs (1986) described an indifference curve along which combined sickness, pain, and restricted-activity-day composite measures of suffering are weighted equally undesirable. Viscusi and Evans (1990) improved on the concept of building utility functions that depend on health status. Their study of workplace injury and disability suggested that the injury-value figures used for deferred risk reductions should take into account the income growth of those affected by the safety regulations, thus leading to an adjustment that serves to mute much of the role of discounting.

The best practical early application of utility analysis was provided by Weinstein, Pliskin, and Stason (1977) in their assessment of quality-of-life considerations after coronary artery bypass surgery. Quality-of-life outcome measures include pain at rest, pain with minimal activity, pain with mild activity, pain with strenuous activity, and no pain. Quite predictably, a potential surgical patient places a higher utility value on no pain if he or she avoids exercise. A utility function to value outcomes was specified as a function of life-style and life expectancy. The data are highly subjective, but reliance on imperfect analysis provides more insights than analytical nihilism. A Rand Corporation analyst (Keeler 1989) reported that the lifetime subsidy of the average citizen to the sedentary life-style person is $1,900. Life style choice is a critical issue for many medical decisions from birth (Garber and Fenerty 1991) to old age (Paiement, Wessinger, and Harris 1991; Max, Rice, and MacKenzie 1990).

Cost-effectiveness analysis is more frequently completed because intangible benefits need only be estimated, not valued. Cost-effectiveness analysis requires only that all benefits be expressed in commensurate units so that the cost of achieving a specified level of benefits might be minimized. Cost-effectiveness analysis is not any simpler than cost-benefit analysis if multiple varieties of benefit are specified (lives, years, pain), except that in doing cost-benefit analysis one must also value intangible benefits.

NET-PRESENT-VALUE ANALYSIS: DISCOUNTING

The uneven distribution of costs and benefits over time poses little conceptual difficulty for the analyst. One simply reduces the stream of future costs and benefits to net present value by discounting. The most common rationale for discounting social programs to present value reflects the uncertainty of the future: A benefit in hand is worth two in the future (Robinson 1990; Lipscomb 1989). In contrast, health economists have downplayed the business-sector rationale for discounting, which is the time value of money. In the business sector uncertainty is always incorporated through the use of decision trees.

Most studies offer a sensitivity analysis of the impact of discounting on cost per year of life saved: $31,300 for heart transplants discounted at 10 percent (but $27,200 if they are discounted at 5.0 percent), or $50,600 for liver transplants discounted at 10 percent (but $44,000 if they are discounted at 5.0 percent) (Evans 1986). A discount rate of 10 percent produces a discount factor of 0.3855 after 10 years and 0.0085 after 50 years. In other words, benefits accruing a decade from now are worth just under two-fifths as much as comparable benefits accruing today; benefits accuring 50 years from now are worth one-eighty-fifth as much as comparable benefits accruing today. Present value of lifetime treatment costs are a function of expected life expectancy. Baker (1991) estimates that discounting over 3.6 years terminal breast cancer had a present value of $11,444 in 1984 dollars, whereas maintenance of breast cancer cases discounting over 9.25 years had a present value of $211,409.

The discount rate is designed to reflect the opportunity cost of postponing benefits or expenditures for an uncertain future. Arrow and Lind (1970) posited that the yield on private investment can be properly regarded as the appropriate opportunity yield for public investment only if the subjective cost of risk bearing is the same for the average taxpayer as it is for the private investor. Musgrave (1969) indicated that the benchmarks should be a function of the source of financing; private consumption has a higher discount rate than public investment. What is most frequently misunderstood by noneconomists is that inflation is only one part of the rationale for discounting. Even if all benefits were adjusted for the projected rate of inflation, discounting would still be necessary to account for the social rate of time preference. Discounting future years of life implies no utilitarian value judgment. It only presumes that benefits and costs must be juxtaposed and measured in commensurable dollar units at a single given discount rate. Choice of a discount rate is of no consequence for a short-lived program with benefits and costs concentrated within one to two years.

Selection of the rate of discount is a crucial parameter in most net-present-value calculations. For example, Jackson et al. (1978) reported that elective hysterectomy is only justified on tangible cost grounds if the discount rate is under 4 percent. Waaler and Piot (1970) reported in a cost-effectiveness analysis of tuberculosis-control measures that discount rates greater than 6 percent favor case finding and treatment, whereas a lower discount rate would favor a vaccination program. Discount-rate selection is crucial for evaluating screening programs that yield benefits 20 to 60 years in the future. A prediction that technology will become more cost-increasing in the future argues for selection of a lower discount rate in order to make lifesaving more valuable in future years. This viewpoint is supported by the suggestion that technology is reaching a state of diminishing returns where even an optimistic 50 percent reduction in the three leading causes of death (cardiovascular disease, cancer, and motor vehicle accidents) would add less than one year of life for people aged 15 to 65 (Tsai, Lee, and Hardy 1978). There are three basic varieties of discount rates: (1) the corporate discount rate if the private sector borrowed the funds, (2) the government borrowing rate on bond issues in the marketplace, and (3) the social discount rate to enable programs and procedures with benefits far in the future to prove more acceptable.

The social discount rate (Pigou 1920) is probably the most often used because of the strength of the intergenerational equity argument. For example, a $25-million one-shot project in 1996 with a payoff of $75 million in the year 2016 has a positive net present value only if the discount rate is 6 percent or less. The typical social discount rate is on the order of 4 to 6 percent. However, a bias against the value of future generations might still remain apparent to some futurists if they realized that at a 5 percent discount rate, 30 deaths in 2066 are exactly equivalent to 1 death in 1996. To those political scientists and welfare economists concerned with ethical issues, any discount rate will have some slight bias in favor of present generations (a counterargument might be Keynes's rejoinder that "in the long run we are all dead").

Opportunity-cost principles argue for a high discount rate. The true cost of a health care investment is the return that could have been achieved if the resources had gone elsewhere in the private sector. For Mishan (1976), the relevant comparison is not the expected rate of return but the expected rate of return net of the subjective costs of risk bearing. The first option, the corporate discount rate, is obviously overinflated since it includes both a risk premium and a markup for corporate taxes. In order to achieve equivalent after-tax investor earnings, a corporation must offer stockholders a 10 percent return (that is, a 15 percent before-tax gross return) to compete with a riskless municipal bond returning 7.25 percent. Operationally, the second choice, government borrowing rates, serves as the upper bound in most analyses. Given the implicit assumption that the discount rate is not changing over time, the most prudent course of action is to perform a sensitivity analysis of the net present value under a range of discount rates. If a sensitivity analysis can demonstrate that selection of a discount rate does not affect the recommendations, then the tenuousness of the assumption will not be a source for concern (Robinson 1990).

The last discounting issue that must be considered is the selection of an appropriate downward adjustment to reflect the degree to which the medical price index exceeds the consumer price index (CPI). Klarman, Francis, and Rosenthal (1968) were the first to incorporate a net discount rate adjusted downward by 1 to 2 percent to reflect the extent that growth in medical prices exceeded the growth in the CPI. Jackson et al. (1978) utilized a downward adjustment of 5 percent to reflect the excess of medical inflation relative to inflation in the general economy. This net-discount-rate factor reflects the value of direct health-service forgone costs (benefits) that would also have increased by the excess of the medical price index over the CPI. If cost-containment programs were to bring the medical inflation rate to parity with the CPI, then this adjustment would be unnecessary.

APPLICATIONS OF COST-BENEFIT ANALYSIS TO THERAPEUTIC TREATMENT

Both analysts and decision makers disagree over how to value the intangible benefits of health programs. Most decision makers find the valuation process in cost-benefit analysis difficult and do not trust analyses that depend on gross approximations, small samples, and a poor data base. These decision makers are willing to violate the efficiency criteria and invest more in hospitals and physicians than society receives as a return on the dollar. Society might profit from having a more healthy skepticism concerning therapeutic treatments. Many therapies will exhibit dramatic benefits on introduction and require no cost-benefit analyses. For example, the dramatic 90 percent decline in the fatality rate from heart block exhibited after introduction of cardiac pacemakers in 1968 is a classic example of a clearly cost-beneficial new treatment mode. However, as Lewis Thomas (1977) observed, modern medicine increasingly creates "halfway" technologies like bypass surgery or heart transplants and "complex" technologies like hemodialysis. Thomas reserved the label of a truly "sophisticated" technology for therapeutic treatments that eliminate the disease and restore the patient to prior health status. Consequently, a therapy like coronary artery bypass surgery is not sophisticated because it does nothing for the disease (arteriosclerosis). It has been assessed as having a low cost-effectiveness ratio because it does little to prolong life, but it almost always reduces chest pain for the 95 to 98 percent of patients surviving the operation (Weinstein, Pliskin, and Stason 1977).

Somewhere between 10 and 20 percent of new treatments might be prime candidates for cost-benefit studies to decide whether the benefits are worth the costs to society. A smaller percentage of established therapies might also deserve the same cost-benefit analysis. The policy issue is seldom one of cost-beneficial yes or no, but rather an issue of frequency. Obviously, if clinicians start treating more nonserious cases, the frequency of treatment skyrockets. For example, prophylactically treating slightly symptomatic conditions of appendectomy (Neutra 1977) or completely asymptomatic conditions of disease without consequence (for example, cholecystectomy; Ingelfinger 1968) will dramatically decrease the benefit-to-cost ratio. It has been estimated that a program to treat asymptomatic silent gallstone carriers (15 million) would cost at least $45 billion (Fitzpatrick, Neutra, and Gilbert 1977). One of the intangible benefits of doing an economic evaluation is that it may suggest to the medical community the benefits of decreasing overutilization by increasing the degree of discrimination through improved clinical interpretation skills. This policy is good medicine and good economics. For example, Neutra (1977) suggested that decreasing the removal rate of normal appendices will lead to slightly lower rates of perforation and other complications. One study in China reproted reported a mere 0.2 percent mortality rate from nonsurgical treatment of appendicitis (China Medical Group 1974).

Very few complete cost-benefit studies have been published. Many times a limited cost-benefit analysis will lead to the most socially cost-effective clinical decision rules. For example, Schoenbaum et al. (1976) suggested that a single rubella vaccination at 12 years or at two ages would be better than the typical norm of a single vaccination for all children at an early age. Berwick, Keeler, and Cretin (1975) suggested that hypercholesterolemia screening and treatment for children is more cost-beneficial than treatment and/or screening in adult years. This study also considered the issue of whether childhood screening is best done on the umbilical cord, all school-age children, or high-risk school-age children. The study suggested that selection of the discount rate determines whether the screen should be as liberal as 238 mgm for normal nonfamilial children or as conservative as 252 mgm for 10-year-old high-risk familial hypercholesterolemics. Sometimes the selection of a decision rule depends on how many intangible benefits are loaded into the analysis. For example, prevention of Down's syndrome (mongolism) is a cost-beneficial screening venture for women over 40, but the screening for women aged 35 to 39 is justified only if more disastrous psychological sequelae for the parents are postulated following the birth of an abnormal child.

Cost-benefit analysis can provide the justification for new or mandatory screening and treatment programs. Layde, Allmen, and Oakley (1979) reported a benefit-to-cost ratio of two ($4 billion/$2 billion) for a new multitiered alpha-fetoprotein screening program for detecting neural defects for a theoretical cohort of 100,000 American women. The mock analysis was necessary because the only existing data came from a small sample in Scotland. The study neglected many ethical issues and intangible benefit problems with a test that has only a 64 percent sensitivity—that is, the failure to identify an abnormality in a screened woman may result in more costly psychological sequelae than if the child had not been tested and declared healthy *in utero*.

Cost-benefit analysis can also be used to support expansion of an existing treatment program. Ward (1977) reported that an $8-billion hypertension-control program would return a benefit to society of $10 billion. The suggestion that 6.1 million Americans with diastolic blood pressure above 105 mm undergo drug therapy was the by-product of a 1967–69 controlled clinical trial on treatment effectiveness of males visiting Veterans Administration facilities. The two problems with hypertension control are the side effects of the drugs (dizziness, impotence, and malaise) and the difficulty of maintaining a high degree of patient compliance in nonexperimental situations. Finnerty et al. (1971) reported that patient compliance was 84 percent in the experimental situation but only 16 percent if the patient did not receive the ''red-carpet treatment.'' Before the nation spends $8 or $12 billion on hypertension control, it seems reasonable to require that we make sure that the technology is effective (will not fail under normal conditions).

Frequently, the economic analyst is asked to perform a cost-benefit evaluation on a questionable treatment or mandatory screening program. For example, the Farber and Finkelstein (1979) cost-benefit study of mandatory premarital rubella-antibody screening dampened the initial enthusiasm for the program. In some cases the evaluators need only look at the touted benefits in a more scientific fashion, with a randomized controlled trial, to conclude that the treatment has zero benefits. For example, the New York University 1973 study group, finding that hyperbaric oxygen provided no benefits for the elderly, eliminated enthusiasm for the treatment that had been stimulated by an unscientific study published in a nationally acclaimed journal in 1969 (Jacobs, Winter, and Alvis 1969). The oxygen "treatment" cost $2,500 per week in 1970. The easy acceptance of a faulty, but profitable, treatment seems to be rather unprofessional if one views medicine as a science. For example, the time lag between general acceptance and proof of zero benefits was seven years in the case of gastric freezing as a cure for ulcers (1962 to 1969) and five years for internal mammary artery ligation surgery (1956 to 1961). The duration of the acceptance of faulty treatments was much longer in the early 1900s. For more than a quarter of a century, physicians tried to cure constipation with surgery (1906 to 1933) and to treat menopausal symptoms with ptosis surgery (1890 to 1928) (Barnes 1977).

Currently, the issue of unnecessary surgery is a major problem for public and private insurance companies. After cesarean section, the hysterectomy is the most common surgical operation, costing an average of $12,000 per case. The Blue Shield medical director (Widen 1991) estimated that one-third or more of hysterectomies are unnecessary. In his Blue Shield sample 30 percent of the hysterectomies were in women of childbearing age with no sign of malignancy. These operations were attributed to small fibroid tumors that typically never require radical surgery and 98 to 99 percent of the time stop growing at the onset of menopause. Providers collect cash for unnecessary surgery, while the surgery has serious psychological and medical aftereffects on the victim. Two methods to curtail unnecessary surgery (guidelines and mandatory second-opinion programs) will be discussed at the end of this chapter.

Health education, which has been assailed by skeptics, is a popular current example of a new approach to improving the effectiveness of medical care. Table 11.1 presents the results of a limited benefit-cost comparison of four approaches to increasing patient compliance to antihypertensive medications. The study sample included 402 patients randomly assigned to experimental and control groups. The emphasis of the study concerned the efficacy of utilizing a triage process, whereby patients are subdivided into groups more predisposed to benefit from a given health education approach. The benefits of the triage method for achieving medication compliance clearly outweigh the cost only in the case of the highly depressed patients (24.3 percent of the sample), as defined by responses to five of the seven items used in the depression-scale questionnaire. The benefit-to-cost ratio for this group (2.2) compares favorably with the average benefit-to-cost ratio of 1.24 for hypertension control for persons in the age range of 35 to 65 (option 4). In other words, triaging only the 24 percent highly depressed subpopulation and providing family-member reinforcement is more cost-beneficial than giving everyone the special health education intervention. Previous studies demonstrating a cost-benefit ratio in the 1.1 to 1.3 range may not stand the test of time in claiming a statistically significant ratio above the 1.0 level when applied to a larger population or to a nonexperimental population that will be less susceptible to the Hawthorne effect. Individuals are known to change their behavior more dramatically under experimental conditions due to the mere fact of being under concerned observation.

Edelson (1990) simulated the impact of various antihypertensive medications

Table 11.1
Simple Benefit-to-Cost Comparisons of Triage Options versus the Option Not to Triage in Achieving Improved Medication Compliance among Hypertensives

Option	Triage	Type of Patients	IHC[a]	Health Education Intervention(s)	Benefit-Cost Ratio
1	Yes	High Level of Depression	65-26	Family Reinforce-ment (FR)	2.20[b]
2	Yes	Medium Level of Depression	58-33	FR + Message Clarification	1.15
3	Yes	No Depression	65-35	FR + Message Clarification	1.33
4	No	All Patients	60-32	FR + Message Clarification	1.24

Source: Eastaugh and Hatcher 1982.
[a]IHC = Increase in number of high compliers with treatment versus control per hundred patients.
[b]Only option 1 has a significantly better ratio for triaging in comparison to not triaging.

in persons aged 35 to 64 for two decades of therapy (1990–2010). The projected cost per year of life saved ranged from $72,100 for captopril to $10,900 for propranolol. Developing a simulation based on an insufficient data base can prove inaccurate (Holmes, Rovner, and Rothert 1989). For example, Kinosian and Eisenberg (1988) reported that the cost per year of life saved in lowering cholesterol was $17,800 for oat bran and $117,400 for cholestyramine resin packets. Subsequent data collection suggested that oat bran is a failure as a strategy; and primary prevention had favorable cost-effectiveness ratios only in selected subgroups based on high cholesterol levels and other established risk factors (Goldman et al. 1991). Economic analysis is very self-financing; for example, the nation avoided wasting $15 billion trying to reduce cholesterol levels for healthy people in the 200–240 mg/dl range.

APPLICATIONS OF COST-EFFECTIVENESS ANALYSIS

The purpose of cost-effectiveness analysis in the therapeutic arena is to identify the preferred alternatives. Physician preoccupation with survival probabilities must not preclude measurement of quality-of-life factors in performing a cost-effectiveness analysis. Cost-effectiveness analysis still requires that intangible factors be measured; however, they do not have to be valued. Typically, the search for preferred alternatives involves comparisons of less invasive treatment versus radical surgery—for example, simple versus radical mastectomies; medical treatment versus bypass surgery; medical treatment versus doing a vagotomy for common duodenal ulcers; pyloroplasty versus antrectomy surgery for intractable duodenal ulcers; and internal urethrotomy versus uteral reimplantation for vesicoureteral reflux. In some cases the preferred alternative depends on treatment location—for example, home dialysis versus facility-based dialysis. Lee (1990) reported that half the inpatient cardiac catheterizations could be done on an outpatient basis, saving the customer $580 in charges per patient.

A second generalization concerning cost-effectiveness analysis is the paramount relevancy of the patient—for example, "The patient is not advantaged by having an innocent murmur confirmed as innocent by echocardiography" (Fitzgerald 1988). A third generalization is that many "cost-effectiveness studies" are in fact efficacy or effectiveness studies having nothing to do with cost or cost effect (Valenzuela, Criss, and Spaite 1990; Califf and Wagner 1989). Increasingly, studies are well done and appropriately labeled (e.g., Showstack 1989). Mandelblatt and Fahs (1988) reported that early detection of cervical neoplasia saved $5,907 and 3.7 years of life per 100 Pap tests, for a net program cost of only $2,874 per year of life saved. Randolph and Washington (1990) reported that the leukocyte esterase test saved over $9,700 per cohort of 1,000 sexually active males screened for chlamydia. Sensitivity analysis demonstrated that this test had the lowest cost per cure ($51) and the lowest overall cost per cohort of the three tests studied.

Thrombolytic therapy refers to treatment with drugs, which may be either natural or synthetic products, that are used to reestablish coronary blood flow after a myocardial infarction. The two most widely used products are streptokinase (SK), derived from a microorganism, and synthetic tissue plasminogen activator (TPA). Thrombolytic therapy has been increasingly used in the last several years as data have been collected to demonstrate that such therapy can lead to increased coronary blood flow and improved myocardial function. The arrival of the synthetic TPA had been eagerly awaited since it was hoped that it would have enhanced activity and reduced toxicity. The toxicities of these compounds are related to changes in the blood clotting system that can lead to severe hemorrhages. When this bleeding occurs within the brain, it may often be fatal. Tempering this anticipation, however, was the very substantial cost difference between the two products. Rapaport (1989) stated that SK was $78 at his institution (SF General Hospital), versus $2,268 for TPA. These figures are comparable to other reports. In comparing these costs, however, one must also consider the effect that a difference in efficacy would have in drugs used to treat a common, often fatal disease, AMI. The significance of these differences in efficacy might depend on what measures of outcome are used to evaluate these drugs. One obvious consideration would be a difference in outcome as measured by survival; a second would be a difference in quality of life based upon differences in functional status, or as a surrogate, differences in ventricular function. In this analysis I shall concentrate on the effect of survival. Since a patient may live for years after an AMI however, one could anticipate that such differences in functional status could have important cost implications.

In this analysis we shall concentrate on small differences in survival (that were not demonstrated to be statistically significant) that have been encountered in some clinical studies. One can use $2,000 as the difference in direct cost of the drugs. The value of life lost will be analyzed over a range of values. In estimating the value of premature death, one must consider the mean ages (54 to 59) in participants in several studies of these agents.

Is it worth it to spend an extra $2,000 on day one for the TPA as an alternative to the SK? Yes, if at some future date TPA were found to enhance survival probability by 1.325 percent. In this example, the 57-year-old individual presumed to live an additional 7.0 years (less than the average life expectancy for a healthy 57-year-old) would earn at average 1991 wages $31,000 a year, or a total of $150,921 discounted at 10 percent. This quick calculation takes a restricted discounted future earnings perspective to valuing a life (in contrast to the more refined willingness-to-pay approach we shall take in chapter 13). The generic point to consider is that for very modest differences in survival the cost ratios can begin to favor the drug with the higher direct cost. TPA has yet to prove that it has a better survival rate than SK. Data on the efficacy of TPA and SK are still being accumulated. In one study by White et al. (1989) 270 patients were randomized to receive either SK or TPA. The mortality at 30 days was 3.7 percent in the TPA group and 7.4 percent in the SK group ($p > .20$). At nine months the mortality was 8.9% in the SK group and 5.9% in the TPA group ($p = 0.34$). The effects on ventricular function, a primary endpoint, were almost identical with the two drugs. The authors corrcetly pointed out that the study lacked sufficient power to determine whether this difference in mortality was genuine. A large European GISSI–3 study (Gruppo Italiano 1992) evaluated 41,299 patients who were randomized to receive either SK or TPA and then either heparin (an anticoagulant) or no heparin. The mortality rates were 9.0 percent for TPA versus 8.6% for SK. The rates for the combined endpoint (death or severe myocardial injury) were 23.1 percent for TPA versus 22.5% for SK.

We should now examine the policy lessons we can draw from this example. In many respects the clinical and economic lessons go hand in hand. There needs to be a greater general awareness that what appear to be relatively small differences in efficacy between competing therapies may have major ramifications in terms of lives saved and dollars spent. The standard of "equivalency" between therapies should reflect these realities. Currently there is no regulatory basis for using cost in drug approval. One could certainly argue that this should change, but this seems unlikely, at least in the near future. Of more concern is the effect that an accelerated drug approval process may have on our current ability to make the types of estimates discussed in this section. The regulations for the approval of drugs for debilitating or life-threatening illnesses state:

FDA has determined that it is appropriate to exercise the broadest flexibility in applying the statutory standards, while preserving appropriate guarantees for safety and effectiveness. These procedures reflect the recognition that physicians and patients are generally willing to accept greater risks or side effects from products that treat life-threatening or severely debilitating illnesses, than they would accept from products that treat less serious illnesses. These procedures also reflect the recognition that the benefits of the drug need to be evaluated in light of the severity of the disease being treated. (21 C.F.R. 312.80; Subpart E regulations, FY 1989)

The disease or condition under study should, when both its incidence and the likelihood of severe adverse outcome are considered together, be of sufficient importance to warrant a detailed clinical study of competing therapies. In essence this is a statement that the overall effect of therapy is likely to compare favorably in a cost-benefit analysis across a range of possible options. It should be noted that the benefit of such a study is cumulative over the projected useful lifetime of the therapy (Asbury 1986).

Cost-effectiveness analyses usually report either costs per unit of desired benefit achieved or units of tangible benefits per dollar expended. However, in some analyses the need for computing any ratio is obviated by the lack of any differential in effectiveness between treatment modes. In such cases the lower-cost mode is preferable. One randomized study (Hill, Hampton, and Mitchell 1978) of the cost-effectiveness of home care versus hospital care in the coronary-care unit (CCU) for heart-attack victims (mild cases, originally seen at their homes) found no statistically significant difference in the six-week mortality between the two groups (13 percent). Another controlled trial (Hampton and Nicholas 1978) that randomly allocated mobile coronary-care units (MCCU) and routine ambulances to answer emergency calls found no differential in prehospital coronary mortality rates (47 percent). Despite the comments on high costs of CCUs and MCCUs, and in view of the concern for lack of substantially improved outcomes following the public expenditure of more resources for such technologies, groups of cardiologists continue to support the more institutionalized modes of therapy. Coincidentally, the cardiologists derive higher fees from hospital utilization. The prudent decision maker might suggest that CCUs and MCCUs should continue to be utilized in carefully controlled pilot-study settings until effectiveness can be clearly established. One does not want to impede innovation if a period of trial and improvement can produce a more cost-effective alternative.

DECISION ANALYSIS, PHYSICIAN INVOLVEMENT AND BAYES THEOREM

Many physician-directed cost-effectiveness analyses ignore larger social issues in considering questions of whether a given procedure during an operation is worth the effort. For example, Skillings, Williams, and Hinshaw (1979) rejected the concept of routine operative cholangiography since the technique detected only two unsuspected cases of ''silent'' gallstones at an average cost of $6,612.

The authors rejected operative cholangiography if performed either routinely or for isolated silent small stones in the gallbladder. This study ignored the issues of false positives (reported diseased when in fact healthy) yielding unnecessary surgery and mortality associated with increased time under anesthesia. However, including these negative benefits would only reinforce the case against operative cholangiography. Alon, Turina, and Gattiker (1979) performed a randomized trial and cost-effectiveness analysis of bypass patients treated under bubble oxygenators and membrane oxygenators. The more expensive membrane oxygenator brought no lasting benefits beyond the second postoperative day and was therefore only recommended for extended open-heart procedures on high-risk patients. In some cases an analysis is touted as a cost-benefit analysis, when in fact it does not technically even qualify as a cost-effectiveness analysis. For example, a myringotomy with tube insertion was labeled cost-benefical compared to the possibility of a forgone tympanoplasty simply because the relative fees were $75 and $925, respectively (Armstrong and Armstrong 1979).

Nonclinicians are not familiar with the cascades of hypotheses to be tested in the severely ill teaching hospital patient (Eddy 1989). Physicians do not live in a world of perfect knowledge concerning certain probabilities (Haug 1989). Bayes theorem is the operating axiom implicit in most clinical decision making: Statistical inference concerning probabilities is associated with individual events (tests, clinical results) or qualitative statements (judgments, guesses) and not merely with sequences of events (as in frequency theories developed by statisticians studying only plants). An economist may have an easier time describing his or her body with exact numerical probability, but the tendency for most members of the human race is to describe things in qualitative categories (likely, unlikely, and in between). Conventional use of simple categories of probability is acceptable for a Bayesian diagnostic system in the academic medical center because the target conditions have a relatively high prior probability. For example, Chard (1991) studied pelvic infection to compare the effects of quantitative and qualitative probability estimates on the diagnostic accuracy of Bayes theorem. For the commoner conditions (prior probability greater than 20 percent), the use of a two- or three-category system was virtually equivalent to the use of exact probability. However, uncommon conditions (with prior probability under 3.0 percent) were completely ignored by the qualitative system.

Decision-analysis techniques incorporate the probabilities (assessed from data or expert opinion) of chance events and the values a patient or decision maker assigns to the benefits and risks to yield prescriptive thresholds (e.g., above or below this level, one would do X course of action). Decision analysis continues to be limited by the difficulties inherent in eliciting and quantifying willingness-to-pay dollar valuation for health-status improvements (or deterioration). One increasingly popular alternative, threshold analysis, attempts to derive the thresholds that physicians actually use to guide their choices (Eisenberg et al. 1984). Unfortunately, there is no statistical method to compare the summary measure of thresholds that is derived from the distribution of doctors' thresholds (or patients' thresholds). Young et al. (1986) suggested two methods of developing a summary measure of the thresholds for groups of physicians. The first method, the unweighted mean of the midpoints, indicates confidence limits of means and standard t-tests to compare different groups (e.g., cardiologists have higher thresholds than family practitioners). The second method, the weighted standard error of the mean, involves the determination of confidence intervals and weighted regressions to compare weighted means of the midpoints of threshold ranges. Future research should compare thresholds derived by either of the two methods to the more familiar prescriptive thresholds obtained in decision analysis to ascertain which technique holds more promise in health care.

One study in 1985 compared the expert-opinion decision-analysis approach to the prescriptive-threshold-analysis approach in the case of coronary bypass surgery. Decision-analysis criteria were compared to the care strategy proposed by 61 randomly selected board-certified cardiologists (Manu and Runge 1985). The 61 cardiologists surveyed demonstrated a fairly inaccurate factual knowledge regarding the probabilities involved in the diagnostic process. As a group, the 61 cardiologists performed suboptimally relative to decision analysis, under-utilizing coronary angiography and overusing radionuclide exercise imaging for patients with unequivocally positive EKG stress tests. In addition, the intuitive thresholds for the use of angiography had little association with the judged probability of severe coronary artery disease. Unfortunately, valid and reliable decision-analysis models exist for only a few dozen therapeutic and diagnostic situations. Decision-analysis models, when updated with better-quality expert opinion, can be utilized to educate practitioners and to calibrate and improve practitioner decision-making guidelines.

POLICY CONSIDERATIONS

Cost-benefit analysis should increasingly assist government and third-party insurance carriers in inhibiting the financing of halfway technologies that provide palliative relief but not a definitive treatment. If it is politically difficult to underfinance therapies that are not cost-beneficial, then government can intervene on the development side to limit technological diffusion to a few well-evaluated pilot studies. If the evaluation suggests that the treatment mode is definitive and worth the price tag, then the new technology should diffuse through the medical sector.

An example of a complete and technically competent cost-effectiveness analysis is the comparison by Piachaud and Weddell (1972) of medical versus surgical removal of varicose veins. Fifty men and 200 women were allocated at random to either surgery or injection-compression sclerotherapy. Direct costs were four times higher for the surgical group. The treatment in the medical group involved seven clinic visits, in comparison to the surgical treatment that required three to four days of hospitalization and two clinic visits. The time cost to the patient was 100 hours for surgery and 30 hours for medical treatment. The opportunity cost to the economy was 31 workless days for surgery and 7.5 days for medical therapy. After three years of follow-up, there existed no clinical basis for selecting either mode of therapy. There may be many treatments or procedures in medicine that, like varicose vein surgery, are effective, but less cost-effective than a recently developed alternative. The widespread disdain for randomized experimentation and the general acceptance of existing techniques among the physician community might retard the research and development of more efficient and equally effective alternatives.

Economic evaluation and decision analysis do not merit the unmitigated pessimism of Ransohoff and Feinstein (1976), who characterized them as a "computerized Ouija board." As Albert (1978) pointed out, the true role of evaluation in medicine lies between the pessimism of the Ouija board and the naive optimism of a "new Rosetta stone." The direct value of economic evaluation is that it can erode some of the areas of the unknown that surround the benefit-to-cost assumptions implicit in the behavior of physicians and administrators. Evaluation should be viewed as a consumerist cause if it forces those in power to be explicit about valuation assumptions in cost-benefit calculations and the resource cutoff level required in cost-effectiveness ranking decisions. The indirect benefit of economic evaluation is that it might teach health professionals to apply their craft only to the point where the marginal benefits equal the marginal costs. The credulity of economists and regulators has been taxed by the disorderly diffusion of every new unproven technology. A possible intangible benefit of the evaluation process lies in the hope that cost-effective clinical decision-making principles will seep into the subconscious cognitive process of American physicians and result in a less costly style of medical care.

It would take a high degree of naive optimism to suggest that economic analysis can produce a matrix of relative benefits measured in quality-of-life points. Will quality improvements be cost-increasing, cost-decreasing, or self-financing, with the cost savings counterbalancing the cost increases? The conventional wisdom is that quality is cost-increasing. However, doing things right the first time should potentially diminish the cost of services per patient. Doing things incorrectly, unnecessarily, or repetitively is what costs money. Consider an example in the context of ordering diagnostic tests. If a large-enough number of tests are ordered on a healthy person, just because of random variation one or more false-positive results will emerge. The experience will lead the patient on an anxiety-provoking, costly journey through unnecessary follow-up tests and procedures, only to eventually discharge him or her free of disease (provided the hospital did not add an iatrogenic infection). This situation was labeled the "Ulysses syndrome" by Rang (1972) in memory of an individual who took a detour and was pulled into a series of unnecessary tests and dangerous adventures. If the frequency of diagnostic and therapeutic misadventures is trimmed, the resulting cost savings can more than outweigh the costs of investments in quality-control systems and continuing education.

Higher hospitalization costs per case do not always generate superior patient outcomes when studied over a time horizon of several months. Garber, Fuchs, and Silverman (1984) compared the differences between faculty and private/ community services within a university medical center for several DRGs. In a 12-month time frame the faculty service created higher levels of expense but did not improve patient survival relative to community physicians. Almost 30 percent more of the patients on the faculty service survived hospitalization, but at the end of 12 months the survival curves for the 48 pairs of matched patients were identical in both settings. In summary, the diagnostic system is rife with uncertainty, ambiguity, chance, and risk. How well a clinician copes with uncertainty will, to a large extent, determine the cost and quality of care he or she can provide.

It is impossible to do a cost-benefit analysis of a hospital (Greer 1988). Rather, hospitals should be viewed as flexible collections of medical technologies, where the benefit-cost possibilities of each technology need to be assessed separately. From the forgoing discussion it is clear that economists should be encouraged to address themselves to clinical applications of normative economic techniques (cost-benefit analysis, cost-effectiveness analysis, and decision analysis). Aside from public health applications of cost-benefit analysis to polio and syphilis, few complete studies have been conducted to date. Many studies avoid the issue of valuation and perform limited cost-effectiveness analyses, and in the other cases the retreat is to provide only societal cost estimates of the impact of a disease or condition (Institute of Medicine 1989).

In view of the uncertainties implicit in any technological assessment effort, one might question whether medicine should lock itself into an expensive and unproven therapy, such as bone marrow transplants, as a type of standard treatment. A sliding fee schedule could be employed to make the utilization of expensive marginal technologies less profitable for the physicians. In order to create a positive incentive for physicians to evaluate and get experience with a new test or treatment, the fee could increase as the service is proven to be more valuable. This concept of a technology evaluation-sensitive fee schedule was suggested by Gaus and Cooper (1978). Another possible positive planning solution to stimulate less costly behavior may be the allowance of replacement-cost reimbursement for depreciation at projected (higher) market prices if the hospital introduces cost-reducing technologies or tests and/or phases out cost-increasing equipment and services of unproved efficacy (Roper et al. 1988). The coercion implicit in rate regulation inevitably adds to bureaucracy and creates some barriers to innovation. Society should fear also any movement toward technology prohibition that creates disincentives for scientific inquiry merely because the economy cannot afford the implementation costs of every resulting procedure. The nation must strike some sort of balance between the relative risks of disorderly diffusion versus orderly slow diffusion of new technologies, treatments, and tests (Antman, Schnipper, and Frei 1988).

THE FEDERAL ROLE

The Omnibus Budget Reconciliation Act of 1989 (Pub. L. 101–239), enacted in December 1989, added Title IX to the Public Health Service Act. This title established the Agency for Health Care Policy and Research (AHCPR) to enhance the quality, appropriateness, and effectiveness of health care services, and access to such services. The AHCPR is to achieve its goals through the establishment of a broad base of scientific research and through the promotion of improvements in clinical practice and in the organization, financing, and delivery of health care services. AHCPR published guidelines in three areas in 1991: urinary incontinence, pain management, and prostate surgery. Section 911 of the act (42 U.S.C. 299b) established within the AHCPR the Office of the Forum for Quality and Effectiveness in Health Care. Through this office the agency is arranging for the development and periodic review and updating of clinically relevant guidelines that may be used by physicians, educators, and health care practitioners to assist in determining how diseases, disorders, and other health conditions can most effectively and appropriately be prevented, diagnosed, treated, and managed clinically. AHCPR will publish additional guidelines in 1992 concerning cataracts, sickle cell, prevention of pressure sores, depression, AIDS, low back pain, knee replacements, and acute myocardial infarction (MI). The guidelines must be (1) based on the best available research and professional judgment; (2) presented in formats appropriate for use by physicians, health care practitioners, providers, medical educators, medical review organizations, and consumers of health care; and (3) presented in forms appropriate for use in clinical practice, educational programs, and reviewing quality and appropriateness of medical care (AHCPR 1991). Other AHCPR guideline panels will report in the areas of gallbladder disease, cesarean sections, and diarrhea in children. Gallbladder care could be cost-decreasing as increasing numbers of the 460,000 cholecystectomies done on an inpatient basis annually are done by the outpatient laparoscopic technique.

Because of the federal budget deficit problems it is doutful that the AHCPR will ever achieve a $200-million budget in three years (Perry and Pillar 1990). A number of preliminary reports have been published in the areas of back pain (Deyo, Cherkin, and Conrad 1990), cataracts (Steinberg 1990), total knee replacement (Freund et al., 1990), acute myocardial infarction (Pashos and McNeil 1990), and prostate disease (Wennberg 1990).

The Pew Memorial Trust is also supporting a number of technology-assessment studies. The Pew study by Leape (1989) suggested that consensus of expert opinion, disseminated by means of guidelines, offers the best opportunity to identify and eliminate unnecessary surgery. Leape suggested a limited long-run effectiveness of mandatory second-surgical-opinion programs. Lindsey and Newhouse (1990) confirmed the same negative opinion of mandatory second-opinion programs. Future research will evaluate the effectiveness of the guideline strategy for preferred practice patterns (PPPs). We can ask in 10 years: Did the guidelines

Table 11.2
**Estimated Fiscal Year 1991 Incremental Medicare Cost Impact of Cost-increasing
Technologies in Existing Cases in PPS Hospitals**

Technology	Amount (in Millions)		
	Low	High	Best
Electrophysiologic studies	11.3	22.5	16.9
Implantable defibrillators	65.0	127.1	96.0
Lead replacements	7.2	18.4	12.8
Implantable infusion pumps	1.8	3.5	2.7
Laser angioplasty	3.7	6.8	5.3
Low osmolar and nonionic contrast agents	5.3	37.1	21.1
Magnetic resonance imaging (MRI)	8.2	15.1	11.7
Monoclonal antibodies for sepsis	45.0	150.0	97.5
Pacemakers (advances)	15.2	19.1	17.1
Percutaneous transluminal angioplasty	1.7	3.3	2.5
Percutaneous transluminal coronary angioplasty	20.6	28.5	20.6
Positron emission tomography (PET)	5.8	16.2	11.0
Single photon emission computed tomography (SPECT)	2.1	15.1	11.7
Thrombolytic agents	27.5	36.3	31.9

Source: ProPAC (1991), 58.

help control costs (or enhance quality)? Congress is clearly interested in a number of the cost-increasing technologies listed in table 11.2 (ProPAC 1991).

Medical innovation will rapidly inflate the number of new technologies requiring economic assessment. The number of academic medical centers with free-electron lasers has tripled in the past two years. In the late 1990s bloodless surgery will be possible through advances in laser technology. Expensive research will continue on cancer treatment (monoclonal antibodies, tumor necrosis factor) and also on implantable infusion pumps (for arthritis, diabetes, and cardiovascular disease). Are private research and development (R & D) funds sufficient? Should we have a public payment policy that insulates and supports health-related R & D at the expense of other sectors of the domestic economy? Many medical suppliers report that the Medicare prospective payment system (PPS) has precipitated a slight decline in new-product development and research. PPS is not the main cause. Nondefense R & D was on the decline in the economy until 1988. Computers and health care are the only two components of the domestic economy where R & D funding has outpaced inflation. From 1979 to 1988 spending on domestic R & D declined 29 percent in real dollars (Eastaugh 1990).

Little-ticket items may get more expensive. A proven technology like Swan-Ganz pulmonary artery catheterization may only be worth the risks for certain risk groups (Zimmerman 1991). New experimental methods to estimate cardiac function at the bedside may soon substitute for Swan-Ganz, including the nuclear stethoscope, transthoracic electrical impedance, and three-dimensional Doppler color-flow mapping. None of these techniques were subject to an evaluation of efficacy before being eventually evaluated from a cost-effectiveness and cost-benefit framework. With the help of the AHCPR (1991) and the Pew Foundation, the 1990s could provide some answers to basic questions: How do we educate physicians for technology-assessment studies? How do we link technology assessment and outcomes management? How do frontline managers and physicians balance ethical and economic issues in making utilization decisions? How do we select patients for bilary lithotripsy, MRI, or bypass surgery?

Hiatt (1990) and the Institute of Medicine (1989) documented how shifts in financing health care services or research programs can drive (or retard) their rate of diffusion. But will the causal relationship be a two-way street in the future? One should avoid the absolute assertion that "technology developments are unlikely to impact financing reforms themselves." If we define technology in a broad sense, financing reforms may be partially driven by technology (e.g., teleradiology or microchip medical record implants within the patient). Such technology makes capitation payment a more viable undertaking. Moreover, new joint ventures in technology development between subspecialty groups may naturally suggest financing reforms. For example, if cardiac surgeons or oncologists bind together as joint-venture partners to assure both stable R & D cash flow and quality care, they may naturally form research PPOs (RPPOs, preferred provider organizations doing patient care and research). Such specialty groups can advertise their superior quality-of-care statistics to HMOs, PPOs, consumer groups, and managed-care plans.

REFERENCES

Abt, C. (1977). "The Issue of Social Cost in Cost-Benefit Analysis of Surgery." In J. Bunker, B. Barnes, and F. Mosteller (eds.), *Costs, Risks, and Benefits of Surgery.* New York: Oxford University Press.

Acton, J. (1973). *Evaluating Public Programs to Save Lives: The Case of Heart Attacks.* Rand Corporation Report R–950-RC. Santa Monica, Calif.: Rand Corporation.

Agency for Health Care Policy and Research (AHCPR). (1991). *Bibliography and Project Summary.* Agency for Health Care Policy and Research, DHHS, Rockville, Maryland.

Albert, D. (1978). "Decision Theory in Medicine: A Review and Critique." *Milbank Memorial Fund Quarterly* 56:3 (Summer), 362–400.

Alon, L., Turina, M., and Gattiker, R. (1979). "Membrane and Bubble Oxygenator: A Clinical Comparison in Patients Undergoing Bypass Procedures." *Herz* (German) 4, 56–62.

Antman, K., Schnipper, L., and Frei, E. (1988). "Crisis in Clinical Cancer Research:

Third-Party Insurance and Investigational Therapy.'' *New England Journal of Medicine* 319:1 (July 7), 46–48.

Armstrong, B., and Armstrong, R. (1979). ''Tympanostomy Tubes: Their Use, Abuse, and Cost-Benefit Ratio.'' *Laryngoscope* 89:3 (March), 443–449.

Arrow, K., and Lind, R. (1970). ''Uncertainty and the Evaluation of Public Investment Decisions.'' *American Economic Review* 60:3 (June), 364–378.

Asbury, C. (1986). *Orphan Drugs, Medical vs. Market Value*, Lexington Books.

Bailey, M. (1989). *Reducing Risks to Life: Measurement of the Benefits*. Washington, D. C.: American Enterprise Institute.

Baker, M., Kessler, L., Urban, N., and Smucker, R. (1991). ''Estimating the Treatment Costs of Breast and Lung Cancer.'' *Medical Care* 29:1 (January), 40–49.

Barnes, B. (1977). ''Discarded Operations: Surgical Innovation by Trial and Error.'' In J. Bunker, B. Barnes, and F. Mosteller (eds.), *Costs, Risks, and Benefits of Surgery*. New York: Oxford University Press.

Becker, G. (1964). *Human Capital*. New York: National Bureau of Economic Research.

Begg, C., and McNeil, B. (1985). ''Response: To the Use of the Polychotomous Model.'' *Medical Decision Making* 5:1 (Spring), 123–126.

Berry, R., and Boland, J. (1977). *The Economic Cost of Alcohol Abuse*. New York: Free Press.

Berwick, D., Keeler, E., and Cretin, S. (1975). ''Screening for Cholesterol: Costs and Benefits.'' Report from the Center for the Analysis of Health Practices, Harvard School of Public Health.

Boss, L., and Gukes, F. (1992). ''Medicaid Coverage of Screening Tests for Breast and Cervical Cancer.'' *American Journal of Public Health* 82:2 (February), 252–254.

Callahan, D. (1991). *An Ounce of Prevention*. San Francisco: Jossey-Bass.

Califf, R., and Wagner, G. (1989). *Acute Coronary Care*. Boston: Martinus Nijhoff.

Callahan, D. (1990). ''Rationing Medical Progress: The Affordable Way to Health Care.'' *New England Journal of Medicine* 322:25 (June 21), 1810–1811.

Chard, T. (1991). ''Qualitative Probability versus Quantitative Probability in Clinical Diagnosis: Study Using a Computer Simulation.'' *Medical Decision Making* 11:1 (January–March), 38–41.

Chassin, M., Kosecoff, J., and Park, R. (1990). *The Appropriateness of Selected Medical and Surgical Procedures: Relationship to Geographical Variations*. Ann Arbor, Mich.: Health Administration Press.

China Medical Group. (1974). ''Some Problems in Nonoperative Treatment of Acute Appendicitis.'' Report of the Acute Abdominal Conditions Research Group. *China Medical Journal* 2, 21–40.

Cleary, P., Epstein, A., Oster, G., and Morrissey, G. (1991). ''Health-related Quality of Life among Patients Undergoing Percutaneous Coronary Angioplasty.'' *Medical Care* 29:10 (October), 939–950.

Cohen, D. (1989). *Health, Prevention, and Economics*. New York: Oxford University Press.

Coile, R. (1991). ''Cost-tips, Computer-docs, and minty fresh air.'' *Healthcare Forum Journal* 34:5 (September/October) 69–70.

Cooper, B., and Rice D. (1976). ''The Economic Cost of Illness Revisited.'' *Social Security Bulletin* 39:1 (February), 21–36.

Demlo, L. (1990). ''Measuring Health Care Effectiveness: Research and Policy Implications." *International Journal of Technology Assessment in Health Care* 6:2 (April), 288–294.

Deyo, R., Cherkin, D., and Conrad, D. (1990). "The Back Pain Outcome Assessment Team." *Health Services Research* 25:5 (December), 733–738.

Eastaugh, S. (1991). "Valuation of the Benefits of Risk-free Blood: Willingness to Pay for Hemoglobin Solutions." *International Journal of Technology Assessment in Health Care* 7:1 (Winter), 51–59.

Eastaugh, S. (1990). "Financing the Correct Rate of Growth of Medical Technology." *Quarterly Review of Economics and Business*, 30:4 (Winter) 54–60.

———. (1983). "Placing a Value on Life and Limb: The Role of the Informed Consumer." *Health Matrix* 1:1 (Spring), 5–21.

Eastaugh, S., and Hatcher, M. (1982). "Improving Compliance among Hypertensives: A Triage Criterion and Cost-Benefit Implications." *Medical Care* 20:8 (August) 1001–1017.

Eddy, D. (1990). "Clinical Decision Making: From Theory to Practice." *Journal of the American Medical Association* 263:2 (January 19), 441–443.

———. (1989). "Confidence Profile Method: Bayesian Method for Assessing Health Technologies." *Operations Research* 37:2 (March–April), 210–228.

Edelson, J. (1990). "Long-Term Cost-Effectiveness of Various Initial Monotherapies for Mild to Moderate Hypertension." *Journal of the American Medical Association* 263:3 (January 19), 407–413.

Eisenberg, J., Schumacher, H., Davidson, P., and Kaufman, L. (1984). "Usefulness of Synovial Fluid Analysis in the Evaluation of Joint Effusions: Use of Threshold Analysis and Likelihood Ratios to Assess a Diagnostic Test." *Archives of Internal Medicine* 144:4 (April), 715–719.

Ershoff, D., Mullen, P., and Quinn, V. (1989). "Randomized Trial of a Specialized Self-Help Smoking Cessation Program for Pregnant Women in an HMO." *American Journal of Public Health* 79:2 (February), 182–187.

Evans, R. (1986). "Cost Effectiveness Analysis of Transplantation." *Surgical Clinics of North America* 66:8, 603–616.

Evans, R., Larsen, R., and Burke, J. (1986). "Computer Surveillance of Hospital-acquired Infections and Antibiotic Use." *Journal of the American Medical Association* 256:8 (August 29), 1007–1011.

Farber, M., and Finkelstein, S. (1979). "A Cost-Benefit Analysis of a Mandatory Premarital Rubella-Antibody Screening Program." *New England Journal of Medicine* 300:15 (April 12), 856–859.

Finkler, M., and Wirtschafter, D. (1991). "Cost-effectiveness and Obstetrics Services." *Medical Care* 29:10 (October), 951–963.

Finnerty, F., et al. (1971). "Reasons for Poor Clinic Attendance." *Clinical Research* 19:10 (October), 500–510.

Fitzgerald, F. (1988). "Questions about the Cost-Effectiveness of Echocardiography." *Consultant* 28:7 (July), 2–4.

Fitzpatrick, G., Neutra, R., and Gilbert, J. (1977). "Cost-Effectiveness of Cholecystectomy for Silent Gallstones." In J. Bunker, B. Barnes, and F. Mosteller (eds.), *Costs, Risks, and Benefits of Surgery*, 246–261. New York: Oxford University Press.

Foote, A., and Erfurt, J. (1991). "Benefit to Cost Ratio of Work-Site Blood Pressure

Control Programs.'' *Journal of the American Medical Association* 265:10 (March 13), 1283–1286.

Freund, D., Dittus, R., Fitzgerald, J., and Heck, D. (1990). ''Assessing and Improving Outcomes: Total Knee Replacement.'' *Health Services Research* 25:5 (December), 723–726.

Fromm, G. (1965). ''Civil Aviation Expenditures.'' In R. Dorfman (ed.), *Measuring Benefits of Government Investments*, 172–230. Washington, D.C.: Brookings Institution.

Fuchs, V. (1986). *The Health Economy*. Cambridge, Mass.: Harvard University Press.

Garber, A., and Fenerty, J. (1991). ''Costs and Benefits of Prenatal Screening for Cystic Fibrosis.'' *Medical Care* 29:5 (May) 473–489.

Garber, A., Fuchs, V., and Silverman, J. (1984). ''Casemix, Costs, and Outcomes: Differences between Faculty and Community Services in a University Hospital.'' *New England Journal of Medicine* 310:23 (May 17), 1231–1237.

Gaus, C., and Cooper, B. (1978). ''Technology and Medicare: Alternatives for Change.'' In R. Egdahl and P. Gertman (eds.), *Technology and the Quality of Health Care*, 225–236. Germantown, Md.: Aspen.

Giaque, W., and Peebles, T. (1976). ''Application of Multidimensional Utility Theory in Determining Optimal Test-Treatment Strategies for Streptococcal Sore Throat and Rheumatic Fever.'' *Operations Research* 24:5 (September–October), 933–950.

Glass, N. (1973). ''Cost Benefit Analysis and Health Services.'' *Health Trends* 5:1 (January), 51–60.

Goldman, L., Weinstein, M., Goldman, P., and Williams, L. (1991). ''Cost-Effectiveness of HMG-CoA Inhibition for Primary and Secondary Prevention of Coronary Heart Disease.'' *Journal of the American Medical Association* 265:9 (March 6), 1145–1151.

Graveley, E., and Littlefield, J. (1992) ''Cost-effectiveness Analysis of Three Staffing Models for the Delivery of Low-risk Prenatal Care.'' *American Journal of Public Health* 82:2 (February), 180–184.

Green, D. (1990). ''Streptokinase Equal to TPA.'' *Nature* 344:6 (March 15), 183.

Greer, A. (1988). ''State of the Art versus State of the Science: Diffusion of New Medical Technologies.'' *International Journal of Technology Assessment in Health Care* 4:1 (January), 5–26.

Grogono, A., and Woodgate, D. (1971). ''Index for Measuring Health.'' *Lancet* 2:7738 (November 1), 1024–1029.

Gruppo Italiano. (1992). ''GISSI-3: A Factorial Randomized Trial of Alteplase vs. Streptokinase and Heparin vs. No Heparin among 41,299 Patients with Acute Myocardial Infarction.'' *Lancet* 339: 8796 (March 28), 753–781.

Hackler, J., and Hiller, F. (1990). ''Family Consent to Orders Not to Resuscitate: Reconsidering Hospital Policy.'' *Journal of the American Medical Association* 264:10 (September 12), 1281–1283.

Hampton, J., and Nicholas, C. (1978). ''Randomized Trial of Mobile Coronary Care Unit for Emergency Calls.'' *British Medical Journal* 10:6120 (April 29), 1118–1122.

Hardy, A., Rauch, K., Echenberg, D., Morgan, W., and Curran, J. (1986). ''Economic Impact of the First 10,000 Cases of AIDS in the United States.'' *Journal of the American Medical Association* 255:2 (January 10), 209–211.

Harrison, R., and Payne, B. (1991). "Developing Criteria for Ordering Common Ancillary Services." *Medical Care* 29:9 (September), 853–877.

Haug, P. (1989). "Revision of Diagnostic Logic Using a Clinical Data Base." *Medical
Decision Making* 9:2 (April–June), 84–90.

Hiatt, H. (1990). *Medical Lifeboat: Will There Be Room for You in the Health Care
System?* New York: Harper and Row.

Hill, J., Hampton, J., and Mitchell, J. (1978). "A Randomized Trial of Home-versus-
Hospital Management for Patients with Suspected Myocardial Infarction." *Lancet*
1:8069 (April 22), 837–844.

Holmes, M., Rovner, D., and Rothert, M. (1989). "Methods of Analyzing Physician
Practice Patterns in Hypertension." *Medical Care* 27:1 (January), 59–68.

Ingelfinger, F. (1968). "Digestive Disease as a National Problem: Case V—Gallstones."
Gastroenterology 55, 102–110.

Institute of Medicine. (1989). *Effectiveness Initiative: Setting Priorities for Clinical Conditions.* Washington, D.C.: NAS Press.

Jackson, M., LoGerfo, J., Diehr, P., Watts, C., and Richardson, W. (1978). "Elective
Hysterectomy: A Cost-Benefit Analysis." *Inquiry* 15:3 (September), 275–280.

Jacobs, E., Winter, P., and Alvis, H. (1969). "Hyperoxygenation Effects of Cognitive
Functioning in the Aged." *New England Journal of Medicine* 281:13 (October
2), 753–757.

Johannesson, M., Jonsson, B., and Borg, L. (1992). "Willingness to Pay for Antihypertensive Therapy." *Journal of Health Economics* 10:4 (March), 451–463.

Jonsen, A. (1988). "Bentham in a Box: Technology Assessment and Health Care Allocation." *Law and Medicine in Health Care* 14:2, 172–174.

Kahneman, D., Slovic, P., and Tversky, A. (1982). *Judgment under Uncertainty: Heu-
ristics and Biases.* New York: Cambridge University Press.

Kanouse, D., Winkler, J., and Kosecoff, J. (1989). *Changing Medical Practice through
Technology Assessment: An Evaluation of the NIH Consensus Development Program.* Ann Arbor, Mich.: Health Administration Press.

Keeler, E. (1989). "The External Costs of a Sedentary Lifestyle." *American Journal of
Public Health* 79:8 (August), 975–981.

Kinosian, B., and Eisenberg, J. (1988). "Cutting into Cholesterol: Cost-Effective Alternatives." *Journal of the American Medical Association* 259:15 (April 15),
2249–2254.

Kitzhaber, J. (1990). "The Oregon Basic Health Services Act." State capital monograph,
Salem, Oregon.

Klarman, H. (1974). "Application of Cost-Benefit Analysis to the Health Services and
the Special Case of the Technologic Innovation." *International Journal of Health
Services* 4:3 (Fall), 325–352.

———. (1967). "Present Status of Cost-Benefit Analysis in the Health Field." *American
Journal of Public Health* 57:11 (November), 1948–1953.

———. (1965). "Syphilis Control Programs." In R. Dorfman (ed.), *Measuring Benefits
of Government Investments*, 367–410, Washington, D.C.: Brookings Institution.

Klarman, H., Francis, J., and Rosenthal, G. (1968). "Cost Effectiveness Analysis Applied to the Treatment of Chronic Renal Disease." *Medical Care* 6:1 (January–
February), 48–54.

Klein, R. (1991). "On the Oregon Trail: Rationing Health Care." *British Medical Journal*
337:1 (January 5), 5.

Krischer, J. (1976). "The Mathematics of Cleft Lip and Palate Treatment Evaluation: Measuring the Desirability of Treatment Outcomes." *Cleft Palate Journal* 13:4 (April), 165–180.

Lamm, R. (1990). "High-Tech Health Care and Society's Ability to Pay." *Healthcare Financial Management* 45:9 (September), 21–30.

Layde, P., Allmen, S., and Oakley, G. (1979). "Maternal Serum Alpha-Fetoprotein Screening: A Cost-Benefit Analysis." *American Journal of Public Health* 69:6 (June), 566–573.

Leaf, A. (1989). "Cost Effectiveness as a Criterion for Medicare Coverage." *New England Journal of Medicine* 321:13 (September 28), 898–900.

Leape, L. (1989). "Unnecessary Surgery." *Health Services Research* 24:3 (August), 351–407.

Lee, J. (1990). "Feasibility and Cost-saving Potential of Outpatient Cardiac Catheterization." *Journal of the American College of Cardiology* 15:2 (February), 378–384.

Lindsey, P., and Newhouse, J. (1990). "Cost and Value of Second Surgical Opinion Programs: A Critical Review of the Literature." *Journal of Health Politics, Policy, and Law* 15:3 (Fall), 543–570.

Linton, A., and Naylor, C. (1990). "Organized Medicine and the Assessment of Technology." *New England Journal of Medicine* 323:21 (November 22), 1463–1467.

Lipscomb, J. (1989). "Time Preference for Health in Cost-Effectiveness. *Medical Care* 27:3 (March) S233–S253.

Mandelblatt, J., and Fahs, M. (1988). "Cost-Effectiveness of Cervical Cancer Screening for Low-Income Elderly Women." *Journal of the American Medical Association* 259:16 (April 29), 2409–2413.

Manu, P., and Runge, L. (1985). "Testing Stable Angina: Expert Opinion versus Decision Analysis." *Medical Care* 23:12 (December), 1381–1390.

Max, W., Rice, D., and MacKenzie, E. (1990), "The Lifetime Cost of Injury." *Inquiry* 27:4 (Winter), 332–342.

Mechanic, D. (1989). "Social Policy, Technology, and Rationing of Health Care." *Medical Care Review* 46:2 (Summer), 113–123.

Mishan, E. (1976). *Cost-Benefit Analysis.* New York: Praeger.

Musgrave, R. (1969). "Cost-Benefit Analysis and the Theory of Public Finance." *Journal of Economic Literature* 7:3 (September), 797–806.

Mushkin, S. (1962). "Health as an Investment." *Journal of Political Economy* 70:5 (October), 129–157.

Neuhauser, D. (1991). "Parallel Providers, Ongoing Randomization, and Continuous Improvement." *Medical Care* 29:7 (July Supplement), JS5–JS9.

Neutra, R. (1977). "Indications for the Surgical Treatment of Suspected Acute Appendicitis: A Cost-Effectiveness Approach." In J. Bunker, B. Barnes, and F. Mosteller (eds.), *Costs, Risks, and Benefits of Surgery*, 277–307. New York: Oxford University Press.

Newcomer, L. (1990). "Defining Experimental Therapy: A Third-Party Payer's Dilemma." *New England Journal of Medicine* 323:24 (December 13), 1702–1704.

Osberg, J., and DiScala, C. (1992). "Morbidity Among Pediatric Motor Vehicle Crash Victims: Effectiveness of Seat Belts." *American Journal of Public Health* 82:3 (March), 422–425.

Paiement, G., Wessinger, S., and Harris, W. (1991). "Cost-effectiveness of Prophylaxis in Total Hip Replacement." *American Journal of Surgery* 161:5 (May), 519–525.

Pashos, C., and McNeil, B. (1990). "Consequences of Variation in Treatment for Acute MI." *Health Services Research* 25:5 (December), 717–722.

Pauly, M., and Held, P. (1990). "Benign Moral Hazard and the Cost-Effectiveness Analysis of Insurance Coverage." *Journal of Health Economics* 9:3 (December), 447–461.

Perry, S., and Pillar, B. (1990). "National Policy for Health Care Technology." *Medical Care Review* 47:4 (Winter), 401–418.

Piachaud, D., and Weddell, J. (1972). "The Economics of Treating Varicose Veins." *International Journal of Epidemiology* 1:3 (Autumn), 287–299.

Pigou, A. (1920). *The Economics of Welfare*. London: Macmillan.

Prospective Payment Commission (ProPAC). (1991). *Report to the Congress*. Washington, D.C., March.

Randolph, A., and Washington, A. (1990). "Screening for Chlamydia in Adolescent Males: A Cost-based Decision Analysis." *American Journal of Public Health* 80:5 (May), 545–550.

Rang, M. (1972). "The Ulysses Syndrome." *Canadian Medical Association Journal* 106:2 (January 22), 122–127.

Ransohoff, D., and Feinstein, A. (1976). "Is Decision Analysis Useful in Clinical Medicine?" *Yale Journal of Biology and Medicine* 49:2 (May), 165–179.

Rapaport, E. (1989). "Thrombolytic Agents in Acute Myocardial Infarction." *New England Journal of Medicine* 320:12 (April 22), 861–864.

Redelmeier, D., and Tversky, A. (1990). "Discrepancy between Medical Decisions for Individual Patients and Groups." *New England Journal of Medicine* 322:16 (April 19), 1162–1164.

Relman, A. (1990). "Is Rationing Inevitable?" *New England Journal of Medicine* 322:25 (June 21), 1809–1810.

Rice, D. (1966). *Estimating the Cost of Illness*. Health Economics Series no. 6. Washington, D.C.: U.S. Government Printing Office.

Rice, D., Hodgson, T., and Kopstein, A. (1985). "The Economic Costs of Illness: A Replication and Update." *Health Care Financing Review* 7:1 (Fall), 61–80.

Rizzo, J. (1992). "Supply and Demand Factors in the Determination of Expenditures." *Health Services Research* 26:6, 708–722.

Robinson, J. (1990). "Philosophical Origins of the Social Rate of Discount in Cost-Benefit Analysis." *Milbank Quarterly* 68:2 (Summer), 245–265.

Roper, W., Winkenwerder, W., Hackbarth, G., and Krakauer, H. (1988). "Effectiveness in Health Care: An Initiative to Evaluate and Improve Medical Practice." *New England Journal of Medicine* 319:18 (November 3), 1197–1202.

Russell, L. (1985). *Is Prevention Better Than Cure?* Washington, D.C.: Brookings Institution.

Scheffler, R., and Andrews, N. (1989). *Cancer Care and Cost: DRGs and Beyond*. Ann Arbor, Mich.: Health Administration Press.

Schelling, T. (1986). "Economics and Cigarettes." *Preventive Medicine* 15:5 (September), 549–560.

———. (1968). "The Life You Save May Be Your Own." In S. Chase (ed.), *Problems in Public Expenditure Analysis*, 127–162. Washington, D.C.: Brookings Institution.

Schoenbaum, S., Hyde, J., Bartoshesky, L., and Crampton, K. (1976). "Benefit-Cost Analysis of Rubella Vaccination Policy." *New England Journal of Medicine* 294:6 (February 5), 306–310.

Schwartz, W., and Aaron, H. (1990). "The Achilles Heel of Health Care Rationing." *New York Times*, July 9, 28.

Shortliffe, E. (1991). "Medical Informatics and Clinical Decision Making." *Medical Decision Making* 11:4 (October-December), S4-S14.

Showstack, J. (1989). "Cyclosporine for the Use of Hospital Resources for Kidney Transplant." *New England Journal of Medicine* 321:16 (October 19), 1086–1092.

Sisk, J. (1990). "Introduction to Measuring Health Care Effectiveness." *International Journal of Technology Assessment in Health Care* 6:2 (April), 181–184.

Skillings, J., Williams, J., and Hinshaw, J. (1979). "Cost-Effectiveness of Operative Cholangiography." *American Journal of Surgery* 137:1 (January), 26–30.

Spiegelhalter, D., and Knill-Jones, R. (1984). "Statistical and Knowledge-based Approaches to Clinical Decision-Support Systems, with an Application in Gastroenterology." *Journal of the Royal Statistical Society* 147:1 (Series A), 35–77.

Steinberg, E. (1990). "Variations in Cataract Management: Patient and Economic Outcomes." *Health Services Research* 25:5 (December), 727–732.

Stewart, A., Ware, J., and Johnston, S. (1975). "Construction of Scales Measuring Health and Health-related Concepts from the Dayton Medical History Questionnaire." In *The Conceptualization and Measurement of Health in the Health Insurance Study*. Santa Monica, Calif.: Rand Corporation.

Thomas, L. (1977). "On the Science and Technology of Medicine." *Daedalus* 106:1 (Winter), 35–46.

Tomlinson, T., and Brody, H. (1990). "Futility and the Ethics of Resuscitation." *Journal of the American Medical Association* 264:10 (September 12), 1276–1280.

Tsai, S., Lee, E., and Hardy, R. (1978). "The Effect of a Reduction in Leading Causes of Death: Potential Gains in Life Expectancy." *American Journal of Public Health* 68:10 (October), 966–971.

Valenzuela, T., Criss, E., and Spaite, D. (1990). "Cost-Effectiveness Analysis of Paramedic EMS in the Treatment of Prehospital Cardiac Arrest." *Annals of Emergency Medicine* 19:12 (December), 1407–1411.

Viens-Bitker, C., Fery, E., and Blum, C. (1989). "Cost of Allogenic Bone Marrow Transplantation in Four Diseases." *Health Policy* 12:4, 309–317.

Viscusi, W., and Evans, W. (1990). "Utility Functions That Depend on Health Status: Estimates and Economic Implications." *American Economic Review* 80:3 (June), 353–374.

Waaler, H., and Piot, M. (1970). "Use of an Epidemiological Model for Estimating the Effectiveness of Tuberculosis Control Measures." *Bulletin of the World Health Organization* 43, 1–16.

Walker, A., and Whynes, D. (1992). "Filtering Strategies in Mass Population Screening for Colorectal Cancer." *Medical Decision Making* 12:1 (January-March), 2–7.

Ward, G. (1977). "National High Blood Pressure Program." Report from The National Institutes of Health to the Congressional Office of Technological Assessment.

Warner, K., and Luce, B. (1989). *Cost-Benefit and Cost-Effectiveness Analysis in Health Care: Principles, Practice, and Potential*. 2d ed. Ann Arbor, Mich.: Health Administration Press.

Weinstein, M., Pliskin, J., and Stason, W. (1977). "Coronary Artery Bypass Surgery:

Decision and Policy Analysis.'' In J. Bunker, B. Barnes, and F. Mosteller (eds.), *Costs, Risks, and Benefits of Surgery*, 342–371. New York: Oxford University Press.

Weisbrod, B. (1968). ''Income Redistribution Effects and Benefit-Cost Analysis.'' In S. Chase (ed.), *Problems in Public Expenditure Analysis*, 177–209. Washington, D.C.: Brookings Institution.

Welch, H., and Larsen, E. (1989). ''Cost Effectiveness of Bone Marrow Transplantation.'' *New England Journal of Medicine* 321:13 (September 21), 807–812.

Wennberg, J. (1990). ''Status of the Prostate Disease Assessment Team.'' *Health Services Research* 25:5 (December), 709–716.

White, H., Rivers, J., Jacobs, H. et al. Team (1989). ''Effect of Intravenous Streptokinase as Compared with that of Tissue Plasminogen Activator on Left Ventricular Function After First Myocardial Infarction.'' *New England Journal of Medicine* 320:13 (March 22), 817–821.

Widen, A. (1991). ''Illinois Plan Calls for Cut in Hysterectomies.'' *Consumer Exchange* 11:9, 1–2.

Young, M., Eisenberg, J., Williams, S., and Hershey, J. (1986). ''Comparing Aggregate Estimates of Derived Thresholds for Clinical Decisions.'' *Health Services Research* 20:6 (February 1), 763–780.

Zimmerman, F. (1991). ''When Is Pulmonary Artery Catheterization Worth The Risks?'' *Postgraduate Medicine* 89:2 (February), 169–174.

12 The Role of Medical Technology Assessment

Saving money will require a reduction in the number of beds and in the number of employees in the hospital; not their redeployment to provide yet another untested treatment. We need a leaner, trimmer health care economy.

—John E. Wennberg, M.D.

Medline Research Service does not list the word "health" in its index. In a teaching hospital there is no such thing as a healthy patient. A healthy patient is one who has not been sufficiently worked up at high cost. Come to a teaching hospital as a Medicare patient with the complaint of "stiff hands in the morning" and we will send you to rheumatology for a workup to discover Lupus in one case per 1,000 screened.

—John G. Freymann, M.D.

If humans are distinguished from other primates by their need to take drugs, then physicians must be distinguished by their need to order tests.

—William Osler, M.D.

Medical technology assessment is becoming an increasingly important topic for physicians and health policy makers (Institute of Medicine 1989). Formal training in cost-effective clinical decision making for residents and medical students is a potential alternative to further coercive federal cost-containment efforts (Fuchs and Garber 1990). If further regulatory ventures are to be avoided, and the dual goals of cost containment and quality are to be achieved, physicians should be taught in their formative clinical years to apply parsimony and efficiency principles in ordering tests and treatments. Many published physician reports misuse basic concepts (e.g., cost-effectiveness; Doubilet, Weinstein, and McNeil 1986). This chapter examines the question of whether exposure to such instruction changes attitudes among medical students electing to take a course on decision analysis and health economics. Further research is needed as to the timing and content of the most cost-effective means of promoting cost-effective clinical decisions. Ethical and social issues raised by cost-benefit and cost-effectiveness applications are also discussed. This chapter examines clinical protocols, physician profiles, and McNeil's (1985) innovative approach to preferred practice patterns (PPPs). Marcus Merz, president of Preferred One in St. Paul, has continued developing a professional consensus around PPPs, disseminating information to physicians, and accomplishing slow incremental improvements in practice patterns. PPPs are a more equitable approach to supply-side improvements in resource allocation than demand-side age-based rationing (O'Malley 1991; Levinsky 1990). Improving physician habits is better than telling Granny Doe that she is too old to have medical care.

The need for more cost-effective clinical decision making is clear when one considers the burden of a demand inflation in tests and procedures. In 1991 dollars the nation annually spends $5.4 billion on 280 million blood cholesterol tests, $4.5 billion on 230 million urinalysis tests, $7.4 billion on 126 million sequential multiple analyzer (SMA) tests, $3.2 billion on 115 million blood counts, $4.2 billion on 49 million chest X-rays, $2.6 billion on 35 million ultrasound exams (for pregnancy and for heart and gallbladder problems), $2.7 billion for 32 million annual electrocardiograms, $1.8 billion on 26 million endoscopy exams, and $1.8 billion for 6.6 million stress/treadmill tests. Utilization review and prior-certification programs have done little to slow the inflation rate in demand and dollars for these tests and procedures. Media coverage has helped foster the explosion in patient demand for repeat cholesterol tests. One could speculate that adoptions of Medicare physician fee schedules in 1992 for certain procedures like endoscopy may dampen the volume for those procedures. Even little-ticket expenditures like Pap tests are a $1.0-billion item if we perform 46 million annually. Ultimately education based on the evolution of cost-effective preferred practice patterns is the number one tool we have to control physician ordering habits.

A cost-effective medical staff should strive to trim overuse of new procedures; e.g., if only 60 percent of the 490,000 cholecystectomies were performed with the laparoscope and without the laser (saving $900 per case), the cost savings would exceed $264 million in 1992. This is a conservative estimate if clinicians could identify more than 60 percent of the cases *ex ante* as receiving no improved outcomes from laser surgery compared to the less expensive traditional electro-coagulation. Cost-effective providers should trim overreliance of disposable items, e.g., switching to reusable surgical staple removers can save the typical 300 bed hospital $100,000 a year.

The medical staff should promote efficient sequential scheduling of tests: order only sodium and potassium electrolytes (cost $14), and not the full panel of electrolytes ($40), if these two tests are sufficient. If there is no suggestive evidence from the peripheral smear don't order unnecessary tests like iron studies or multiple vitamin levels for anemic patients. Other cost reduction ideas include reducing the flow of anesthesia from five to two liters per minute thus saving $8 per hour and not eroding the quality of care. Nearly half of the basic pre-operative tests (electrolytes, CBC, PT/PTT) need not be done if previous testing was normal within the past year, and no clinical indication for retesting exists. FAX machines have improved the information flow between the hospital and physicians offices, thus decreasing the amount of repeat testing.

This chapter will outline the need to avoid chasing the wild goose: don't spend $9 million for routine liver-function tests of patients on disulfiram to detect only one case of hepatitis. Consumerism should also play a part in the cost-effective medical staff. Make the consumer king, e.g., teach diabetics to use pocket insulin-dosage computers to enhance independence and self-esteem, and save money by reducing the rate of hospital admissions among brittle diabetics. Often what is less costly is better for the patient: use a $19 pulse oximeter to get the same basic information as arterial blood gases—thus saving $75 and reducing the discomfort for the patient (as long as acidosis or CO_2 retention are not suspected). The style of medical practice is moving toward cost-effective clinical decision making. Most nephrologists do not order a metabolic workup for the first kidney stone. Pulmonary specialists order spirometry rather than expensive more complete pulmonary function testing for the pre-operative chronic emphysema patient.

DEFINING THE ISSUES

Nonmedical technology is typically not controversial. Everyone is for it, and it usually is cost-decreasing. In contrast, medical technology has moved into the public eye as a culprit in rising health care costs (Anderson and Morrison 1989). However, there is a wide range of opinions as to whether technology, on balance, is a major or minor source of rising costs. Technology can sometimes be cost-decreasing, although this is less frequently the case in the medical sector of the economy. One wonders whether technology explains 5 or 40 percent of the cost-inflation problem. For Wilensky (1990) and other data analysts, technology has been implicated as a substantial cause of increased cost (30 to 40 percent) through increasing intensity of services and utilization. Other economists suggest that technology plays a more minor role in rising health care expenditures. What could society remove or ration to make a substantial reduction in the $700-billion annual health care bill?

If the cost problem were technology driven, would not the sectors of the medical economy that are high-tech grow the most? The data do not support this hypothesis. Even with 865 magnetic resonance imaging (MRI) facilities set up in the last seven years, one cannot argue that imaging technologies have driven up the cost of health care. Indeed, diagnostic imaging has increased from 3.1 to 3.5 percent of health care expenditures. Substitution for old techniques and prudent utilization controls to hold down variable costs have made MRI a costly burden. Many technologies would perform more cost-effectively with the aid of more stringent utilization review, for example, fiber optics. Inappropriate utilization makes a technology less cost-effective.

Some medical technologies appear cost-decreasing, such as visualizing gallstones with ultrasound and crushing the stones with lithotripsy. This is also clearly quality-enhancing in comparison to traditional exploratory surgery. Unfortunately, the public is not well versed in life-cycle costing or the risks of old-style invasive medicine (with iatrogenic infections and prolonged lengths of stay). The media tend to focus excessive attention on initial capital outlays rather than on long-run cost-benefit and cost-effectiveness. The public reads that MRI technology costs $1 to $2 million more than traditional X-ray equipment, or that IBM is trying to bring a $20-million compact synchrotron to market in the 1990s, and concludes that health care costs must be 90 percent technology driven. This is simply not true. Much of the administrative technology that hospitals have added since 1984 is cost-decreasing in pharmacy or nursing (e.g., automated nurse-scheduling systems to create workload-driven staffing patterns).

Clinicians also have an incomplete understanding of life-cycle costing, product maturity, and development. Some physicians find technology a convenient bogeyman to blame for increasing health care costs. If technology and demanding patients are tagged as 90 percent of the cost-control problem, then organized medicine proceeds to lobby for higher fee schedules, claiming that its members, as professionals, are not getting enough money for their value. Advocates for either price competition or tight fee schedules reverse the perspective and ask if consumers are getting enough value for their money. Many agree with Wilensky (1990) that consumers and third-party payers need better-funded high-quality assessments of the costs, risks, and benefits of medical technology. The argument that technology cannot be evaluated because it presents a "moving target," constantly improving and efficiently circumscribing the indicators for clinical usage, is not to be believed. As Wilensky (1990) suggested, careful analysis is especially needed in those grey areas where technology attempts to improve quality-adjusted life years (QALYs) without extending life expectancy.

A number of classic writings by physicians have called for such economic analysis. Lewis Thomas in his classic popular book *The Medusa and the Snail* (1979) argued that we have too much of a technological imperative for acquisition of expensive halfway technologies that do little to benefit patients. The financing revolution of the 1980s, with DRG price controls and the proliferation of alternative delivery systems, did not eliminate or slow this technological imperative. One could speculate that in the longer run the current focus on cost containment may skew what products are brought to market to those that are cost-decreasing or likely to be reimbursed (Soumerai 1990).

Technology assessment proceeds in sequential stages (Eddy 1990). Physicians dominate the first stage of analysis, examining short-term safety and descriptive analysis (e.g., does the new technique or procedure yield improvements?). Statisticians dominate the second stage of technology assessment with a middle-term study of efficacy utilizing the randomized controlled clinical trials. Diagnostic efficacy studies report sensitivity and specificity (outlined in the middle of this chapter). Economists, operations researchers, and policy makers dominate the third stage of technology assessment: clinical cost-effectiveness (is it less costly than the alternative options at achieving a prescribed package of "effects," e.g., X percent less pain or Y percent less morbidity?) and long-run cost-benefit (does the ratio of benefit to cost exceed one, counting all costs and benefits to society?). Since cost-benefit analysis should include intangible benefits (e.g., pain reduction) to be comprehensive, it is necessary to shadow-price patients' willingness-to-pay preferences regarding a given medical technology. The activity of shadow-pricing the hard-to-measure items in a cost-benefit study is the subject for the next chapter.

ECONOMICS AND MEDICINE

Future physicians must realize that cost-benefit analysis and cost-effectiveness analysis are tools that can produce better-informed decisions. However, as we have seen in chapter 11, these two analytical techniques have occasionally been oversold in the health sector because of the multiplicity of dimensions of health-service output and the difficulty of comparing disparate types of health benefits. Economic techniques should not be sold as value-free mathematics. However, without such analysis, decision making will remain ad hoc, with the assumptions hidden and the value judgments implicit. Some decision makers may want their values and assumptions to be kept secret and free from refutation, rather than to be made public and explicit.

The congressional Office of Technology Assessment's evaluation of cost-effectiveness and cost-benefit applications in the health field concluded that the conceptual and practical limitations of the techniques are such that they should not be considered definitive tools that produce "correct" decisions (U.S. Congress, OTA 1980). For example, construction of a hospice may not be justified merely by the projected medical cost savings, but the humanitarian intangible benefits (bereavement support, and so on) might more than justify the investment. According to the Office of Technology Assessment report, the analyst's role is one of information generation and decision assistance, because limited resources typically preclude valuation of intangible benefits.

As we observed in chapter 11, regulators and politicians have not been effective at rationing the availability of new hospital technologies. Traditionally, once the supply is in place, we deal ineffectively with rationing decisions. For example, Rettig (1978) documented a classic case of the physician community's inability to cope with ethical issues in the rationing of renal dialysis care after Shana Alexander published the November 1962 *Life* magazine article, "They Decide Who Lives, Who Dies." The American tradition has been to make local selective choices through critical-care committees rather than to implement an "all or none" rationing decision; that is, everyone is allowed access or no one is allowed access, as with most European countries. A legal scholar in Boston wrote a hypothetical Supreme Court decision for the year 2002 that upheld the concept of a national lottery for distribution of artificial hearts (Annas 1977). The author pointed out that American society cannot accept "all or none" rationing.

Economic evaluations often consider questions of whether a procedure or treatment should be done more or less frequently. For example, Cole (1976) reported that performing one million prophylactic hysterectomies would save $1.4 billion (mostly in the form of 35,000 prevented cases of cancer), but cost $2.9 billion. The congressional study on unnecessary surgery estimated the cost of excess and inappropriate elective surgery at $4 billion in 1976 (U.S. Congress 1976).

Since the reader may not have conceptualized excess utilization in graphic terms, Figure 12.1 illustrates three possible scenarios for medical treatment production functions. Curve *AB* represents a cost-beneficial treatment mode such as heart pacemakers. If the technology were inappropriately utilized or prophylactically prescribed for an indiscriminately large fraction of the population, the assessed technology could move along the curve into the region *BC* where benefits do not justify costs. Hypothetical curve *DE* might represent the benefit-cost range when surgeons perform only 110,000 coronary artery bypass operations annually, but the treatment may appear unjustified (region *EF*) if the operative incidence increases to 180,000 annual bypass cases. Brott, Labutta, and Kempczinski (1986) suggested that many of the 60,000 annual carotid endarterectomies may be medically unnecessary. The number of endarterectomies increased 74 percent in the Cincinnati area from 1980 to 1984. In 1984 half of the procedures were performed in patients with asymptomatic carotid disease, at a combined stroke or death rate of 5.3 percent. This rate was higher than the 3.0 percent suggested rate for prophylactic carotid endarterectomies. Brott, Labutta, and Kempczinski (1986) called for a more conservative (less surgical) treatment of asymptomatic cases and future randomized clinical trials to assess the benefits of medical treatment (antiplatelet agents and risk-factor reduction) versus surgical treatment. The third hypothetical curve *GH* is an example of a treatment mode that is never cost-beneficial (for example, gastric freezing for ulcers; Miao 1977). Unfortunately, the public had to endure the fad from the introductory usage stage at point *G* (1962) to peak popularity at point *H* (1968) before the faulty treatment mode (gastric freezing) was finally discredited (1969).

ETHICAL AND SOCIAL ISSUES

In the United States we allow any individual who can afford it to buy any technology, and we selectively finance transplants and less effective technologies from the public treasury. Questions of cost-benefit and resource limitations do disturb some American physicians and prompt the medical community to ask how we can afford dialysis and transplants during resurgence of polio and other childhood diseases. In contrast to England, America has said that a citizen should not be barred from the opportunity to receive tertiary-care services if he or she

Figure 12.1
Three Hypothetical Production Functions of Total Treatment Benefits as a Function of Total Costs

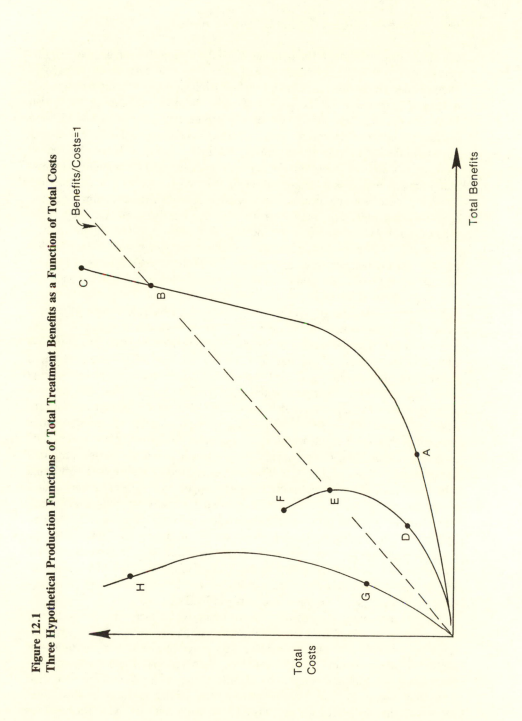

can afford them. Although England has made the slogan "health care as a right" operational by funding all primary- and secondary-care service activities, frequently individuals are not allowed to buy even proven technologies that are judged too expensive for the society. One of the demands during the British hospital strikes in the mid–1970s was that private-pay patients not be allowed to have medically unnecessary services performed (Eastaugh 1983). For the 91 percent of the British population utilizing the British National Health Service as their primary provider, publicly funded bypass surgery and heart and renal transplants are now available for those willing to wait two to four months. In America, obtaining most basic medical services is done through a process similar to the search for any other consumer good (that is, the family plans and budgets for the purchase), but obtaining very expensive new services is very often a matter of chance. It is possible that this situation reflects consumer preferences, in that the American consumer may value the assurance that comes with knowing that the nation can provide the utmost care for a given individual following the onset of a catastrophic disease (Institute of Medicine 1991).

Economic evaluation of common diseases will probably continue to receive more critical assessment than innovations for rare diseases that pose a less significant net financial burden in spite of the higher unit costs. An innovation like coronary bypass surgery has attracted the attention of the health-services research community in the United States because expenditures have rocketed from zero to $8 billion per year within a single decade. Economic-impact considerations should be a critical determinant in selecting the procedures for randomized clinical trials (RCTs). Neuhauser (1979) pointed out the dangerous limitations that short-sighted ethical considerations impose if they become the sole determinant of RCT experimentation. He argued that in some cases proposed sham operations (for example, telling the patient the operation was performed when in actuality it was not) should not be stopped by the local human-subject committee of the hospital. For example, internal mammary artery ligation therapy was exposed by eight pairs of sham operations as an ineffective multimillion-dollar mode of treatment. Neuhauser suggested an appropriate reward for the eight patients who saved our economy and the public chest: "Each should receive $1 million tax-free and be flown to the White House to shake hands with the President." The economy may be wasting tens of billions of dollars on unnecessary care because of the failure to perform RCTs.

The less tangible quality-of-life benefits comprise an increasing proportion of medical care benefits (Mushkin 1989). For example, elective surgical expenditures are properly intended to achieve less tangible goals than mortality- or morbidity-rate reduction, such as relief of disability, pain, and disfigurement. Such quality-of-life factors are to be identified, then quantified in terms of their equivalent social costs by shadow-pricing, and finally balanced against commensurate shadow prices for quantity of life. Advocates of the willingness-to-pay approach suggest the maximization of lives saved as the social objective function.

The willingness to pay surveys summarized in chapter 13 have an analog called willingness to accept. We have asked the maximum amount that an individual is willing to pay (WTP) for a program or service, but one could also ask the minimum amount that an individual is willing to accept (WTA) to forgo the service or program. Hanemann (1991) has demonstrated that holding income effects constant, the smaller the substitution effect (fewer substitutes for the service or product) the greater the disparity between WTP and WTA. If future economic conditions prompt a contraction in the social welfare programs (e.g., New Zealand 1992), more economists may be surveying the WTA issue. The divergence between WTP and WTA survey results may be an example of the Will Rogers rule: the public knows more about limits than the economists or the politicians. Consumers make mistakes because they are provided with imperfect information, so individuals' willingness to pay will sometimes be underestimated (e.g., vaccinations) and other times overestimated (e.g., laetrile).

Valuation problems still tend to plague most analyses. Subjective questions concerning valuation and effectiveness are largely a product of the values and occupation of the respondent. For example, computerized axial tomography (CAT) scanner effectiveness to a radiologist is measured by whether the pictures are clearer and the information is more detailed. The economist must represent the public interest and ask whether CAT scanning yields a better diagnosis, resulting in better treatment and ultimately improving patient outcome. The radiologist's definition of effectiveness might argue for 7,000 CAT scanners, with each hospital replacing its CAT machines every few years because of marginal improvements (e.g., they "read spines 0.5 percent better").

A central dilemma that the economic analyst faces is the unsubstantiated thesis of ever-improving technology—that is, the assumption that any evaluation will be obsolete when completed since medical science is improving so fast. Yet another problem faced by the analyst attempting to do a prospective study is refusal by the physicians to pursue randomized controlled trials if any hint of inferiority among the alternatives can be raised as a "red herring" to prevent the experiment. However, difficult decisions will increasingly need to be made concerning the allocation of scarce resources. Contrary to the conventional wisdom, the majority of Americans would like to place a dollar value on human life. According to a 1981 national Harris Poll, 52 percent of the American public believed that government and the courts must attempt to place an economic value on human life. Only 34 percent of the national sample of the population disagreed with the need to put a dollar value on life, and 14 percent responded "not sure" or "it depends" (American Public Health Association [APHA] 1981)

Value judgments increasingly will have to be made by the courts. For example, should patient X be provided with chloromycetin if the drug is known to correlate weakly with fatal anemia? Taking the drug increases the risk of dying from aplastic anemia from 1 in 500,000 to 1 in 40,000. How shall we decide when changing a probability distribution constitutes "causing" an event? This question has been raised in a wide range of circumstances, from auto safety to the case of swine flu vaccination side effects.

CONSUMER COST ISSUES

The growth in third-party financing of medical care has frequently been criticized for funding excessive and/or inappropriate therapies. One postulated negative effect of health insurance is the increased financing of useless technologies like gastric freezing for ulcers. Another postulated negative by-product of the growth in health insurance is the utilization of treatments to an excess (see points C, F, and H in Figure 12.1). The growth in health insurance coverage provided health care institutions with the wherewithal to expand service capability and produce service at the point where the cost exceeds the benefit. As health insurance becomes more comprehensive and the consumer's out-of-pocket cost falls to zero, health-service institutions continue to provide care beyond the point where marginal cost is equal to marginal benefit (Q_2) up to point Q_3 (see figure 12.2). The situation is somewhat analogous to that of the consumer who visits an automobile showroom and asks the dealer to select a car for him, price being no object. Because the dealer's profit margin is higher if he provides a Mercedes rather than a Mustang, the customer will never see the Mustang.

The present American economy cannot afford a Mercedes for every consumer (point Q_3). In defense of production at point Q_3 is the argument by the American medical establishment that it must do the utmost for each patient irrespective of cost. Many economists argue that society can barely afford the Mustang unless we decrease utilization rates by increasing the coinsurance paid by patients. Future physicians should realize that relaxing the degree of clinical discrimination and increasing the quantity of care provided per illness episode (intensity) will be curtailed by professional review organizations (PROs) and private utilization review efforts. Moreover, doing the utmost for everybody will save a few lives but at an ever-diminishing rate. Production of Q_3 minus Q_1 additional units of medical service ignores the opportunity cost of spending that money on housing or pollution control. Some analysts would hope that every dollar wasted in the medical economy is a dollar not utilized on defense or nuclear power. However, it is the broader health economy of prevention and public health that is being squeezed by the growth in the medical economy.

ECONOMIC AND DECISION-THEORY TOOLS FOR REDUCING "LITTLE-TICKET" EXPENDITURES

A consideration to be dealt with in technology assessment is that there is more to cost containment than simply preventing the purchase of $500,000 machines. Many health planners assume that the cost problem will disappear only if society can control the purchase of "big-ticket" items and so reduce the availability of expensive therapeutic treatment approaches. A number of studies in the 1970s

Figure 12.2
Hypothetical Marginal Benefit and Marginal Cost Curves

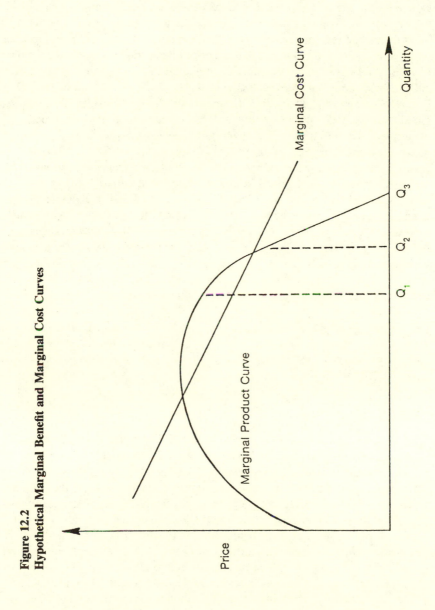

(Maloney and Rogers 1979) suggested that "little-ticket" items, such as laboratory tests and diagnostic procedures, comprise the bulk of the cost-crisis iceberg. Diagnostic charges account for over 25 percent of total hospital expenditures, and diagnostic testing costs have been increasing at almost double the rate of total hospital costs. The efficiency and increased costs of performing more diagnostic tests are central issues in the public debate about rising medical costs. Twentyfold variations in the number of diagnostic tests utilized by groups of interns did not measurably affect the outcome following care for a cohort of patients with ambulatory hypertensive disease (Daniels and Schroeder 1977). Providers continue to study little-ticket item volume. Consider the complete blood count (CBC), the laboratory test most often ordered in the emergency department. The $10 to $20 CBC test lacks the necessary specificity or sensitivity to benefit most emergency-room patients (Young 1986). Because absolute differential counts are more accurate than differential percentages, the clinician can rapidly enhance the data gained from any white blood count (WBC) and differential at no extra marginal cost. The absolute count of each leukocyte cell type is easily calculated from the total WBC count and the differential percentages reported by the lab. A little thinking can save a lot of little-ticket expenses for the patient and society. Santos, Starich, and Mazzaferri (1989) demonstrated how sequence, which test is done first, has important cost implications for diagnosing thyroid disease. Two decades earlier John Knowles (1969) was one of the first physicians to link the cost and efficiency issues:

One should ask how many renal arteriograms in patients with hypertension have resulted in the surgical or medical cure of the patients' hypertension. . . . Increasingly we shall be asked to answer such questions, for our resources are not infinite nor is our share of the Gross National Product.

TESTING SPECIFICITY AND SENSITIVITY

In considering the cost-effectiveness value of diagnostic tests, clinicians and medical students should be encouraged to examine three issues: (1) the reliability of test interpretation among physicians, (2) the specificity of the test, and (3) the marginal costs and benefits of additional testing. With respect to the reliability issue, there is wide disagreement among physicians over what constitutes a significant change in diagnostic test results for the same patient (Skendzel 1978). The previously cited study by Daniels and Schroeder (1977) indicated a strong but not statistically significant correlation between poor clinical outcome and laboratory costs, suggesting that physicians who tend to be less competent use the laboratory more. A growing body of evidence indicates physician confusion in the interpretation and application of information contained in diagnostic tests (Eastaugh 1981). This confusion tends to result in suboptimal patient care and high medical costs.

Obviously, diagnostic tests do not disclose the presence or absence of disease.

They are merely tools to detect the presence or absence of particular signs or symptoms from which the presence or absence of a specific disease may be predicted. The following diagram illustrates the two-step sequence from testing to diagnosis:

(1)   (2)

Diagnostic test → The sign or symptom → Disease is present

is + or −   or absent

There are two points of potential slippage, each with its own implications, in the diagnostic testing procedure. Type-one breakdowns are often due to inadequate technology, which translates into an inability to detect the target sign or symptom with adequate accuracy. It follows that these breakdowns often can be remedied by improving technology. Type-two breakdowns occur when the presence or absence of the target sign or symptom has a low predictive value for the presence or absence of disease. These breakdowns are inherent in the test and usually cannot be remedied.

Sensitivity and specificity analysis have traditionally been used to measure the efficacy of diagnostic tests. These values are determined by performing the test on two selected groups of subjects, those with disease and those without disease. They answer the questions: Given that the patient has the disease, how likely is he or she to have a positive test? Conversely, given that the patient does not have the disease, how likely is he or she to have a negative test? Sensitivity and specificity are rarely both 100 percent because diagnostic tests measure biologic variations that are then used to predict disease. These variations are usually distributed over a range of values roughly conforming to a normal curve. The curves representing the range of laboratory values of the diseased and the nondiseased populations overlap. The more overlap, the greater the trade-off between sensitivity and specificity.

Better specificity usually brings with it the trade-off of increases in the false-negative rate (eroded sensitivity). Determination of the patient sample size required to measure the false-negative rate to the researchers' specified degree of precision in two group-comparison studies varied from 62 for a sensitivity of 0.80 to 298 for a sensitivity of 0.95 and a sample size of 1,552 for a sensitivity of 0.99 (Wears and Kamens 1986). Such sampling concerns are important in projecting research costs and in estimating the smallest increase in false-negative rates that a study of a given size is likely to detect.

Diagnostic tests are used for at least three purposes: discovery, confirmation, and exclusion. Discovery tests must have high sensitivity and are used to detect disease in patients who seem healthy. Confirmation tests must have high specificity and are used to verify disease in situations of strong suspicion. Sometimes it is better to avoid the confirmation test (e.g., a biopsy) and treat all highly suspect cases with the therapy (e.g., the antiviral drug adenine arabinoside for herpes virus encephalitis [HVE]). Braun (1980) demonstrated that it is better on the average to avoid the risk of brain biopsy and directly administer the drug on the basis of other tests. Exclusion tests must have high sensitivity and are used to rule out disease in situations of suspicion, but are too expensive to use for discovery purposes. A test can be used for one, two, or all three purposes. Physicians and medical students should be encouraged to develop strategies utilizing combinations of tests that allow the achievement of both high sensitivity and high specificity.

Rather than optimize the two attributes, many doctors simply maximize sensitivity or specificity in terms of the consequences of error and harm to the patient. For example, in disease type A, a false-negative diagnosis is disastrous and a false-positive diagnosis is of little consequence. Maximum test sensitivity would therefore be selected. Hypothyroidism, most venereal diseases, and pheochromocytoma are examples of type-A diseases (Pestotnik 1990; Washington, Browner, and Korenbrot 1987). In disease type B, a false-negative diagnosis is of little consequence and a false-positive diagnosis is disastrous. Maximum test specificity would therefore be selected to protect the patient. Examples of type-B diseases are multiple sclerosis and oat-cell carcinoma. Falsely telling patients that they have serious, terminal diseases could result in psychological harm. In disease type C, both false negatives and false positives are of little consequence. Examples of type-C diseases are rheumatoid arthritis and chronic dermatitis. In type-D disease, both false positives and false negatives are disastrous. Maximum test specificity and sensitivity must be achieved simultaneously, leading to numerous costly confirmatory procedures. Examples of type-D diseases are prostate cancer, acute myocardial infarction and leukemia (Paushter and McNeil 1990). Another strategy to deal with uncertainty is dependent upon the characteristics of the available therapies (Kassirer 1989). When a therapy is high in effectiveness but low in risk, considerable diagnostic uncertainty can be tolerated, and, as a result, testing can be minimized. A sore throat or pharyngitis illustrates this approach. The inflammation may be bacteriological or viral in origin. However, the underlying cause is often irrelevant. The regimen of choice—antibiotics—will clear up the more dangerous pathogens (streptococcus) if they are present and, at the same time, cause little harm if they are not. In contrast, therapies that are low in effectiveness and high in risk require reducing uncertainty to a minimum through aggressive diagnostic testing (and procedures). This situation is illustrated by the classic ischemic heart attack. Many questions must be answered and the answers integrated before a choice can be made between carotid arteriography or managing the patient medically. How likely is the arteriogram to produce serious complications? What is the probability of finding a surgically treatable lesion? If a treatable lesion is found, what are the risks of the operation? What is the patient's attitude toward the immediate risk of death or disability posed by arteriography or operation? What is the prognosis if the patient is treated medically? What are the risks of anticoagulant therapy?

SPECIFICITY AND FETAL MONITORING

The importance of the specificity or false-positive issue has been raised recently in the context of fetal monitoring and renovascular disease screening among hypertensives. The direct annual costs of electronic fetal monitoring in 1990 were $240 million, but the indirect costs to both mother and child could exceed $800 million annually. The benefits of fetal monitoring are to be found in the degree to which early detection of fetal distress prevents mental retardation or death. The poor specificity of this diagnostic tool gives rise to many false-positive indications of fetal distress and contributed to 100,000 additional unnecessary cesarean sections in 1990 (costing $660 million). Future controlled clinical trials are necessary to determine whether there is a "best" mode of monitoring among the five (internal electronic monitoring, external electronic monitoring, diagnostic amniocentesis, scalp sampling, and ultrasonography). Banta and Thacker (1979) pointed to the need to acknowledge increased risk to the mother associated with pelvic infections or death from unnecessary operations. In addition, estimated costs of $160 million are associated with the risk of infant hemorrhaging, respiratory distress, and infection at the site of the electrode.

The popularity of cesarean deliveries increased dramatically from 6 percent in 1972 to 25 percent of all births in 1990. According to many experts in the field, cesarean deliveries (C-sections) and electronic fetal monitoring are being overutilized. Leveno et al. (1986) studied 35,000 deliveries in Dallas and found that continuous electronic monitoring of the fetal heart rate led to a significant increase in C-sections, but with no improvement in health to the babies. C-sections obviously do harm to the health status of the mother, with more trauma and more resulting days off work. Regt et al. (1986) reported in a study of 65,600 deliveries at four Brooklyn hospitals that private physicians performed significantly more C-sections than doctors treating clinic patients, without improving the outcome for most babies. Demographic factors that have been related to higher rates of C-sections, such as percentage of teenagers, medically complicated pregnancies, and low birth weight, were all controlled for in these studies. Nonetheless, private patients had substantially higher C-section rates than clinic patients.

Payment incentives obviously feed the inflation in C-section rates and fetal monitoring utilization. Patient charges for C-sections are typically 90 to 120 percent higher than for a normal vaginal delivery. One might suggest that if providers were paid the same rate regardless of whether the delivery required a C-section or not, the C-section rate would decline substantially. However, the payment rate would have to be higher for hospitals treating more teenagers and poor patients, so as not to discriminate unfairly against hospitals with a high rate of necessary C-sections. Employers are already beginning to institute more stringent claims review and quality audits. Some employers and insurance plans in Maryland and California are beginning to deny payment for C-sections deemed unnecessary.

Stafford (1990) outlined a long list of ideas to curtail the rate of cesarean sections, including lowering the payment rate, physician education, public education, and medical malpractice reform. The productivity focus outlined in Eastaugh (1992) can assist in the curtailment of excess utilization. Preferred practice patterns also exist in the productivity arena. In a number of hospitals, better staffing of the obstetrics service, with the help of provider education efforts, can cut the C-section rate in half. If the obstetrics service is more effectively staffed with nurse extenders, the doctor has more time to shepherd a mother through a difficult delivery. But if the service is inefficiently staffed (too few expensive people, not enough nurse extenders) it is more profitable and clinically easier to cut the process short by going straight to the cesarean incision into the abdominal wall. In emergency situations the cesarean section must be performed, but too many physicians do mandatory C-sections to any mother that has previously had a C-section. New surgical techniques since 1972 have left the mother's abdominal muscle stronger and have reduced the need for repeat C-sections. If the obstetrics team really considers the patient as most important, it will optimize the rate of vaginal births to reduce morbidity, mortality, and expense. The rate of repeat C-sections may be too high at 80 percent in HMOs and 70 percent in teaching hospitals, but the repeat rate is much too high in nonteaching community hospitals (92 percent; Stafford 1990). However, habit and other factors, such as doing the C-section at the first sign of fetal distress, may keep the C-section rate high (Goyert et al. 1989).

A potential explanation for why fetal monitoring became so popular in a matter of months might center around what Foltz and Kelsey (1978) called "the nation's ideology to support the maximum utilization of new technologies." Two clinical trials by Haverkamp et al. (1979, 1976) of the effectiveness of electronic fetal monitoring versus basic nurse monitoring found no significant differences. Our medical technology is all too quick to accept new diagnostic techniques that have been founded on faulty evaluations or have poor specificity in the average hospital. Two examples are the CEA (carcinoembryonic antigen) test for colonic cancer and the NBT (nitro-blue tetrazolium) test in the diagnosis of bacterial infection. Both tests were promoted to medical students in 1973, then found to be substantially less effective by 1975–76 (Ransohoff and Feinstein 1978).

Another case of the importance of considering the costs associated with poor test specificity was provided by McNeil and Adelstein (1975). The effect of high sensitivity but poor specificity in the primary screening modality for detecting renovascular disease among hypertensives ($83 intravenous pyelogram plus $100 renography) can be improved by subsequent arteriography at a cost of $375 (1975 prices). This subsequent angiogram increases the specificity to a perfect 100 percent, but the new information is hardly worthwhile since case finding is not associated with improved survival figures, and surgical treatment following the angiogram was found to be no more efficacious than medical treatment prior to testing (McNeil 1977). However, improved specificity and case finding through pulmonary angiography ($300) and perfusion lung scanning ($125) have been demonstrated to be worth the 40 percent increased costs for diagnosis of pulmonary embolism in young patients. More clinical guidelines for cost-effectiveness must be developed (Field and Lohr 1991).

MARGINAL COSTS AND BENEFITS OF ADDITIONAL TESTING

Having addressed the reliability and specificity issues in cost-effectiveness analysis, we turn to the issue of marginal costs. Neuhauser and Lewicki (1975) performed a marginal cost analysis on the value of doing a fifth or sixth sequential stool guaiac, in reaction to the recommendation by Gregor (1969) and the American Cancer Society (Leffall 1974) that six guaiacs be done on all persons over 40 years of age to detect asymptomatic colon cancer. Even with a diagnostic test of high sensitivity (92.67 percent), the marginal cost of the sixth test ($47.1 million per cancer case detected) was 20,000 times the average cost per case discovered. Although six sequential stool guaiacs, followed by barium enemas for all positive guaiacs, will identify virtually all "silent" colon cancers, is it worth $47.1 million to detect that one rare case when the resources could be used elsewhere? Physicians are too oriented toward citing simple average costs ($4 for the first stool guaiac and $1 for each subsequent guaiac) to recognize the devastating implications that the recommendation of up to six guaiacs could have on medical costs. For example, physicians would neglect the 41 percent of total diagnostic costs devoted to diagnosing incorrectly (false-positive) colon cancer and then ruling out presence of the disease with a $100 barium enema. Maximization of specificity (the minimization of false positives) has the added benefit of reducing needless patient anxiety, in addition to the tangible benefits of reducing unnecessary care, iatrogenic morbidity, and mortality.

Subsequent analysis with more recent data on specificity and sensitivity suggested that Neuhauser and Lewicki (1975) overestimated the $47.1 million marginal cost of finding one colon cancer case on the sixth stool guaiac. The actual marginal current cost may be much lower (Brown and Burrows 1990), and the effective marginal cost question will be answered with the publication in 1992 of the Arthur Walker study in Newcastle, England. However, the generic point raised by Neuhauser and Lewicki is still correct in the 1990s context. Professional groups tend to overorder frequent repeat tests (Bengtson 1990). To paraphrase the work of Duke University health economist David Eddy, when the American Cancer Society suggests annual mammograms for young women, it neglects to consider (1) intangible costs of the high false-positive rates (harming the psyche of thousands of healthy women) and (2) the direct costs of $1.3 billion in additional expense to find 280 additional early cancer cases per year. These costs could be avoided if young women received mammograms every three years (not annually).

Policy makers have a need for more accurate data on costs of specific conditions over the life cycle of individuals including cancer (Scheffler and Andrews 1989) and other conditions (Leader and Moon 1989; Anderson, Steinberg, and Whittle 1990; Kahn 1990). For example, Roos, Wennberg, and Malenka (1989) evaluated the long-run life-cycle effectiveness of individuals having a transurethral resection of the prostate (TURP) with those having an open prostatectomy. The authors showed a higher rate of second prostatectomy surgery after the initial

TURP than after the alternative operation in all three countries studied. TURPs are therefore less effective in overcoming urinary obstruction than the open operation. Wennberg (1989) outlined the need for more of these types of longitudinal population-based studies. (We surveyed examples of Wennberg's small-area-variation [SAV] studies in chapter 3.)

Longitudinal life-cycle analysis sometimes demonstrates that the highly criticized surgical option is not inferior to medical treatment. Califf (1989) outlined three factors associated with improved relative effectiveness of coronary artery bypass surgery from 1973 to 1989: a worsening prognosis with medical therapy, more severe coronary disease, and quicker operative scheduling. However, Gersh (1989) indicated that in patients at low risk, medical therapy is still the more cost-effective alternative. In patients at high risk, based on clinical anatomic and functional characteristics, the bypass surgery prolongs survival when compared with medical therapy alone. We shall survey the trade-offs of sensitivity and specificity in making a diagnosis in the next section.

BALANCING SENSITIVITY AND SPECIFICITY

Goldman (1988) offered a decision model for predicting myocardial infarction (MI) in emergency departments. If the ECG test is normal, a more detailed evaluation of pain may be called for (the ECG Electrocardiographic Monitoring for MI has a true-positive rate of 0.58 and a false-positive rate of 0.05). Alternatively, if the ECG is abnormal, the decision-making treatment can progress without further workup and history. The clinician is selecting a test that has the greatest likelihood of increasing or decreasing the probability that the patient has a specific problem. To rule in a disease, a test with a high positive likelihood ratio (the ratio of the true-positive rate to the false-positive rate, which is 11.6 for the ECG) is most efficient (Sklar 1989). By the same logic, consider a second example. A child with stridor who is not coughing and is drooling has a very high likelihood of epiglotitis (Mauro, Poole, and Lockhart 1988). The positive likelihood ratio for a diagnosis of epiglotitis in a child with drooling and no coughing is a whopping 74 (true-positive rate of 0.67/false-positive rate of 0.009). When the positive likelihood ratio is so high (over 10), confidence in ruling in a disease or condition is high even if the prevalence of epiglotitis is very low in the emergency-department population.

What if the test result had been negative in the first example? The negative likelihood ratio (1 minus sensitivity/specificity) is much more dependent on sensitivity. The ECG for myocardial infarction has a negative likelihood ratio of 0.44, which means that a negative ECG result for MI does not really lower the odds very much. As Goldsch and Sox (1988) indicated, if the odds of a MI are 0.10 before the ECG test, the odds will be 0.044 after a negative test. This may not be enough of a reduction in odds in the mind of the attending physician to eliminate the need for additional expensive tests for cardiac enzymes. Other examples of tests with a low negative likelihood ratio include the physical exam for epiglotitis (0.33) and the anemia physical exam for pallor (0.61 negative likelihood ratio).

Parkan and Holland (1990) made a preliminary attempt to describe a linear programming approach to finding optimal clinical strategies when event probabilities are not known, but their value ranges are available. Linear programming (Schrage 1991) offers a simple approach to balancing trade-offs between sensitivity and specificity. Wharton School professor Hershey (1991) offered the easier and more powerful parametric programming approach, which yields optimal values in the same units as the original utility scale. Medicine deals with uncertain probabilities, and if the number of states whose probabilities are uncertain increases, one can use Hershey's method to do pairwise analysis, varying two states simultaneously until all states are included. Strategies that never reach optimality for any such pair can safely be rejected until optimal solutions are found.

The puzzle of finding an optimal strategy varies with confidence limits, degrees of uncertainty, and anatomic complexity. The statistics for sensitivity and specificity can get complex when three to eight potential anatomic sites of disease are involved in a CAT scan. Global sensitivity (all nodal sites collectively) varies with the anatomic distribution of the disease in the reference population.

One final problem in assessing new tests or techniques concerns the issue of substitutability. New diagnostic procedures can seldom be judged 100 percent accurate, perfect substitutes for the old methods. For example, CAT scanning may be considered by physicians to be cost-effective simply because it replaces other costly, painful, and invasive diagnostic procedures. However, CAT scans did not have sufficient substitutability to more than compensate for the cost add-on of new volume (Eastaugh 1981). A second technology, magnetic resonance imaging (MRI), was sold by Evans (1984) and others as a substitute for CAT. Even without a DRG payment rate for MRI, the machine grew in popularity and seldom reduced neighboring CAT volume by more than 25 percent per capita. Therefore, imaging technologies increased to more than 3.5 percent of the health budget in 1991. A third diagnostic tool has now been initiated in over 70 hospitals, positron emission tomography (PET). PET scanners have established scientific value, but the undocumented clinical value must undergo a rigorous cost-benefit analysis. A randomized trial in the 70 medical centers may establish the diagnostic value of PET scanners in the treatment of patients (Reiman and Mintun 1990). Reliance on rate regulation will never answer the question of whether the nation needs 4, 40, or 140 PET scanners. All three imaging technologies have reduced the need for exploratory surgery, but they are also overused. Inappropriate utilization will be a future topic in this chapter. Fewer physicians make claims that the new technology will replace the old, and we can be thankful that anti-cost-effectiveness (ACE) physicians with the attitude that more tests always mean more information and therefore a better diagnosis (Knoebel 1988) seem to publish less frequently.

THE TUNNEL OF TECHNOLOGY AND COSTLY MARGINAL INFORMATION GAINS

We live in an information age. Doctors are not unlike other professionals in wanting the most marginal information gain (MIG) as an agent for their clients. Unfortunately, benefits are often mainly to the physician's curiosity ("an interesting question answered" or "rare zebra case found and ready for publication") rather than to the health care benefit of the patient. Attending physicians also receive a financial benefit from overtreating or overtesting their patients. One study described a treatment style that runs independent of patient needs. Rifkin, Zerhouni, and Gatsonis (1990), after reporting a disappointingly low predictive value of MRI scanning for nodal involvement in cancer staging, suggested that this diagnostic strategy may be questionable if the marginal information gain to the physician is outweighed by the more specific information (but discomfort to the patient) to be gained by surgical biopsy. If providers did not operate clinics and hospitals like tunnels of technology, maximizing costs, we would have less need for cost-benefit and cost-effectiveness analyses in health care.

Despite the tighter reimbursement climate in the 1980s, more and more community hospitals purchased expensive medical technologies. The percentage of community hospitals having MRI increased from 3.1 percent in 1984 to 17.7 percent in 1991. The percentage of community hospitals having organ transplantation nearly tripled, from 4.4 percent in 1984 to 11.2 percent in 1991. The percentage of community hospitals having CT scanners increased from 47.9 percent in 1984 to 68.9 percent in 1991. The percentage of community hospitals having Extra-corporeal Shock Wave Lithotripsy (ESWL) went from zero in 1984 to 7.6 percent in 1991. The percentage of community hospitals having open-heart surgery increased from 11.8 percent in 1984 to 15.9 percent in 1991.

RISING IMPORTANCE OF BIG-TICKET TECHNOLOGIES

Scitovsky (1985) examined the effects of changing medical technologies on medical costs by comparing treatment patterns for a number of common illnesses at four points in time (1954, 1964, 1971, and 1981). While the results from 1954 to 1971 indicated that little-ticket items like lab tests and X-rays were driving up the cost of care, the big-ticket new and expensive technologies appeared to be the major inflationary factor. New modes of treatment and big-ticket technologies significantly increased the cost of myocardial infarction and breast cancer cases. For example, in 1981 dollars, treatment involving streptokinase infusion cost $19,206 per case, compared to $47,564 for bypass surgery and $10,094 for "conventional care." The increased reliance on an existing big-ticket technology, delivery by cesarean section, significantly increased the average cost of maternity care. Hospital costs of a delivery by cesarean section were 2.4 times higher than the costs of a vaginal delivery, and nonhospital costs were 52 percent higher.

Scitovsky's results are consistent with other findings. Showstack, Stone, and Schroeder (1985) studied 10 diagnoses at one San Francisco teaching hospital for the years 1972, 1977, and 1982. They concluded that little-ticket laboratory tests did not contribute substantially to rising costs, and new imaging techniques were commonly substituted for traditional invasive procedures. The authors concluded that the primary driving force behind rising hospital costs were intensive treatments for the critically ill, provision of surgery to patients admitted with acute myocardial infarction, delivery, and newborn respiratory distress syndrome. Among the 10 diagnoses studied, only for acute myocardial infarction patients did the use of imaging procedures increase substantially (2 percent cardiac catheterization in 1977 and 40 percent in 1982).

Little-ticket items still contribute to the rising cost of medical care. For example, the annual change in the number of lab tests per case increased 7.1 percent for mastectomy cases, 4.4 percent for conventional-care myocardial infarction cases, and over 3.0 percent per year for appendicitis and vaginal delivery. Test usage per patient increased more than 3.0 percent per year for a number of nonhospitalized patients: duodenal ulcer, pneumonia, and complete (adult) physical exam (Scitovsky 1985). Attempts to trim little-ticket items also occur in radiology and the emergency room. For example, Clinton (1986) argued that application of more rigorous specific clinical indications will lead to continued major declines in the number of unnecessary chest radiographs performed.

PHYSICIAN INVOLVEMENT OR INCREASED FEDERAL INTERVENTION?

The existence of growing federal regulation in the health field is a by-product of the observation that the imperfect private sector has been of little help in selecting the programs and services that are to be available as a reimbursable expense in the clinical armada. Consequently, as a matter of public policy, the congressional Office of Technology Assessment (U.S. Congress OTA 1978) suggested a sequence for evaluating medical technology: Consider efficacy, cost-effectiveness, cost-benefit, and then safety. Efficacy is concerned with measuring the benefit of a technology under ideal conditions of use—for example, at the Mayo Clinic and Johns Hopkins Hospital. Cost-effectiveness is a measure of the relative benefits and costs to society of various technologies applied to the same problem area under average conditions of use. Consequently, a technology can have efficacy in the best hospitals but be cost-ineffective for general use. Cost-effectiveness is measured by the ratio of costs to tangible benefits, expressed as cost per person-year saved or cost per quality-adjusted person-year saved or cost per disability-year prevented.

The estimation of direct benefits is usually a simple process of measuring what costs are forgone as a result of the consumption of the service under evaluation. One frequently mentioned caveat to the problem of benefit estimation is double counting, or overestimating the benefit of eliminating one disease if there is a simultaneous presence of multiple diseases. Weisbrod (1961) was one of the first to recognize that patients who avoid one cause of death (cancer) may have a higher susceptibility to another competing cause of death (heart disease). The bias in the benefit-estimation process is to overstate the benefits projected from reducing the prevalence or incidence of any single disease category—that is, the whole is smaller than the sum of the individual parts. The estimation of intangible benefits is also a major problem in most studies. One of the most overlooked intangible benefits is the patient reassurance factor. However, if the false-positive rate is too high, the intangible negative benefit of unnecessary patient distress could outweigh the net amount of patient assurance.

Physician involvement in the process of doing cost-benefit or cost-effectiveness research is crucial (Agency for Health Care Policy and Research [AHCPR] 1990). Construction of a decision tree is the first step in most cost-effectiveness analyses designed to assist in the selection of alternative approaches to patient care. It allows the practitioner to incorporate the predictive values obtained from appropriate therapeutic procedures into a wider framework. This analysis is not purely mechanical and requires input from a group of experienced clinicians. The twin problems of ''dirty'' data and unreasonable assumptions could be eliminated if heavy-handed regulators allowed clinicians to have more input in the design phase, funded better epidemiological studies, and sponsored more randomized controlled clinical trials.

EDUCATION PROGRAMS FOR PHYSICIANS

Physician education programs have as their goal apprising doctors of the appropriate use of tests, procedures, and treatment options. Educational efforts come in a number of formats, offered in combination, including didactic lectures, order-form restructuring, cost feedback, concurrent or retrospective protocol review, and other retrospective medical-record audits. The didactic course approach typically makes four basic points: (1) Do what must be done in a cost-effective way (e.g., home health care or ambulatory surgery), (2) perform a cost-benefit assessment of the case management alternatives, (3) avoid the unnecessary/outmoded/duplicative procedures, and (4) encourage preventive and health promotion activities. On this last point, Bartlett (1985) reported that health promotion can do more than reduce future illness; it can also reduce duration of stay, patient anxiety, and complications. Didactic examples work best if they are targeted to areas of interest for future practice. Historically, the problem with most didactic educational programs is that by themselves they tend to produce only short-run changes in behavior.

Restructuring the excessively convenient patient order forms was one of the first nondidactic approaches to be utilized successfully. For example, Wong et al. (1983) found didactic programs to be ineffective in reducing test usage unless the order form was redesigned to alter the test selection process. If the physician has to take an action beyond simply checking the entire row of boxes, fewer medically unnecessary tests are performed. Eisenberg and Williams (1983) decreased lab overuse by no longer allowing standing orders (i.e., a test would be done multiple times per day until discharge, whether the test was medically necessary or not). Under their program, all test orders only become good for the day they are written.

The medical staff of Boston City Hospital reduced the volume of common labor-intensive lab tests 28 to 45 percent by requiring doctors to enter their reason for ordering each specific test on the test request form. This suggests that clinicians have the cognitive knowledge to select tests more efficiently but need a continuing reminder of the importance of cost-effective selection. Moreover, placing responsibility for parsimony on the physicians prevents resentment over perceived limits on physicians' exercise of clinical judgment. Detsky et al. (1986) confirmed this second point by showing that there is no intrinsic reason why teaching hospitals need to order more tests per case—that is, there is no pure teaching effect.

A second nondidactic educational approach involves simply attaching a copy of the patient's cumulative bill to the last progress note (McPhee 1984). Berwick and Coltin (1986) tested the effectiveness of cost feedback versus two other forms of feedback (didactic teacher feedback and yield feedback flags on abnormal test results). Studying internists' usage of 12 common blood tests and roentgenograms over four months, the authors concluded that test usage declined across the board 14.2 percent. Other studies have reported comparable success from pharmacy feedback, with the review process reducing ineffective, irrational, or excessively costly drug-prescribing habits. Expert systems such as computerized algorithms to monitor drug usage patterns can save money and reduce morbidity. Pestotnik's (1990) expert system for spotting inconsistencies changed or started therapy in 125 of the 420 identified alerts.

There are few clinical trials documenting the long-run effectiveness of feedback techniques. Chassin and McCue (1986) reported results from one educational quality-assurance program assigned randomly across 120 study and control-group hospitals. Education concerning acceptable indications for X-ray pelvimetry reduced usage by 33 percent more in the study hospitals. Some of the more innovative chiefs of medical staff have initiated protocol development as a third alternative approach to cost-containment education. Within their institutions, protocol development has not always been a smooth developmental process. Protocols could be used for case management by hospital administrators, or even by the federal government. The primary challenge for the chiefs of staff is to keep their fellow physicians happy or, if not happy, at least not too unhappy. Wachtel et al. (1986) designed protocols at Brown University's largest teaching hospital for four medical conditions (chest pain, stroke, pneumonia, and upper gastrointestinal hemorrhage). The protocols were implemented on 64 experimental patients who were compared to 64 control-group (nonprotocol) patients. The protocols resulted in a 15 percent reduction in total charges per case (and reductions as high as 35 percent for EKGs and 20 percent for lab tests). The benefit of altering clinician behavior by using protocol standards developed by the medical staff could be substantial. However, other analysts have suggested that the medical staff should simply develop a brief manual with test characteristics or EKG information. For example, Marton, Tul, and Sox (1985) studied test usage among three intervention groups (detailed manual, manual plus feedback, and feedback) and found the most significant declines in utilization among the mixed-strategy intervention (manual plus feedback).

One should not come away from this brief survey of protocols with the opinion that few conditions have been studied (Mohr et al. 1986). Decision analysts and clinicians have developed protocols for over 1,860 conditions; over 1,000 were developed in Pittsburgh alone. While protocol development clearly works best if it is done by those who will use the protocols, there are conceptual problems with protocols. The failure of researchers to incorporate all aspects of a clinical problem into the protocol is analogous to the attempts of a blind man to ascertain the nature of an elephant by inspecting its trunk alone (Kassirer 1986). Some protocols may cover 80 to 99 percent of their specific elephants, but the risks and benefits of all possible outcomes must be assessed. The challenge for those who promulgate protocols is to encompass the whole problem and avoid both the wild-goose chase and the sometimes inappropriately "cheap" strategy of watch and wait. Three Institute of Medicine studies (1990, 1989, 1985) endorsed greater reliance on explicit review criteria, and the AMA has its own directory of practice parameters (Kelly and Swartwout 1991).

HOSPITAL PRACTICE PRIVILEGES

Fewer than 1,000 physicians had their licenses suspended or revoked for inappropriate or unnecessary practice behavior in 1990. The federal professional review organizations (PROs) took sanction actions against fewer than 200 physicians during 1990–91. However, as hospitals win court cases related to staff-privilege decisions based on quality or efficiency concerns, hospital managers and medical staff are getting more selective about which physicians they allow admitting privileges. Self-serving members of the medical staff may want to close the doors on their hospital's medical staff in a crowded marketplace and force the institution to cease taking new applications from potential competitors. In negotiating compensation agreements with hospital-based physicians, management clearly likes the leverage to negotiate from a large pool of potential replacement clinicians. All types of physicians have potential anticompetitive reasons for closing their segment of the medical staff (raising antitrust legal concerns); but hospital managers and trustees are more interested in the composition of their medical staff and their cost behavior relative to levels of payment.

Institutions may no longer allow physicians who erode the financial standing of the institution through imprudent, wasteful use of hospital resources to admit patients. Hospitals that allow inefficient doctors to admit patients may go so heavily into debt that their survival is unlikely. In 1990–91 almost one-third of

Figure 12.3
Two Dimensions of Utilization Review before and after the Initiation of
Prospective Payment

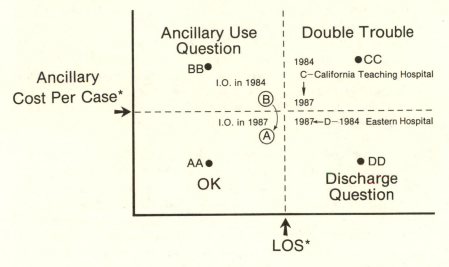

*Corrected for Case-mix differences between institutions. A third dimension of utilization review would monitor physician billings.

all hospital clinical departments were closed to new medical staff appointments; most of these were internally reviewing whether certain clinicians should not have their privileges renewed (legally it is easier not to renew privileges than actually to revoke privileges). The percentage of physicians with admitting privileges at any hospital has been declining each year since 1982, according to AMA survey statistics. Almost half of the physicians only have privileges at one hospital. Any physicians losing their practice privileges at one hospital will have a tough time establishing a relationship with other local hospitals. Inefficient ordering and treatment habits are a liability for the individual doctor in a market in which fees increasingly are paid prospectively (i.e., inefficiency is not reimbursed by a pass-through of costs for the hospital) and in which hospital privileges are in short supply. The practice-profile cost per case experience of a doctor should be appropriately adjusted for DRG mix and case severity to make any data-based credentialling process fair (i.e., for medical-staff membership). Physicians can be analyzed on whether they are inefficient on two basic dimensions: length of stay and ancillary cost per case (figure 12.3). (The third dimension, appropriate admissions, discussed by Wennberg 1989; Siu, Manning, and Benjamin 1990, suggested that 24 percent of admissions are inappropriate.)

If the individual physician is "double trouble" on both dimensions, the total cost per case (adjusted for case mix) will be high. Many midwestern hospitals have been particularly effective at trimming lengths of stay relative to the national average since 1983. By point of contrast, West Coast hospitals historically tend to be very efficient on length of stay. However, West Coast investor-owned hospitals have tended to generate particularly high ancillary costs per case. Such behavior was rewarded in an era of cost reimbursement or full-charge payment, when the profit margins were highest in the area of ancillary tests. The hospital CFOs' best physicians were the ones who ordered the most ancillary tests per case (earning the hospital more money). However, now the medical staffs have had to unlearn all the lessons of the 1969–83 ''maximization of reimbursement'' period (outlined in chapters 1 and 2) and become more efficient (move from point B to point A in figure 12.3). The medical staff is sometimes provided a break-even-point analysis by product line to serve as a yardstick for target areas to trim cost behavior.

The concept of strategic product-line groupings (SPGs) is used in many hospitals (Eastaugh 1992). The intent of table 12.1 is to provide the medical staff with sensitivity estimates as to how much one has to trim in the other three areas if, for example, the clinicians running SPG 7 decide that they cannot improve length of stay (options 8 or 9) or adjust behavior in radiology (options 1–3 and 5). Such estimates are highly dependent on the blend of variable and fixed costs for the specific hospital under study. Therefore, the analysis must be done at each hospital every one to three months. In studying two of the hospitals sampled in chapter 1, Tables 1.4–1.7, McNeil (1985, 18) indicated that there was

enormous variability in the fixed-variable cost ratios of tests done in chemistry labs, ranging from under 20 percent variable cost for some to over 90 percent for others. Information on the distribution of tests in the ''highly fixed'' cost category compared to those in the ''highly variable'' cost category should be useful in the design of educational programs for cost containment.

The challenge for physicians and managers is not to break even on every product line. There will always be some cross-subsidization in the hospital sector. The real challenge is to have all parties work toward common goals: quality care, institutional financial health, and enough retained earnings to keep the hospital/ doctor workshop state-of-the-art. One must balance this last goal against the broader social goal of not having too much wasteful excess capacity or excess patient admissions (chapter 3).

PREFERRED PRACTICE PATTERNS

Checklist protocols and decision rules are but one approach for the medical staff to define preferred styles of behavior. McNeil (1985) reported on the preferred practice pattern (PPP) study of Massachusetts General Hospital, Brigham Hospital, and New England Medical Center. The study team identified nine diseases or procedures, ranging from carotid endarterectomies to gastrointestinal bleeding. The physicians were of the opinion that quality was equally good

Table 12.1

Cost-Behavior Profile for Strategic Product-line Grouping 7 (SPG 7 Consists of 16 DRGs Produced by 13 Attending Physicians)

Option	LOS[a] Length of Stay	InhalationTherapy,[b] IVs, and Misc. Therapy[c]	Lab[c]	Radiology
1	-15%	0	0	0
2	-10%	-27%	0	0
3	-10%	-10%	-23%	0
4	-10%[d]	-10%	-10%	-18%
5	-5%	-20%	-24%	0
6	-5%	-20%	-10%	-19%
7	-5%	-16.8%	-16.8%	-16.8%
8	0	-27%	-22%	-39.7%
9	0	-29.8%	-29.8%	-29.8%

[a]The semivariable and variable cost savings from reduction in LOS are distributed as follows: 45.0 percent in forgone "hotel" costs, 27.1 percent in forgone nursing services, 13.3 percent in forgone therapy (inhalation therapy, IVs, medications, recovery room, OR, anesthesia, etc.), 8.5 percent in forgone lab tests, and 6.1 percent in forgone radiologic services.

[b]For this hospital and this strategic product-line grouping 7, the example is only atypical to the extent that overutilization of inhalation therapy was a major problem identified in peer review audits. Requiring a 27 percent aggregate reduction in inhalation therapy could be easily accomplished by a 75 percent reduction in usage by 4 of the 13 doctors offering this SPG, with no change in behavior required of the other 9 doctors (who were already utilizing 24 to 32 percent less inhalation therapy than the group average).

[c]Utilization per diem.

[d]The cost savings from a 5 percent drop in LOS equal a 27 percent drop in therapy per diem (for the reduced number of per diems remaining after the LOS reduction), which is equivalent to a 43 percent drop in lab tests per diem and a 59 percent drop in radiology usage per diem.

across all three hospitals, in which case the research question became measuring the efficiency of utilization (a concept originally pioneered by Neuhauser in the 1960s) across the three hospitals. By looking across all cost items, the study group identified a lowest-cost, high-quality PPP based on the approach that it is best to have the "least resource usage for the same quality output." Detailed chart reviews were undertaken to assess the comparability of the patients, adjust for case severity, and ascertain the vagaries and errors in the discharge coding.

Many hospitals have eschewed equally careful concern for discharge abstract data or patient severity and have developed crude profit-and-loss statements by DRG, groups of DRGs, and physician. The idea of profit-and-loss statements is only as good as the data (clinical and cost accounting). Good data can yield good PPP analysis. Needless to say, the phrase "preferred practice pattern" is more popular among clinicians than the more inflexible label "standard proto-col." However, without valid cost-accounting information and a severity mea-sure, the analysis will be less than useful for many hospitals. Horn, Horn, and Moses (1986) reported that 37 percent of the physicians at one medical center would have errors, up or down, of more than $10,000 in the apparent impact of the clinician on the hospital's profit and loss, depending on whether one incorporated the severity measure into the analysis. An amazing 14 percent of physicians would be labeled under- or overutilizers of hospital resources relative to a $30,000 threshold of accuracy. For example, doctors with a terrible profit-and-loss profile could actually be efficient, but all the most severe cases within a given DRG might be channeled their way in the referral process. These results may pertain to a typical medical center, but the need to adjust individual per-formance for patient severity may not exist at most nonteaching hospitals.

Many clinical outliers will discuss details of their PPP and their individual performance relative to the PPP standard with the various utilization review committees. Judgments of individual practice habits will always involve some degree of uncertainty. For example, if doctor X appears to prophylactically order inhalation therapy in varying amounts, the exact amount of unnecessary and controllable inhalation therapy may be difficult to determine from the medical record. Deliberate deviations from the PPP standard of care should be docu-mented in the medical record such that the objective observer could follow the reasoning behind certain clinical decisions. The medical staff can make appro-priate documentation of records a precondition for membership and determine whether a given individual offers a pattern of deception to defend his or her inefficient performance relative to the PPP yardstick.

In 1991 a few hospitals began to make medical-staff membership decisions on the basis of cost profiles and forecast sales quotas as to how much volume the individual would "harvest." If the sales-quota concept seems a bit aggressive, more radical approaches may come in the future. At the extreme, some hospitals may one day require that independent contractors (called physicians) pay the hospital a security deposit or rent in order to admit patients (e.g., the way some car mechanics pay their garage). If the physician is cost-effective from the hospital's viewpoint, the deposit or rent is returned to the physician. However, if the "body mechanic" wastes resources of the firm (the garage or hospital) that he or she controls but does not own, then the professional (mechanic or doctor) must make good on any cost overrun. Unlike the imperfect garage analogy, one would want to take account for case severity and outliers (e.g., not penalizing the doctor for serving AIDS patients). However, if the physician harms the hospital's financial health on a regular basis, after repeated attempts at behavior modification, all or part of the rent or security deposit would be retained by the hospital. (This idea was originally suggested to the author by a garage mechanic and a Nobel Prize winner in economics, which may or may not offer proof that great minds think alike when it comes to professional fees.) The current payment system is clearly unfair for hospitals in that business risk is borne by the hospital, yet it is the physician's behavior that dictates the amount of risk.

TEACHING MEDICAL STUDENTS

The purpose of this section is to outline one approach to teaching cost-effective clinical decision making and to measure the degree of attitudinal change produced by a brief course in this area. The elective course was offered to third-year medical students at Cornell Medical College. As medicine has grown more technological, the decision process has also become more statistically complex. Unfortunately, the recent medical school graduate's statistical knowledge has not kept pace with the growth in medical science. In one early study at four Harvard teaching hospitals, only 20 percent of fourth-year medical students, 15 percent of internal-medicine residents, and 20 percent of attending physicians correctly responded to a question that required the application of elementary statistical analysis to diagnostic test results (Cassells et al., 1978).

A potential benefit of injecting economic content into the medical school curriculum is that the new clinicians might informally utilize cost-effective clinical decision-making principles to provide equivalent quality of care at less cost. The Association of American Medical Colleges, the American Hospital Association, and the American Medical Association House of Delegates have all endorsed cost education for physicians during the undergraduate and postgraduate educational process.

Socioeconomic courses often take a back seat to the "hard sciences." One would hope that the progressive social and economic course content of residency and medical school programs will not fall to the budget ax. If we are to make intelligent decisions on how to improve the quality of care and contain the cost of services, it is our responsibility to discover the most effective means of training physicians to make economical decisions. The hope is that formal training in decision analysis and economics can yield more rational decisions and perhaps better patient outcomes, or at least more informed choice if economy happens to conflict with the pursuit of the "highest possible" quality of care. The norm for the 1990s may have to be the provision of the best possible patient outcomes within the constraint of a given amount of available resources—for example, 12 percent of gross national product for health care. With the aging of the population, however, this 12 percent may be difficult to achieve.

If some of the principles of cost-effective clinical decision making would permeate into the subconscious cognitive processes of American physicians, a less costly style of medical care might result. Continuing-education programs may affect practicing physicians' behavior, but it might be more cost-beneficial to bring formal discussion of these issues to medical students and help them reflect on their future role as clinicians. Most of the previous effort in this area has concentrated on house staff (AMA 1988). The approaches include identifying those individuals with out-of-line utilization profiles, testing residents with a price list of hospital charges, and asking the young clinician if the marginal information gain (MIG) of the test justified the cost (Eastaugh 1981).

The next section reviews the results of the precourse and postcourse attitude survey of the students. The course had three major themes (Eastaugh 1981). The first basic theme was that physicians must understand the role of cost-benefit analysis in "big-ticket" resource priority decisions and other policy determinations. The second course theme was that physicians should increasingly utilize and participate in cost-effectiveness evaluations to constrain the proliferation of "little-ticket" expenses for tests and procedures. Third, clinicians should be interested in preserving professional autonomy by cooperating with the health policy decision makers rather than being co-opted by the growth in federal intervention. If further regulation is to be avoided and the dual goals of cost containment and improved patient care achieved, health practitioners must be taught to utilize diagnostic tests more appropriately and treatment modes more effectively.

STUDENT ATTITUDE SURVEY

There is inevitably an imperfect link between attitudes and behavior. Nevertheless, attitude shifts are taken as a proxy estimate of program effectiveness because researchers seldom have the option to wait five years and do a prospective field survey to measure shifts in postgraduate clinical behavior. The self-report attitudinal instrument utilized in this study did not rely on a single question to detect the depth or presence of an attitude. Instead, the four basic constructs (interest in reducing costs, concern with decision-science techniques, concern with economics and biostatistics, and advocating maximum consumer information) were measured by a number of questions. Providing four to seven ordinal attitudinal (agree strongly, agree mildly, disagree mildly, disagree strongly) items for each construct aids in minimizing the error that could result from student misinterpretation of single items.

The instrument was constructed so that the responses were anonymous, while allowing for the recognition of individuals before and after the course. The anonymity of the survey response was intended to minimize the potential bias that could occur if respondents were to hide their true attitudes and bend their answers to conform to the attitudes of the instructor. Of the 80 third-year Cornell Medical School students based in New York City during the month in which the cost-effective clinical decision-making course was offered, 56 filled out a precourse questionnaire. Of these 56, 29 elected to take the course and completed a postcourse questionnaire. The two basic research questions involved how the course affected the attitudes of the 29 course takers and how the 27 respondents who elected not to take the course differed from the 29 course participants.

A number of nonparametric statistical tests demonstrated the significant impact of the course on attitudes and the selection bias between course takers and nontakers. The Kolmogorov-Smirnov test (Siegel and Castellan 1989) demonstrated that the sample of course takers was more predisposed to cost-effective clinical decision-making ideas than those electing not to take the course for 6 of the 20 items. Course takers were significantly predisposed to being procon-sumerists (2 items significant at the 0.01 level), mindful of the need for medical cost containment (3 items significant at the 0.05 level), and conscious of the necessity for decision-analysis applications to medicine (1 item significant at the 0.05 level).

In the case of the 29 students who completed questionnaires before and after the course, the Wilcoxon matched-pairs test provided a measure of the significance of attitudinal change. Those completing the course had not significantly shifted their ideas on consumerism and the need for cost containment. However, there was a significant shift with respect to applications of decision analysis to medicine (2 items were significant at the 0.02 level, and 2 additional items at the 0.05 level). Completion of the course also positively affected their respect for health economics (1 item was significant at the 0.01 level, and 2 additional items were significant at the 0.05 level).

The students most in need of a course in this subject area appeared to be the least likely to take the course. Multivariate discriminant analysis provided an accurate prediction of participation (yes, no) in the course. Of the 56 respondents, 78.6 percent were correctly classified, and the two groups were statistically different (chi-squared $= 4.09$, $p < 0.05$, d.f. $= 1$). In order to investigate further the question concerning the dichotomous variable of course selection, a probit model was tested for the 20 agree/disagree items. One of the early applications of this maximum-likelihood technique in the health field was provided by Finney (1972). In our situation the model was statistically significant in explaining the course selection (chi-squared $= 51.78$, $p < 0.05$). The two items significant at the 0.01 level were "Patients should have convenient access to their medical record" and "Physicians should answer the patient in a quantitative probabilistic fashion if the patient asks for such specific information." The only other statement responses significant at the 0.05 level were "Appropriate applications of statistical tools in differential diagnosis can significantly lower medical costs" and "Understanding of statistical tools is necessary to properly interpret diagnostic test results." The results seem to argue for making the course a requirement since the students most in need of decision-science materials are the least likely to select such a course voluntarily.

TEACHING RESIDENTS: CLASSWORK AND ECONOMIC GRAND ROUNDS

A number of studies have evaluated the impact of resident and intern educational intervention on concurrent behavior. For example, Davidoff, Goodspeed, and Clive (1989) studied the impact of a probabilistic reasoning class on test-ordering behavior in three types of hospitals. Medical interns were randomly assigned to the class or the placebo group. Four months after the class, interns in the class wrote 16 percent fewer orders for "little-ticket" lab tests than the placebo group (significant at the 0.03 level). Differences in test ordering were not explained by changes in case mix, so the class appeared to improve the short-run efficiency of test ordering.

Physicians of all ages must be taught that the *New England Journal of Medicine* "Case Records of the MGH" is a poor standard or yardstick for good medicine. In two decades of reading these case records, this author has "learned" three lessons from this flawed standard: (1) Never trust information provided by other hospitals and clinics (always redo everything), (2) order daily chemistry tests on all patients and expensive manual tests that may someday lead to finding some obscure coincidence (leading to a publication), and (3) diagnostic overkill that leads to an elegant differential diagnosis is more important than patient care. Journals should stop the passive endorsement of fiscally irresponsible habits that offer no substantial marginal benefits to the patient (subject, test case). Inefficient clinical decision making can be as big an incapacitating burden on urban hospitals as the volume of charity care.

Peer pressure can sometimes result in substantial (14.2 percent) cuts in test ordering. For example, the previously cited Berwick and Coltin (1986) study indicated that peer comparison feedback to physicians was the most effective stategy in their HMO. Neither feedback on yield of abnormal tests nor education had any positive effects on curbing utilization of tests. Tierney, Miller, and McDonald (1990) studied the effects of informing physicians on the costs for diagnostic tests at a primary-care medical practice. They reasoned that because physicians are generally unaware of diagnostic test costs, they would order fewer tests if they were reminded of cost at the moment of ordering. All tests in the study were ordered at microcomputer work stations, and the charges for the total tests being ordered were displayed on the screen. During the intervention period there were 14 percent fewer tests per patient in the intervention group, and the charges for tests were 13 percent lower. However, 19 weeks after the intervention ended, the intervention group was only 7.7 percent lower than the control group for test ordering and 3.5 percent less for total charges. In summary, physicians ordered fewer diagnostic tests when they were given information about total test charges.

There is some evidence that younger residents today may be more open to economic grand rounds and cost-conscious decision making than previous studies suggest. In an attempt to assess the impact of chart reviews, feedback, and lectures on residents' ordering behavior, Manheim et al. (1990) randomized residents into two groups: the cost-conscious program-review group and a control group. The authors concluded that a reduction of $391 in charges per patient resulted from lower lengths of stay, and charges were $106 lower in radiology (both statistically significant at the 0.01 level). The lower-cost experimental group's style of care achieved lower patient impairment ratings at discharge (measured by Horn's severity-of-illness measure; see chapter 8), indicating that more efficient care may be quality-enhancing at the one university hospital. The current cost-control climate may be conducive to physician education efforts, whereas physicians were less likely to listen to this "efficiency stuff" during the era of cost reimbursement. Excessive diagnostic testing has many causes: institutional or peer pressure, desire for new knowledge, inadequate physician knowledge of test characteristics, erroneous inferences of test results leading to new tests, diagnostic "overkill," inappropriate tests (the wrong test or right test at the wrong time), medicolegal considerations, monetary incentives, and unique coping strategies for dealing with uncertainty. Two strategies that have proved effective in altering test-ordering behavior include education with regard to test characteristics and cost and feedback of individual and peer-group behavior.

CONCLUSIONS

Health practitioners, especially physicians, must be taught more economics and biostatistics in order to use diagnostic information appropriately and effectively and arrive at the best treatment mode. Duncan Neuhauser has suggested that the Hippocratic oath be rewritten in the 1990s as follows: "I swear by Apollo, the physician, and Aesculapius, and health and all heal and all the Gods and Goddesses that, according to my ability and judgment, *and cost considerations*, I will keep this oath and stipulation." Formal training in decision analysis can be applied to improve patient care in a therapeutic setting as well as to assist medical practitioners in understanding the priority-setting and policy determinations that society will make regarding the future medical practice.

Increasingly, house staffs (residents) and medical students are utilizing the computer for clinical education. New software systems developed in Texas, New Mexico, Massachusetts, and Pennsylvania assist the practicing physician to sort through possible differential diagnoses for 1,000 diseases, based on 1,600 signs and symptoms. Most systems are management tools that can track what is done and sequentially list what further studies are necessary to confirm a diagnosis. The computer interacts with the user by listing disease possibilities and distinguishing features and tests. These programs will also list a number of current approaches to treatment. The computer system is a time saver and aid to quality care—not a robotic competitor to the attending physician. Younger physicians are more familiar with the computer, the concept of cost-utility analysis (Goel and Detsky 1989), and the concept of inappropriate utilization (Kemper 1988). The application of computerized expert systems has had only limited use in the hospital sector, but the applications will expand in the near future (Pestotnik 1990; Safran and Phillips 1989).

Attempts have been made to reform medical education over the past decade. Most of the informational content in medical textbooks is still presented "upside down" in that the student is first informed of the diseases and then told of the probability of various signs and symptoms. Residents and students all too often minimize probabilistic concerns and search for that rare "zebra" condition, as with the search for lupus in the Freymann quote at the beginning of this chapter.

The physician has to take this information and invert the order to go through a process that eventually leads to a diagnosis. A dozen American medical schools are now experimenting with a problem-oriented, computer-enhanced medical curriculum. Originally developed at MacMasters University in Ontario, the problem-oriented approach has spread from New Mexico to Harvard Medical School's New Pathway program.

Criticism of statistical tools usually is based on the subjective estimates included in the formulas, alleging that what appears to be objective analysis is really no better than the examiner's best guess. This criticism will become less justified as decision makers begin to realize that (1) all decisions incorporate subjective estimations and (2) only through disciplined analysis can this subjectivity be evaluated. The recent proliferation of courses in the area of cost education or cost-effective clinical decision making is a healthy trend for those interested in evaluative research and medical cost containment. If we are to contain costs and maintain patient service quality, it is our responsibility to discover the most effective approaches to making economical clinical decisions.

REFERENCES

Aaron, H., and Schwartz, W. (1984). *The Painful Prescription: Rationing Hospital Care.* Washington, D.C.: Brookings Institution.

Agency for Health Care Policy and Research (AHCPR). (1991) "PORT Projects Summary." Agency for Health Care Policy and Research, DHHS, Rockville, Maryland.

American Medical Association. (1988). *Cost-effective Medical Care.* Chicago: Resident Physicians Section, American Medical Association.

American Public Health Association. (1981). "Poll Shows Americans Would Put Dollar Value on Life." *Nation's Health* 20:2 (February), 3.

Anderson, G., Steinberg, E., Whittle, J., Powe, N., and Antebi, S. (1990). "Development of Clinical and Economic Prognoses from Medicare Claims Data." *Journal of the American Medical Association* 263:7 (February 11), 967–72.

Anderson, O., and Morrison, E. (1989). "The Worth of Medical Care." *Medical Care Review* 46:2 (Summer), 121–155.

Annas, G. (1977). "Allocation of Artificial Hearts in the Year 2002: Minerva v. National Health Agency." *American Journal of Law and Medicine* 3 (Spring), 59–76.

Banta, D., and Thacker, S. (1979). *The Premature Delivery of Medical Technology: A Case Report—Electronic Fetal Monitoring.* DHEW, National Center for Health Services Report. Rockville, Md.: U.S. Government Printing Office.

Barrett, B., Parfrey, P., and Vavasour, H. (1992). "A Comparison of Nonionic LOR Agents with Ionic HOA During Cardiac Catheterization." *NEJM* 326:7 (February 13), 431–436.

Bartlett, E. (1985). "Accomplishing More with Less under PPS Using Patient Education." *Healthcare Financial Management* 39:7 (July), 86–94.

Bengtson, J. (1990). "Detection of Restenosis after Elective Percutaneous Transluminal Coronary Angioplasty Using the Exercise Treadmill Test." *American Journal of Cardiology* 65:1 (January), 28–34.

Berkelhamer, J. (1986). "Charges by Residents and Faculty Physicians in a University Hospital Pediatric Practice." *Journal of Medical Education* 61:4 (April), 303–307.

Berwick, D., and Coltin, K. (1986). "Feedback Reduces Test Use in a HMO." *Journal of the American Medical Association* 255:11 (March 21), 1450–1454.

Black, W., and Dwyer, A. (1990). "Local versus Global Measures of Accuracy: Important Decision for Diagnostic Imaging." *Medical Decision Making* 10:4 (October–December), 266–272.

Braun, P. (1980). "The Clinical Management of Suspected Herpes Virus Encephalitis." *American Journal of Medicine* 69, 895–899.

Brott, T., Labutta, R., and Kempczinski, R. (1986). "Changing Patterns in Practice of Carotid Endarterectomy in Large Metropolitan Area." *Journal of the American Medical Association* 255:18 (May 11), 2609–2613.

Brown, K., and Burrows, C. (1990). "The Sixth Stool Guaiac Test: $47 Million That Never Was." *Journal of Health Economics* 9:4 (December), 429–445.

Cahalan, D. (1991). *An Ounce of Prevention*. San Francisco: Jossey-Bass.

Califf, R. (1989). "Evolution of Medical and Surgical Therapy for Coronary Artery Disease: A 15 Year Perspective." *Journal of the American Medical Association* 261:14 (April 14), 2077–2086.

Cassells, W., Schoenberger, A., and Graboys, T. (1978). "Interpretation by Physicians of Clinical Laboratory Results." *New England Journal of Medicine* 299:17 (October 26), 999–1001.

Chassin, M., and McCue, S. (1986). "A Randomized Trial of Medical Quality Assurance." *Journal of the American Medical Association* 256:8 (August 29), 1012–1016.

Clinton, J. (1986). "Chest Radiography in the Emergency Department." *Annals of Emergency Medicine* 15:3 (March), 254–256.

Cole, P. (1976). "Elective Hysterectomy: Pro and Con." *New England Journal of Medicine* 295:5 (July 29), 264–265.

Cropper, M., Evans, W., and Berardi, S. (1992). "Pesticide Regulation: EPA Decision Making." *Journal of Political Economy* 100:1 (February), 175–196.

Daniels, M., and Schroeder, S. (1977). "Variations among Physicians in Use of Laboratory Tests: Relation to Clinical Productivity and Outcomes of Care." *Medical Care* 15:6 (June), 482–487.

Davidoff, F., Goodspeed, R., and Clive, J. (1989). "Changing Test Ordering Behavior: A RCT Comparing Probabilistic Reasoning with Cost Containment Education." *Medical Care* 27:1 (January), 45–58.

Demlo, L. (1990). "Measuring Health Care Effectiveness: Research and Policy Implications." *International Journal of Technology Assessment in Health Care* 6:2 (April), 288–294.

Detsky, A., McLaughlin, J., Abrams, H., Labbe, K., and Markel, F. (1986). "Do Interns and Residents Order More Tests Than Attending Staff?" *Medical Care* 24:6 (June), 526–534.

Doubilet, P., Weinstein, M., and McNeil, B. (1986). "Use and Misuse of the Term 'Cost Effective' in Medicine." *New England Journal of Medicine* 314:4 (January 23), 253–255.

Eastaugh, S. (1992). *Health Care Finance: Economic Incentives and Productivity Enhancement*. Westport, Conn.: Greenwood.

———. (1991). "Valuation of the Benefits of Risk-free Blood: Willingness to Pay for Hemoglobin Solutions." *International Journal of Technology Assessment in Health Care* 7:1 (Winter), 51–59.

———. (1990). "Financing the Correct Rate of Growth in Medical Technology." *Quarterly Review of Economics and Business* 30:4 (Winter), 54–60.

———. (1983). "Placing a Value on Life and Limb: The Role of the Informed Consumer." *Health Matrix* 1:1 (Spring), 5–21.

———. (1981). "Teaching the Principles of Cost-Effective Clinical Decision Making to Medical Students." *Inquiry* 18:1 (Spring), 28–36.

Eddy, D. (1990). "Clinical Decision Making: From Theory to Practice." *Journal of the American Medical Association* 263:2 (January 19), 441–443.

———. (1989). "Selecting Technologies for Assessment." *International Journal of Technology Assessment in Health Care* 5:4 (Fall) 485–501.

Eddy, D., Hasselblad, V., McGivney, W., and Hendee, W. (1988). "The Value of Mammography Screening in Women Under 50." *Journal of the American Medical Association* 259:1512–1519.

Eisenberg, J. (1986). *Doctors' Decisions and the Cost of Medical Care*. Ann Arbor, Mich.: Health Administration Press.

Eisenberg, J., and Williams, S. (1983). "Cost Containment and Changing Physicians' Practice Behavior: Can the Fox Learn to Guard the Chicken Coop?" *Journal of the American Medical Association* 249:22 (May 11), 3074–3076.

Evans, R. (1984). "Computerized Tomography: A Controversy Revisited." *New England Journal of Medicine* 310:18 (May 3), 1183–1185.

Farkas, G. (1992). *Human Capital or Cultural Capital?* Hawthorne, N.Y.: Aldine.

Feldstein, P., Wickizer, T., and Wheeler, J. (1988). "Effects of Utilization Review Programs on Health Care Use and Expenditures." *New England Journal of Medicine* 318:20 (May 19), 1310–1314.

Field, M., and Lohr, K. (1991). *Clinical Practice Guidelines: Directions for a New Program*. Washington, D.C.: National Academy Press.

Finney, D. (1972). *Probit Analysis*. 3rd ed. Cambridge: Cambridge University Press.

Foltz, A., and Kelsey, J. (1978). "The Annual Pap Test: A Dubious Policy Success." *Milbank Memorial Fund Quarterly* 56:4 (Fall), 426–462.

Foote, A., and Erfurt, J. (1991). "Benefit to Cost Ratio of Work-Site Blood Pressure Control Programs." *Journal of the American Medical Association* 265:10 (March 13), 1283–1286.

Fossett, J., Choi, C., and Peterson, J. (1991) "Hospital Outpatient Services and Medicaid Patients' Access to Care." *Medical Care* 29:10 (October), 964–976.

Freund, D., Dittus, R., Fitzgerald, J., and Heck, D. (1990). "Assessing and Improving Outcomes: Total Knee Replacement." *Health Services Research* 25:5 (December), 723–726.

Fuchs, V. (1986). *The Health Economy*. Cambridge, Mass.: Harvard University Press.

Fuchs, V., and Garber, A. (1990). "The New Technology Assessment." *New England Journal of Medicine* 323:10 (September 6), 673–677.

Garrison, L., and Wilensky, G. (1986). "Cost Containment and Technology." *Health Affairs* 5:2 (Summer), 46–59.

Gersh, B. (1989). "Coronary Bypass Surgery in Chronic Stable Angina." *Circulation* 79:6 (June), I46–I59.

Gillespie, K., Romeis, J., Virgo, K., Fletcher, J., and Elixhauser, A. (1989). "Practice

Pattern Variation between Two Medical Schools." *Medical Care* 27:5 (May), 537–542.

Goel, V., and Detsky, A. (1989). "Cost-Utility Analysis of Preoperative Total Parenteral Nutrition." *International Journal of Technology Assessment* 5:2 (April), 111–119.

Goldman, L. (1988). "Chest Pain Clinic to Improve Follow-up." *Annals of Emergency Medicine* 17:8 (August), 867–870.

Goldman, L., Weinstein, M., Goldman, P., and Williams, L. (1991). "Cost-Effectiveness of HMG-CoA Inhibition for Primary and Secondary Prevention of Coronary Heart Disease." *Journal of the American Medical Association* 265:9 (March 6), 1145–1151.

Goldsch and Sox, H. (1988). "Tests in the Evaluation of Chest Pain in MI Patients." *American Heart Journal* 116:2 (August), 523–535.

Goyert, G., Bottoms, S., Treadwell, M., and Nehra, P. (1989). "The Physician Factor in Cesarian Birth Rates." *New England Journal of Medicine* 320:11 (March 16), 706–709.

Gregor, D. (1969). "Detection of Silent Colon Cancer in Routine Examinations." *CA: Cancer Journal for Clinicians* 19:6 (November–December), 330–337.

Hanemann, W. (1991). "Willingness to Pay and Willingness to Accept: How Much Can They Differ?" *American Economic Review* 81:3 (June), 635–647.

Haverkamp, A., Orleans, M., Langendoerfer, S., McFee, J., Murphy, J., and Thompson, H. (1979). "A Controlled Clinical Trial on the Differential Effects of Fetal Monitoring." *American Journal of Obstetrics and Gynecology* 134:4 (June 14), 399–408.

Haverkamp, A., Thompson, H., McFee, J., and Cetrulo, C. (1976). "The Evaluation of Continuous Fetal Heart Rate Monitoring in High-Risk Pregnancy." *American Journal of Obstetrics and Gynecology* 125:3 (June 1), 310–318.

Hershey, J. (1991). "Sensitivity Analysis in Medical Decision Making: Linear Programming." *Medical Decision Making* 11:1 (January–March), 57–60.

Hiatt, H. (1990). *Medical Lifeboat: Will There Be Room for You in the Health Care System?* New York: Harper and Row.

Hirshfeld, J. (1992). "Low Osmolality Contrast Agents: Who Needs Them?" *NEJM* 326:7 (February 13), 482–484.

Horn, S., Horn, R., and Moses, H. (1986). "Profiles of Physician Practice and Severity of Illness." *American Journal of Public Health* 76:5 (May), 532–535.

Institute of Medicine. (1991). *The Changing Economics of Medical Technology*. Washington, D.C.: NAS Press.

———. (1990). *A Strategy for Quality Assurance*. Washington, D.C.: NAS Press.

———. (1989). *Effectiveness Initiative: Setting Priorities for Clinical Conditions*. Washington, D.C.: NAS Press.

———. (1985). *Assessing Medical Technologies*. Washington, D.C.: NAS Press.

Kahn, C. (1990). "Policy Implications of Outcomes Research." *International Journal of Technology Assessment in Health Care* 6:2 (April), 295–297.

Kassirer, J. (1989). "Our Stubborn Quest for Diagnostic Certainty: Cause of Excessive Testing." *New England Journal of Medicine* 320:22 (June 1), 1489–1491.

———. (1986). "The Wild Goose Chase and the Elephant's Relevance." *Journal of the American Medical Association* 256:2 (July 11), 256–257.

Kelly, J., and Swartwout, J. (1991). *Directory of Practice Parameters*. Chicago: Office of Quality Assurance, AMA.

Kemper, K. (1988). "Medically Inappropriate Hospital Use in a Pediatric Population." *New England Journal of Medicine* 318:16 (April 21), 1033–1037.

Knoebel, S. (1988). "Cardiology by the Numbers and Cost-Containments." *American Journal of Cardiology* 61:13 (May 1), 1112–1115.

Knowles, J. (1969). "Radiology: A Case Study in Technology and Manpower." *New England Journal of Medicine* 280:24 (June 12), 1323–1329.

Leader, S., and Moon, M. (1989). "Medicare Trends in Ambulatory Surgery." *Health Affairs* 8:1 (Spring), 158–169.

Leffall, I. (1974). "Early Diagnosis of Colorectal Cancer." *CA: Cancer Journal for Clinicians* 24:3 (May–June), 152–159.

Leveno, K., Cunningham, F., Nelson, S., Roark, M., Williams, M., Guzick, D., Dowling, S., Rosenfeld, C., and Buckley, A. (1986). "A Prospective Comparison of Selective and Universal Electronic Fetal Monitoring in 34,995 Pregnancies." *New England Journal of Medicine* 315:10 (September 4), 615–619.

Levinsky, N. (1990). "Age as a Criteria for Rationing Health Care." *New England Journal of Medicine* 322:25 (June 21), 1813–1816.

Lindsey, P., and Newhouse, J. (1990). "Cost and Value of Second Surgical Opinion Programs: A Critical Review of the Literature." *Journal of Health Politics, Policy, and Law* 15:3 (Fall), 543–570.

Linton, A., and Naylor, C. (1990). "Organized Medicine and the Assessment of Technology." *New England Journal of Medicine* 323:21 (November 22), 1463–1467.

Maloney, I., and Rogers, D. (1979). "Medical Technology—A Different View of the Contentious Debate over Costs." *New England Journal of Medicine* 301:26 (December 27), 1413–1419.

Manheim, L., Feinglas, J., Hughes, R., Martin, G., Conrad, K., and Hughes, R. (1990). "Training House Officers to Be Cost Conscious: Effects of an Educational Intervention on Charges and Length of Stay." *Medical Care* 28:1 (January), 29–41.

Marks J., Koplan J., Hogue J., and Dalmat, M. (1990). A Cost-Benefit/Cost Effectiveness Analysis of Smoking Cessation for Pregnant Women. *American Journal of Preventive Medicine* 6:5 (May), 282–289.

Marton, K., Tul, V., and Sox, H. (1985). "Modifying Test Ordering Behavior in the Outpatient Medical Clinic: A Controlled Trial of Two Educational Interventions." *Archives of Internal Medicine* 145:4 (April), 816–821.

Mauro, R., Poole, S., and Lockhart, C. (1988). "Differentiation of Epiglotitis in Child with Stridor." *American Journal of Diseases of Children* 142:6 (June), 679–682.

McNeil, B. (1985). "Hospital Response of DRG-based Prospective Payment." *Medical Decision Making* 5:1 (January), 15–21.

———. (1977). "The Value of Diagnostic Aids in Patients with Potential Surgical Problems." In J. Bunker, B. Barnes, and F. Mosteller (eds.), *Costs, Risks, and Benefits of Surgery*, 77–90. New York: Oxford University Press.

McNeil, B., and Adelstein, S. (1975). "Measures of Clinical Efficiency: The Value of Case Finding in Hypertensive Renovascular Disease." *New England Journal of Medicine* 293:5 (July 31), 221–226.

McPhee, S. (1984). "Lessons for Teaching Cost Containment." *Journal of Medical Education* 59:9 (September), 722–729.

Merritt, T., Hallman, M., Vaucher, Y., McFeeley, E., Richard, T., and Tubman, J. (1990). "Impact of Surfactant Treatment on Cost of Neonatal Intensive Care: A Cost-Benefit Analysis." *Journal of Perinatology* 10:4 (April) 416–419.

Metz, C., and Shen, J. (1992). "Gains in Accuracy from Replicated Readings of Diagnostic Images: ROC Analysis." *Medical Decision Making* 12:1 (January–March), 60–74.

Miao, L. (1977). "Gastric Freezing: An Example of the Evaluation of Medical Therapy by Randomized Clinical Trials." In J. Bunker, B. Barnes, and F. Mosteller (eds.), *Costs, Risks, and Benefits of Surgery*, 198–211. New York: Oxford University Press.

Mishan, E. (1971). "Evaluation of Life and Limb: A Theoretical Approach." *Journal of Political Economy* 79:4 (July–August), 687–705.

Mohr, D., Offord, K., Owen, R., and Melton, J. (1986). "Asymptomatic Microhematuria and Urologic Disease." *Journal of the American Medical Association* 256:2 (July 11), 224–229.

Mushkin, S. (1989). *Biomedical Research: Costs and Benefits*. Cambridge, Mass.: Ballinger.

Neuhauser, D. (1979). "The Public Voice and the Nation's Health." *Milbank Memorial Fund Quarterly* 57:1 (Winter), 60–69.

Neuhauser, D., and Lewicki, A. (1975). "What Do We Gain from the Sixth Stool Guaiac?" *New England Journal of Medicine* 293:5 (July 31), 226–228.

Norton, L. (1991). "Metastatic Breast Cancer: Length and Quality of Life." *New England Journal of Medicine*. 325:19 (November 7), 1370–1371.

O'Connor, S., and Lanning, J. (1992). "The End of Autonomy?" *Health Care Management Review* 17:1 (Winter), 63–72.

Oliver, R., and Smith, J. (1990). *Influence Diagrams, Belief Nets, and Decision Analysis*. New York: Wiley.

O'Malley, N. (1991). "Age-based Rationing of Health Care." *Health Care Management Review* 16:1 (Winter), 83–93.

Parkan, C., and Holland, L. (1990). "Use of Efficiency Linear Programs for Sensitivity Analysis in Medical Decision Making." *Medical Decision Making* 10:2 (April–June), 116–125.

Paushter, D., and McNeil, B. (1990). "Comparison of MRI and Ultrasonography." *New England Journal of Medicine* 323:10 (September 6), 621–626.

Peddecord, K., Janon, E., and Robins, J. (1988). "Substitution of MRI for Computed Tomography." *International Journal of Technology Assessment in Health Care* 4:4 (Fall) 573–591.

Perry, S., and Pillar, B. (1990). "National Policy for Health Care Technology." *Medical Care Review* 47:4 (Winter), 401–418.

Pestotnik, S. (1990). "Therapeutic Antibiotic Monitoring: Surveillance Using a Computerized Expert System." *American Journal of Medicine* 88:1 (January), 43–48.

Ransohoff, D., and Feinstein, A. (1978). "Problems of Spectrum and Bias in Evaluating the Efficacy of Diagnostic Tests." *New England Journal of Medicine* 299:17 (October 26), 926–930.

Regt, R., Minkoff, H., Feldman, J., and Schwarz, R. (1986). "Relation of Private or Clinic Care to the Cesarean Birth Rate." *New England Journal of Medicine* 315:10 (September 4), 619–624.

Reiman, E., and Mintun, M. (1990). "Positron Emission Tomography." *Archives of Internal Medicine* 150:4 (April), 729–731.

Relman, A. (1990). "Is Rationing Inevitable?" *New England Journal of Medicine* 322:25 (June 21), 1809–1810.

Rettig, R. (1978). "Lessons Learned from the End-Stage Renal Disease Experience." In R. Egdahl and P. Gertman (eds.), *Technology and the Quality of Health Care*, 153–173. Germantown, Md.: Aspen Systems.

Rifkin, M., Zerhouni, E., and Gatsonis, C. (1990). "Comparison of MRI and Ultrasonography in Staging Early Prostate Cancer: Results of a Multi-institutional Cooperative Trial." *New England Journal of Medicine* 323:10 (September 6), 621–626.

Roos, N., Wennberg, J., and Malenka, D. (1989). "Mortality and Reoperation after Open and Transurethral Resection of the Prostate." *New England Journal of Medicine* 320:17 (April 27), 1120–1124.

Safran, C., and Phillips, R. (1989). "Interventions to Prevent Readmission: The Constraints of Cost and Efficacy." *Medical Care* 27:2 (February), 204–211.

Santos, E., Starich, G., and Mazzaferri, E. (1989). "Sensitivity, Specificity, and Cost-Effectiveness of STA in the Diagnosis of Thyroid Disease." *Archives of Internal Medicine* 149:3 (March), 526–532.

Scheffler, R., and Andrews, N. (1989). *Cancer Care and Cost: DRGs and Beyond*. Ann Arbor, Mich.: Health Administration Press.

Schrage, L. (1991). *Linear, Integer, and Quadratic Programming with LINDO*. Redwood City, Calif.: Scientific Press.

Scitovsky, A. (1985). "Changes in the Costs of Treatment of Selected Illnesses, 1971–1981." *Medical Care* 23:12 (December), 1345–1357.

Showstack, J., Stone, M., and Schroeder, S. (1985). "The Role of Changing Clinical Practices in the Rising Costs of Hospital Care." *New England Journal of Medicine* 313:19 (November 7), 1201–1207.

Siegel, S. and Castellan, N. (1989). *Nonparametric Statistics for the Behavioral Sciences*. New York: McGraw-Hill.

Siminoff, L., and Fetting, J. (1991). "Factors Affecting Treatment Decisions for a Life-threatening Illness: The Case of Medical Treatment of Breast Cancer." *Social Science and Medicine* 32:7 (July), 813–818.

Siu, A., Manning, W., and Benjamin, B. (1990). "Patient, Provider, and Hospital Characteristics Associated with Inappropriate Hospitalization." *American Journal of Public Health* 80:10 (October), 1253–1256.

Skendzel, L. (1978). "How Physicians Use Laboratory Tests." *Journal of the American Medical Association* 239:11 (March 13), 1077–1080.

Sklar, D. (1989). "Emergency Department Technicians in a University Hospital." *Annals of Emergency Medicine* 18:4 (April), 401–405.

Soumerai, S. (1990). "Withdrawing Payment for Nonscientific Drug Therapy." *Journal of the American Medical Association* 263:6 (February 9), 831–839.

Stafford, R. (1990). "Alternative Strategies for Controlling Rising Cesarean Section Rates." *Journal of the American Medical Association* 263:5 (February 2), 683–687.

Steinbrook, R., and Lo, B. (1992). "Oregon Medicaid: Will It Provide Adequate Medical Care?" *New England Journal of Medicine* 326:5 (January 30), 340–344.

Thompson, J. (1989). "Experiences at the New MRI Imaging Center." *British Journal of Radiology* 62:2 (February), 134–137.

Tierney, W., Miller, M., and McDonald, C. (1990). "Effect on Test Ordering of Informing Physicians of the Charges for Outpatient Diagnostic Tests." *New England Journal of Medicine* 322:21 (May 30), 1499–1502.

Tomlinson, T., and Brody, H. (1990). "Futility and the Ethics of Resuscitation." *Journal of the American Medical Association* 264:10 (September 12), 1276–1280.

U.S. Congress. (1976). 94th Congress, 2nd Session, Subcommittee on Oversight and Investigations of the Committee on Interstate and Foreign Commerce. *Report on the Cost and Quality of Health Care: Unnecessary Surgery.* Washington, D.C.: U.S. Government Printing Office.

U.S. Congress, Office of Technology Assessment. (1980). *Cost-Effectiveness and Cost-Benefit Analysis in Health Care: Methodology and Literature Review.* Vol. 2. Washington, D.C.: U.S. Government Printing Office.

———. (1978). *Assessing the Efficacy and Safety of Medical Technologies.* Washington, D.C.: U.S. Government Printing Office.

Wachtel, T., Moulton, A., Pezzullo, J., and Hamolsky, M. (1986). "Inpatient Protocols to Reduce Health Care Costs." *Medical Decision Making* 6:2 (April), 101–109.

Washington, A., Browner, W., and Korenbrot, C. (1987). "Cost-Effectiveness of Combined Treatment for Endocervical Gonorrhea." *Journal of the American Medical Association* 257:15 (April 17), 2056–2060.

Wears, R., and Kamens, D. (1986). "A Simple Method for Evaluating the Safety of High-Yield Criteria." *Annals of Emergency Medicine* 15:4 (April), 439–444.

Weisbrod, B. (1961). *Economics of Public Health.* Philadelphia: University of Pennsylvania Press.

Weiss, K., Gergen, P., Hodgson, T. (1992). "Economic Evaluation of Asthma." *New England Journal of Medicine* 326:13 (March 26), 862–866.

Wennberg, J. (1990). "Outcomes Research, Cost Containment, and the Fear of Health Care Rationing." *New England Journal of Medicine* 323:17 (October 25), 1202–1204.

———. (1989). "Hospital Use and Mortality among Medicare Beneficiaries in Boston and New Haven." *New England Journal of Medicine* 321:17 (October 26), 1168–1173.

Wilensky, G. (1990). "Technology as Culprit and Benefactor." *Quarterly Review of Economics and Business* 30:4 (Winter), 45–49.

Wong, E. et al. (1983). "Ordering of Laboratory Tests in a Teaching Hospital: Can It Be Improved?" *Journal of the American Medical Association* 249:22 (June 10), 3076–3080.

Young, G. (1986). "CBC or Not CBC? That Is the Question." *Annals of Emergency Medicine* 13:3 (March), 367–371.

Zaat, J., Eijk, J., and Bonte, H. (1992). "Lab Test Form Design Influences Test Ordering." *Medical Care* 30:3 (March), 189–198.

Zapka, J., Stoddard, A., Maul, L., and Costanza, M. (1991). "Interval Adherence to Mammography Screening Guidelines." *Medical Care* 29:8 (August), 697–708.

13 Benefit Evaluation: The Value of Life and Limb

An economist can tell you the prices of everything, but the value of nothing.
—Will Rogers

American doctors should begin to build up a social ethic and behavioral practices that help them decide when medicine is bad medicine: not simply because it has absolutely no payoff or because it hurts the patient, but also because the costs are not justified by the marginal benefits. To do this we are going to have to develop and disseminate better information; some small fraction of what we now spend on health care could be better spent to determine limits.
—Lester Thurow

Harris Poll reveals that 52 percent of the public think that the government and the courts should place an economic dollar value on life—only 34 percent say No.
—News report, February 1, 1981

Modern medicine increasingly turns to intangible benefits for justification (Bovbjerg et al. 1989). Physicians are realizing the opportunity-cost implications of supporting more high-technology medicine for very rare diseases. The public also realizes that the health economy and the American economy are not limitless. An opportunity for new transplant techniques will, by definition, prevent society from financing some other medical or social program. The objective of cost-benefit analysis is to maximize net benefits (benefits minus costs, appropriately discounted over time). The objective of cost-effectiveness analysis is to rank order the preferred alternatives for achieving a single goal or a specified basket of benefits. Cost-effectiveness analysis is not any easier to perform than cost-benefit analysis if multiple varieties of benefit are specified (person-years, work-loss days, reduced angina), yet in cost-benefit analysis one must value the intangible benefits in commensurate dollar terms (Eastaugh 1991).

Practitioners of cost-benefit analysis are accused in alternating years of either (1) stifling liberal attempts to build better service programs, (2) frustrating conservative attempts to reduce the regulatory burden on industry, or (3) browbeating liberals and conservatives who bring pork-barrel projects with low benefit-to-cost ratios to their home states. Whether the source of pork exists in the social-service sector or the industrial sector, practitioners of cost-benefit analysis are seen as an anathema by many interest groups. Economists have become increasingly skeptical of any political process that encourages waste and ignores careful analysis designed to incorporate all benefits, including intangible benefits, when making resource decisions. When fully identified prices fail to exist (water resources) or price is deemed an ineffective measure of value (health services), an attempt is made to impute value or to shadow-price. In economic sectors where competitive markets fail to operate, such as health care, cost-benefit analysis is an attempt to do what supply and demand forces accomplish in competitive markets (Eastaugh 1983; Callahan 1990).

Analysts and decision makers disagree on how to value the intangible benefits of health programs. Most decision makers find the valuation process in cost-benefit analysis difficult and do not trust analyses that depend on gross approximations, small samples, and a poor data base. These decision makers are willing to violate the efficiency criteria and invest more in hospitals and physicians than society receives as a return on the dollar. Consequently, economic evaluation of new or expensive technologies has become a central issue in the public debate about rising medical care costs.

Cost-benefit analysis must include intangible benefits (e.g., pain reduction) to be comprehensive. It is therefore necessary to shadow-price patients' willingness-to-pay preferences for the given benefits of a given medical technology. This chapter provides an example of shadow-pricing the public value of AIDS-free, disease-free blood products (hemoglobin solutions). A number of other studies have looked at the issue of measuring patients' preferences: one study of transurethral prostate surgery (Barry et al. 1988), a study of magnetic resonance imaging (MRI; Rifkin, Zerhouni, and Gatsonis 1990), a study of medical treatment alternatives for hypertension (Littenberg, Garber, and Sox 1990), and a study of various blood products (Eastaugh 1990). Clinical decisions are based less on paternalism ("Do what the doctor says") and more on technology assessment and the patient's preferences for risk and return (e.g., "No thanks, dear surgeon, as an accountant who never plays tennis or runs I'll skip the surgery you prescribe").

A broader political economy question asks: Do we spend enough for technology assessment? In 1991 we spent only $66 million, or 0.01 percent of the national health budget, on technology assessment. Many analysts think that this figure is too low. If we invested more than one penny per $100 of health care expenses on technology assessment, the efficiency and effectiveness of our sector would improve.

At the present time technology assessment does not provide the individual doctor with a court-sanctioned set of guidelines to make cost or quality trade-offs at the patient's bedside. Lomas et al. (1989) reported that voluntary guidelines from assessment studies are insufficient to compel changes in clinicians' decisions at the bedside. Technology assessment mainly assists reimbursement decisions for what services should be covered by government or the company insurance plan. For example, technology assessment has helped the Health Care Financing Administration save $630 million per year since 1989 by denying hospitals extra payment for using recombinant tissue plasminogen activator (TPA) for patients with a myocardial infarction. It turned out on further study that TPA, at a cost of $2,000 per case, is not necessarily the most effective or cost-effective mode of treatment (Banta and Thacker 1990).

The process of analysis asks explicit questions of valuation that politicians might want to blur, such as why we spend $40,000 to give one executive a bone marrow transplant or bypass operation while forgoing five years of life for 25 ghetto dwellers suffering from rheumatic fever or hypertension. When value judgments are quantified, although some groups dislike this process, unconsciously inaccurate or insidious assumptions are exposed. Public disclosure of the underlying assumptions in a given economic analysis may yield more informed and better quality ex ante "Who shall live?" decisions. Cost-benefit analysis should be an ex ante resource decision rather than an ex post bedside decision of whether to pull the plug. Before we consider the risks within our medical system, a brief health risk assessment of the environment will be presented.

OPINIONS ON RISK ARE NOT MATHEMATICAL

We do not live in a safe world. Cutting one risk typically creates another. For example, if the Soviet Union were to convert the inferior 80 percent of its nuclear generating capacity to coal, over the next four decades the increased traffic from coal trucks, mining accidents, and pollution-induced disease would kill 1.1 to 1.5 million citizens. Many citizens fear nuclear power because unknown fears outrank familiar ones. Breathing or drinking vodka are things a person is familiar with. Consuming radiation from a nuclear accident or eating and drinking dioxin and polychlorinated biphenyls are not familiar experiences. The standard dosage of cosmic radiation at sea level is 2000 times more dangerous to human life than residing in a home 20 miles from an American nuclear power plant. One round trip from New York to Los Angeles has 200 times more risk than living next to an American power plant, according to the April 17, 1987, issue of *Science*. Even the Democratic party's economic advisers, like Yale professor Nordhaus (1990), argue for careful cost-benefit surveys rather than "panicky eco-action."

Risk-assessment models are typically simplistic. The American Environmental Protection Agency (EPA) uses a linear standard risk-assessment model; for example, if 20 out of 1,000 rats get cancer from eating two bowls of dioxin a day, the EPA assumes that half a bowl per day would kill only 5 rats. Sliding down the dosage response curve, the EPA assumes that at 0.006 picograms per day one human in a million would die of cancer. However, the more accurate non-linear models report risk as a decaying exponential function, and government officials in Australia and Canada allow safe doses of dioxin at rates 300 to 500 times the American threshold (standard). Moving to a dioxin standard that is ten times tougher than the Australian threshold would save the American people $1.1 billion in cleanup costs, according to California analyst Dennis Paustenbach at McLaren Environmental Engineering. Formaldehyde has the classic "hockey-stick" dose response curve: It is safe until the dosage exceeds 10 parts per million, but at 15 parts per million 50 percent of the animals get cancer. The American aversion to risk is not based on mathematics or common sense. Moderate content of PCBs in the daily diet has 90 to 98 percent less risk than eating two tablespoons of peanut butter per day. Peanut butter can contain mold-producing aflatoxin, but we do not ban peanut butter because it is an all-American food.

Avoiding a little risk can sometimes create a larger long-run risk. For example, 1960 data suggested that when whooping cough vaccine is given to one million children, 95 will have serious reactions (and a few will die). In the United Kingdom parental pressure caused the National Health Service to withdraw the vaccination requirement. Whooping cough deaths soared, and the requirement was reinstated.

If small risks are often overlooked, large risks of catastrophic expense are highly unpredictable. Fuchs and Zeckhauser (1987) argued for treating catastrophic medical expenses like the demand for firefighting equipment. One does not stand outside a burning building and demand out-of-pocket payments to do the job of firefighting. Fuchs and Zeckhauser argued for collectivizing the burden of catastrophic medical expenses, either in the manner of the United Kingdom (free care) or through public insurance. Unfortunately, the American catastrophic insurance bill that passed in 1988 was never implemented and was repealed in November 1989. We have Medicaid for a number of reasons: social equity, the realization that poverty erodes health status, and that initial endowments of ill health can keep the poor in poverty.

RISK ANALYSIS: EXPERTS DIFFER FROM CITIZENS

The average radiation exposure to residents 1 mile from the Three Mile Island accident (1 millirem) is as risky as 4 extra miles driven in a car or 4 city street crossings. This "bloodless" statistical comparison, while numerically correct, ignores the quality of these three relative risks. Experts worry about the quantity of risk, whereas typical Americans worry about the nature of the risk (whether it is involuntary, controllable, new, unknown, or known). Fear of nuclear radiation, for a citizen of any country, is increased by each of these quality-of-risk factors. In a list of two dozen technologies and behaviors, nuclear power and swimming were ranked first and twenty-fourth in terms of risk by graduate students. However, the probability of morbidity and mortality is much higher for a voluntary behavior such as swimming than it is for a nuclear power accident.

McNeil and Pauker (1982) reported that patients are more willing to take a risk to avoid a sure loss. However, if the same risk is posed in terms of a potential gain, people are less willing to take the risk (e.g., radiation therapy). The effect of a physician's word choice may have a big impact on patient preference, even if all risk elements are statistically unchanged. For example, in lung cancer cases, when the odds were presented in terms of dying, only 18 percent of people chose radiation treatment over surgery. However, if the odds were presented in terms of surviving, almost half of the subjects chose radiation treatment over surgery.

Seen in this context, terminally ill cancer patients seeking laetrile may be victimized, but they are not totally irrational. The terminally ill are risk takers, as is any individual faced with the following situation: A tiger chases you to the bank of a 50-foot river filled with crocodiles; you leap into the water convinced that you can make it safely to the other side. You would never accept such odds if there were no tiger. Many cancer and AIDS patients are faced with this situation daily.

In order to preserve their sense of worth, many physicians also tend to underestimate the risks. The difference is that the physician only observes the risks and outcomes and does not have to live the risks firsthand. Even in the case of elective surgery, with a mere 0.2 percent chance of dying, the typical surgeon understates risk. The surgeon may understate risk for the same reason a truck driver understates risk—it makes working and sleeping easier. A surgeon may look at the small per hour risk and forget that one "healthy" patient dies on the table statewide every nine hours, and even more die postoperatively. Each uncomplicated trip to the operating room may reinforce the idea that one is better than the average surgeon. Analogously, a truck driver may look at the tiny per trip risk and forget that 81 percent of truckers suffer a disabling injury during their career. Any professional, no matter how well educated, tends to look at risk in terms of low-risk short hops. Disabled truckers and surgeons forced into retirement might have something to teach their respective practitioners about tigers, crocodiles, continuing education, and when to quit.

The government makes few macrolevel resource decisions on the basis of cost-benefit analysis. By ignoring the necessity for making cost-benefit judgments for proposed Occupational Safety and Health Administration (OSHA) standards, Congress and the courts have allowed this agency to make a number of extreme decisions. For example, the 1979 proposed OSHA benzene standard of one part per million would benefit society by one life every three years at a cost of $300 to $450 million per life saved. The public does not force Congress to legislate mandatory automobile restraint devices, even though such a program would have a benefit-to-cost ratio that is 3,000 to 6,000 times higher than the benzene standard.

The situations that are most ripe for cost-benefit study are those in which the benefit is incomplete and transient and the costs are high. For example, the cost of $12,000 per course of apheresis treatment for rheumatoid arthritis has been questioned (McCarty 1981). McCarty raised the issue of whether the health economy can afford an additional $1.1 billion dollars or more to provide transient benefits by apheresis. The question is answered clearly only for the small subset of patients facing life-threatening side effects and obvious potential benefit (Jones et al. 1981).

For microdecisions made by the medical community, economic evaluation is frequently held in disrepute because physicians may have the elitist view that cost-benefit analysis is a less satisfactory alternative than ad hoc decisions of hospital committees (Turnbull et al., 1979). The American tradition has been to make local selective choices through critical-care committees rather than to implement an "all-or-none" rationing decision. Under an all-or-none system, as practiced in most European countries, everyone is allowed access or no one is allowed access (Annas 1977). Physicians typically misunderstand the concepts and potential applications of cost-benefit analysis. Attitudes of these professionals are shaped and misshaped by the same sort of colorful but inaccurate portrayal of the topic by the media. For example, throughout the Robert Duvall film *THX–1138*, the king computer states the number of dollar units remaining in the Duvall retention account before the project shuts down and all activity to "save" the individual terminates. The movie thus conveys the viewpoint that approximately 14,000 resource units have been allocated by the economists and the king computer to save the individual, and once that ceiling is attained, the project will be terminated. In real life, as in the film, the public is continually fed an inappropriate definition of both sunk costs and cost-benefit analysis.

Some humanitarians argue that if a small group of individuals report infinitely large intangible benefits, then society should place an infinite value on life. Indeed, in some situations society places the benefits of citizen health above benefit-cost concerns. For example, a June 1981 Supreme Court decision ruled that under the 1970 Occupational Safety and Health Act, OSHA does not have to consider the balance between benefits and costs when implementing regulations. The Reagan administration had argued that cost-benefit analysis should be implicit in any governmental activity. Justice W. J. Brennan interpreted the law as "placing the benefit of worker health above all other considerations save those practical concerns that might make attainment of this benefit unachievable." The OSHA regulations impose on firms a penalty that is in some degree proportional to the presence of unsafe working conditions.

Different groups provide vastly varied estimates of the benefit-cost impact of

OSHA. The value-of-life issues play a major role in congressional budgeting issues. For example, conservatives who wish to abolish the Clean Air Act cited a 1978 study by the National Economic Research Associates, consulting economists, that reported negative $700 million net annual benefits if we that assume life is valued at $560,000. However, supporters of the Clean Air Act reported that under a $1,000,000 estimate of the value of life, the Clean Air Act becomes an attractive proposition with positive annual net benefits of $4.4 billion. The Clean Air Act received renewed life in 1990.

FOUR TECHNIQUES TO VALUE BENEFITS

Some citizens may balk at any value-of-life measurement for religious reasons—that is, they may believe that the process debases the sanctity of life. These individuals would be shocked to learn that for the last two decades public and private agencies have been placing a value on life, ranging from $200,000 by Ford Motor Company to $250,000 by the Federal Aviation Administration and $287,000 by the National Highway Traffic Safety Administration (Hapgood 1980). In the 1990s the figure most frequently used is $1,000,000. The approach taken by these groups involves measuring discounted future earnings (DFE). Forgone earnings as an estimate of indirect benefits are relatively easy to estimate, although some economists would question the assumption that earnings are a suitable measure of social benefit. The resultant biases implicit in measuring benefits in terms of earnings reflect imperfections in the labor market such as racism and sexism. For example, the conclusion that visits to a rheumatology clinic were cost-beneficial only for males merely reflects an artifact of the sex bias in earnings data: Women earn less (Glass 1973). A variant of this approach—subtracting out consumption to yield net output—was considered ill advised, because killing elderly or handicapped individuals would be "valued" as an act that confers a net benefit to society.

The most prevalent assessment approach for researchers in the 1970s was the "willingness-to-pay" (WTP) approach suggested by Schelling (1968). Schelling emphasized the fact that quantity multiplied by price was at best equal to a minimum benefit of health services to the society, since it does not account for the many consumers who would be willing to pay more than the price. The initial WTP studies involved responses to hypothetical questions. However, the bulk of more recent studies have concerned imputed workers' valuation of life based on their willingness to be paid to assume added occupational risk.

There are four basic methods to value life or limb:

1. Paternalistic aggregate-needs assessment
2. DFE observed
3. WTP hypothetical behavior in an opinion survey
4. WTP observed behavior in the labor market (LWTP)

Paternalistic aggregate-needs assessment, the first method of ad hoc valuations, is often practiced by public health professionals acting as "problem" definers—for example, defining mental hygiene cases that "need" deinstitutionalization or defining nutritional status as "inadequate." The definition of what is needed or adequate varies tremendously across time and place. This method is paternalistic in the sense that it takes the aggregate preferences of a single expert or small group of individuals and extrapolates their judgments to other groups of citizens. These techniques are sometimes helpful in making cost-effectiveness decisions within a given discipline (Jones, Densen, and McNitt 1979; Spilker 1991). However, the aggregate-assessment approach has little utility in cost-benefit analysis since each discipline tends to overstate its case. If you bring together 50 experts from 50 separate disciplines, each expert would have you believe that 10 to 20 percent of gross national product should be dedicated to his or her field.

There are a number of strengths and weaknesses for the three remaining valuation methods. Observed WTP measures may be biased by an imperfectly informed wage earner who may bias the responses downward (Moore and Viscusi 1988). Hypothetical WTP (HWTP) measures leave room for individual assessments of the intrinsic intangible benefits. However, the sample sizes are typically small, and the analysis is expensive—that is, the results cannot be derived from secondary data like methods 2 and 4. HWTP surveys are also limited by the usual problems with a survey: response bias, problems with questionnaire phrasing, and so on. Donaldson (1990) provided a good example of a HWTP survey in long-term care.

Discounted Future Earnings

The DFE valuation method has a long history, running back a few hundred years (Fein 1971; Mushkin 1962; Shattuck 1850). Expected earnings replaced income as the relevant measure of indirect benefits in the 1960s (Rice 1966). Cooper and Rice (1976) produced annual tabulations of the present value of lost earnings due to mortality under alternative discount rates and annual estimates of the forgone earnings due to disability. In some cases potential morbidity reduction represents 90 percent of indirect benefits (skin diseases). In other cases potential mortality reduction represents 90 percent of indirect benefits (neoplasms). In many cases the direct benefits of eliminating a disease are a fraction of the indirect benefits (Eastaugh 1983).

There are two basic accounting approaches to DFE studies: the incidence-based approach and the prevalence approach. The incidence-based approach is generally regarded as the superior method for evaluating how much human capital is forgone in the case of chronic or preventable diseases (Hartunian, Smart, and Thompson 1981). A simple example will illustrate the differences between prevalence and incidence-based approaches. Consider an individual experiencing a stroke in 1988 who, over the following eight years, shares the expenses for his medical care with Medicaid, misses some work, and dies in 1996. The traditional prevalence approach assigns the medical expenses and forgone wages to the years in which they occurred and the lost future earnings due to premature death to the year 1996. The incidence-based approach uses present values and assigns all the costs associated with the eight-year duration of the disease to the year of incidence (1988).

Both accounting approaches have comparable drawbacks, depending on the time frame of the relevant policy issue under study. For evaluation of preventive programs or programs aimed at arresting the progression of a chronic illness, federal officials utilize the incidence-based approach. The incidence-based approach provides the better estimate of the cost that may be avoided and, consequently, of the benefits that may be gained by efforts aimed at reducing disease incidence. The traditional prevalance-based viewpoint remains the best of the DFE approaches for decisions concerning the control of current service costs and absenteeism. While the accounting is nice and tidy, the basic flaw of DFE valuation is that it only accounts for society's loss in forgone national income and ignores the person's own value of life, including how much the individual, the direct family, and the overall community value the individual life (Schelling 1968; Mishan 1971; Lipscomb 1990).

One of the major shortcomings of the DFE approach is that to capture fully the intangible costs of losing a life or limb, these attributes must be shadow priced. The results of economists' attempts to shadow-price such nonquantifiable attributes often sound ludicrous: "She will spend $3,000 more per year on alcohol, drugs, and other things to compensate for a lost breast," or "He will forgo sexual experience valued at $40 per encounter, with a frequency of 50 times per year." Even if these costs are a small fraction of the total estimate, one can always discredit the technique by quibbling with the arbitrary price tags.

Hypothetical Measures of Willingness to Pay

The WTP principle in normative economics states that the value of something is simply measured by what people are willing to pay for it. To paraphrase Mishan (1971) in his seminal article on the value of life and limb, economists generally agree as a canon of faith to accept the dictum that each person knows best his or her own interests. Cost-benefit analysis has to operate within the bounds of the individual's deficient information base, congenital optimism, or hypochondria and to accept the expressed consumer preferences as a more relevant measure of benefits than the expert opinions of an educated elite. Experts' presumption that the public is unable to properly assess its interests may be foiled on two counts. First, the observation that people respond in a biased emotional fashion may be irrelevant for policy-making purposes if the bias is unsystematic, since the extremes will cancel each other. Second, one could make the same argument that the public cannot understand the technical details necessary to purchase calculators, cameras, cars, and stereos. The public does not have to understand all the details, as long as a free flow of information creates some small cadre of amateur consultant friends to help guide consumer choice behavior. Providers are improving their capacity to plug patient utilities into the decision analysis (Boyd, Sutherland, and Heasman 1990), survey researchers are more sensitive to elderly respondents (Pearlman and Uhlmann 1988), and development of a quality-of-well-being scale has even extended to AIDS, arthritis, and cystic fibrosis (Kaplan, Anderson, and Wu 1989).

The most often cited early WTP study was done on a sample of 100 Boston residents by Acton (1973). Acton's most publicized question involving public attitude toward risk reduction and heart attacks read as follows:

Let's suppose that your doctor tells you that the odds are 99:1 against your having a heart attack. If you have the attack, the odds are 3:2 that you will live. The heart-attack program would mean that the odds are 4:1 that you live after a heart attack. How much are you willing to pay in taxes per year to have this heart-attack program which would cut your probability of dying from a heart attack in half (i.e., the chances are two per 1,000 you will have a heart attack and be saved by the program this year)?

The median response of $56 suggests that 200 people would chip in $28,000 to save the life of one of the group members in the coming year. The scenario is reasonable because most health programs are risk-reduction efforts. One might also note that a small change in the question, reducing the risk to 0.001, increases the median imputed value of a life saved to $43,000. Both of the two aforementioned questions emphasize the individual's situation. When Acton posed the question in more probabilistic terms, focusing on the 10,000 people living around a hypothetical respondent, the median amounts were reduced by approximately 50 percent for equivalent risk-reduction levels.

The willingness-to-pay approach can be criticized on the grounds that life is probably valued much higher for identified individuals than for members of a hypothetical population. Consumers and physicians tend to value identified individual lives more than statistical anonymous forgone lives, yet physicians are often criticized for placing a substantially higher value on identified individuals than society, with its limited resources, can afford to place on the average citizen.

Labor-Market-Imputed Willingness to Pay

As a general proposition, WTP results may be substantially higher than DFE (Hirshleifer, Bergstrom, and Rappaport 1984). The results in table 13.1 are consistent with this assertion if one considers labor-market WTP studies only (LWTP, studies 10–14 and 16). All of the LWTP studies are based on the presumption that workers perceive the full extent of the risks and have the potential mobility to shift occupations if they do not like a given dictated price for risk taking. Consequently, all of the estimates in table 13.1 should be regarded as very rough approximations. Some perceptions of risk will be reviewed before surveying the specific LWTP studies.

Table 13.1

Value of a Life—Three Basic Approaches: Human-Capital Discounted Future Earnings (DFE), Hypothetical Willingness to Pay from Suggested Consumption Decisions (WTP), and Labor-Market Willingness to Pay (LWTP)

Study	Approach	Data	Value of a Life[a]	Value of a Life in 1992 Dollars
1. Dept. of Defense (1963)	DFE, discounted at 3 percent	U.S. Air Force captain's wages	$135,000 (1962 dollars)	$664,000
2. Dept. of HEW (1967)	DFE, nonmilitary personnel, discounted at 4 percent	a. black male, age 85 b. white male, age 25-29	$396 (1966) $136,121 (1966)	$1,948 $670,000
3. Ford Motor Company (1973)	DFE, study data for federal auto safety officials, discounted at 6 percent	1973 study of the average American DFE, released October 1979 at the Pinto trial	$200,000 (1971)	$788,000
4. Hartunian, Smart, and Thompson (1981)	DFE, discounted at 6 percent	a. male, 25-34 b. female, 25-34	$247,881 (1975) $153,131 (1975)	$711,000 $440,000
5. Schelling (1968)	Hypothetical WTP poll	University-based polling to assess WTP to avoid large risks	$1-$2 million (1967)	$4.6-$9.2 million
6. Acton (1973)	Hypothetical study for a heart-attack ambulance program	a. value to avoid a 0.002 risk of death ($56 mean) b. value to avoid a 0.001 risk of death ($43 mean)	$28,000 (1971) $43,000 (1971)	$109,000 $169,000
7. Blomquist (1979)	WTP based on value drivers place on safety implicit in their demand for seat belts	Seat-belt questionnaire—usage reduces risk from 0.00025 to 0.00010	$257,000 (1975)	$740,000
8. Dardis (1980)	WTP based on consumer demand for smoke detectors, 1974-1979	Implicit valuation from sales and annualized costs for smoke detectors during the five-year period	$101,000 (1976-77)	$259,000

Table 13.1 (Continued)

Study	Approach	Data	Value of a Life[a]	Value of a Life in 1992 Dollars
9. Portney (1981)	WTP assessment of life, home, and environmental quality	Trade-offs implicit in pollution's impact on mortality and housing prices	$355,000 (1977)	$910,000
10. Thaler and Rosen (1976)	LWTP based on actuarial survey of very risky occupations, including all causes of death, not just accidents (no information on actual cause of death)	Observed wages $136 to $260 (mean $176) higher annually to accept an additional death risk of 0.001 per year	$176,000 (1967)	$814,000
11. Smith (1976)	Industrial LWTP risk data (BLS injury data) for hourly workers in manufacturing	a. Observed wages $120-$160 higher annually to accept an additional death risk of 0.00008 per year, 1973, manufacturing. The bias implicit in industrial injury data is that they limit slower causes of death captured in the actuarial data.	$1.5 million (1973)	$5.4 million
		b. 1967, all Industries	$2.5 million (1967)	$11.9 million
12. Viscusi (1978)	Industrial LWTP data controlled for a wide range of occupational characteristics	Industrial risk data, observed wages $60-$180 higher to accept an extra death risk of 0.0001 per year	$600,000-$1.8 million (1970)	$2.4-$7.3 million

Study	Method	Application	Value (year)	Estimate[a]
13. Dillingham (1979)	LWTP based on occupational- and industry-based risk data (wide sample of occupations)	Average observed wages $368 (on average) higher to accept the extra death risk of 0.001 per year	$368,000 (1969)	$1.59 million
14. Olson (1981	Industrial LWTP merged with other occupational data for non-fatal accidents from 70 percent of the industries surveyed by the BLS	a. Average observed annual wages $350 higher to accept an additional risk of 0.000095 per year	$3.2 million (1973)	$11.4 million
		b. Nonunion workers observed annual wages $110 higher to accept an additional risk of 0.00008 per year	$1.4 million (1973)	$5.1 million
		c. Union workers observed annual wages $1,140 higher to accept an extra risk of 0.00014 per year	$8.1 million (1973)	$28.9 million
15. Office of Management and Budget (OMB 1984)	DFE, discounted at 10 percent	Asbestos study	$208,000 (1982)	$402,000
16. Moore and Viscusi (1988)	Industrial LWTP approach like study 11	Observed wages	$5.2-$6.5 million (1986)	$8.6-$11 million
17. Eastaugh (1991)	Hypothetical WTP survey on blood products	Red Cross and George Washington University project	$6.6 million	$7.2 million

aThe "most reasonable" median estimate is reported in most cases; otherwise a range of low and high values is provided.

The world is not a riskless environment. Every product and service used can be shown to be potentially hazardous in some way. For example, in an average month of January, four children died from hazards associated with Christmas toy chests. Should these toy chests be banned? What is the appropriate role for government in this situation? After much reflection, Kass (1975) concluded that the conventional wisdom of "a right to health flies in the face of good sense and serves to undermine personal responsibility." Kass might overestimate the degree to which we can improve the health of the population through personal responsibility and health education, but a riskless society maximizing our safety would surely be a joyless, totalitarian one. Workers have faced occupational risks for centuries, but only in the last century have they extracted a wage premium that is roughly proportional to the measured riskiness of the workplace. An extensive network of insurance reporting systems supplements the industrial accident reporting system of the Bureau of Labor Statistics for fatal and nonfatal incidents. The last five studies in table 13.1 confirm the fact that occupations that are more likely to experience accidents tend to demand a larger risk premium at the bargaining table, presumably to compensate for the expected losses due to injury.

In theory, the LWTP approach provides a valid market measure of the sum total of indirect and intangible benefits. For example, the often-cited Thaler and Rosen (1976) estimate for marginal valuations of safety for select hazardous occupations from the 1967 Survey of Economic Opportunity earnings data extrapolated the value of a life saved to $176,000. Utilizing actuarial data, the authors estimated that on average, workers in certain high-risk occupations demanded an additional $176 a year to accept an extra death risk of 0.001 per year. Thaler and Rosen concluded that a society of workers would together be willing to pay $176,000 (in 1967 dollars) per life saved.

The strength of the Thaler and Rosen study is that they used disaggregate individual actuarial death-rate and wage-rate data by occupation. However, their WTP assessment might be expected to understate the average citizen's WTP, since the data are for 37 very hazardous occupations. The WTP values of those in the very hazardous occupations might represent the viewpoint of the lowest decile of the general population (i.e., these "crazy" individuals have the lowest disutility toward risk in the population and hence value their lives the least). The most basic potential problem with this type of analysis is the assumption that the worker has sufficient information to trade risk for earnings knowledgeably. Better-informed boilermakers and lumbermen might have requested substantially higher wages. The workers might be under the delusion that they are benefiting from thousands of dollars in increased wages per 0.001 increment in risk. Workers might substantially raise the price of risk taking if they had knowledge of the true degree of risk being faced (Eastaugh 1983).

The Thaler and Rosen data provided no information on cause of death nor verification for the assumption that the cause of death was work related. In spite of the fact that Thaler and Rosen included all the relevant disclaimers and expressed little confidence in the precision of their estimate, Bailey (1989) embraced their estimates with total confidence. Given all the disclaimers, it is surprising that Bailey would simply adjust the Thaler and Rosen estimate to allow for inflation, indirect taxes, and special benefit programs (OSHA and workers' compensation) and conclude that $303,000 (in 1978 dollars) was a more reasonable current estimate of the value of a life saved.

A study by Smith (1976) utilizing 1967 data offered the advantages of a more representative range of occupations and controls for the occupation of each worker. Unfortunately, Smith begged the question of allocating the wage compensation for risk between nonfatal and fatal injuries by assuming that more of the compensation was for simple injuries. Smith's definition of a high-risk industry was one with an annual death rate of 16 per 100,000 workers. A low-risk industry had an annual death rate of 8 per 100,000. Smith concluded that workers in high-risk manufacturing industries were willing to receive $1.5 million in pay to forgo saving one industry member's life per annum. The basic problem with the Smith data is that one must assume that job risks in each industry are approximately uniform across occupations within that industry. This assumption may be invalid for many industries.

Subsequent work by Viscusi (1978) reestimated the equations of Smith (1976) using more detailed data for occupational characteristics within an industry. Viscusi's central estimate was roughly half the value of Smith's equation. A later dissertation by Dillingham (1979) replicated the Viscusi study with even more detailed data concerning occupations and risk. His estimates were one-third the central estimate of Viscusi, partially because of the more unfavorable arbitrary allocation of risk compensation between nonfatal injuries and death. Dillingham speculated that previous studies had overstated the variation in risk aversion across occupations.

A study by Olson (1981) disagreed substantially with the work of both Dillingham and Viscusi. The two main advantages of the Olson study relative to studies 10–13 in table 13.1 were that the range of occupations was almost representative of the general economy (not just the most hazardous jobs), and a complex nonlinear risk-wage relationship was estimated. The most significant aspect of the Olson study was that he found a substantial interaction between risk premium and union status. The study year, 1973, represented a peak period for union power in the United States. In this context, the Olson study may have overstated workers' WTP bodily to receive higher wages. The 1973 market situation with lower unemployment and industry operating at above 95 percent capacity might provide workers with the security to value a life above the 1992 level. One might ask: Does the American medical sector ever make decisions with an $8.5-million benefit-to-cost ratio? Yes, in many cases. For example, Himmelstein and Woolhandler (1984) estimated the cost of cholestyramine per myocardial infarction death prevented as $20 million in 1992 dollars.

The WTP study by Blomquist (1979) was based on consumer preference for seat-belt usage (table 13.1, line 7). This hybrid study had some of the attributes of a hypothetical WTP questionnaire in that the consumer responses concerning belt usage were self-reported, but the estimates also incorporated labor-market valuation of the opportunity cost of time. Blomquist imputed a value of life based on belt usage and 13 household parameters. Avoiding injury was part of the rationale for usage, whereas discomfort and time consumption were part of the rationale for nonusage. Blomquist's estimates of the value of life varied from $142,000 to $488,000, with a central estimate of $257,000.

The Moore and Viscusi (1988) LWTP study (table 13.1, line 16) had a range that was very close to that of Viscusi (1978) when expressed in 1992 dollars. The disaggregate studies reporting a relatively low valuation of life (6–10 in table 13.1) avoided one source of bias that hampered studies 11–14, 16, and 17 (table 13.1). These studies, in which analysis was based on aggregate risk assessment for groups rather than on individual risk data, always significantly overestimated the value of a life. To demonstrate this point, consider hypothetical results from a 1982 update of the Olson study. The resulting sample consists of two groups of individuals: (1) 15 percent of the work force in very high risk jobs, defined as an annual extra risk of mortality of 0.0009, and (2) the remaining 85 percent of the sample in zero-risk work situations. The problem with considering only an aggregate risk factor of 0.000135, equal to (0.15×0.0009) plus (0.85×0), is that a reported wage premium of $972 should not be assessed against the 0.000135 risk (yielding a falsely inflated value of life of $7.2 million). In this hypothetical example, the implicit value of life should in fact be calculated as $972 per 0.0009 of extra risk, or $1.08 million per life.

Some individuals may think that the wide range of WTP valuations of life discredits the technique. For example, what would nonunion workers think of a valuation approach that values five nonunion lives as slightly less than one union life? Perhaps these figures reflect positively on the union's ability to act as an agent of the worker and extract the much higher risk premium. One should conclude from this brief survey that improvement in techniques is both possible and necessary. On balance, the public should come to recognize the necessity for making better decisions and hence the necessity to experiment continually with WTP techniques. Two major attempts have been undertaken to reconcile the two styles of WTP studies with the traditional DFE approach (Bailey 1989; Landefeld and Seskin 1982). However, progress has been very slow in developing the theoretical basis for any hybrid technique that could simultaneously capture the positive aspects of both WTP and DFE approaches.

The success of the WTP approach may be somewhat limited, since the methodology is fraught with problems. However, to paraphrase Winston Churchill, the approach is terrible unless you stop and compare it to the alternatives (DFE or doing nothing). The WTP technique generates troublesome questions, but not nearly so troublesome as assuming that a group is merely worth the amount its members can earn, or assuming that political fiat is superior to economic measurement and evaluation. Those who favor political fiat over analysis may take pause to count the number of times pork-barrel projects consumed resources that could have gone to more broadly beneficial projects. Human-service programs and productivity-enhancing projects are generally withering, while breeder reactors and jet bombers increasingly won out in the 1980s despite their net unfavorable cost-benefit ratios.

HYPOTHETICAL WTP SURVEY TECHNIQUES

One central research issue that Arrow (1978), Eastaugh (1983), and others have identified is the timing of a willingness-to-pay evaluation. The issue is whether respondents should be surveyed ex ante under a veil of ignorance concerning their future disease prognosis, or whether the survey should be done ex post on consumers with limited information concerning the prognosis for themselves or members of their socioeconomic group. The problem to be considered is one of response bias, since the ex post WTP responses will surely be highly inflated—that is, the answers will be high because the opportunity costs of those remaining dollars, given the shortened amount of time, are low to the individual about to die. Obviously, people who have a fatal disease may answer with a higher WTP response than the average citizen. However, with some chronic conditions this assertion appears to be false—that is, the general population overstates the burden of all illness more than the actual victims do (Sackett and Torrance 1978). In other words, ex post WTP responses by victims should be adjusted downward because their WTP is based in part on their increased chances of fatality. For example, the WTP for fire protection by store owners on the currently unaffected half of a burning city block would certainly be higher than the WTP of the average store owner in the city. One could not plan a rational public service on the basis of the preferences of respondents undergoing a catastrophe.

Utility preferences need not be linear or independent of wealth. Risk aversion and risk preference can be observed to change over time in the same individual, or concurrently in the same person under different hypothetical situations. However, very few models of lifetime utility functions have suggested a link between individuals' earnings and their WTP for risk reduction (Bailey 1989).

In valuing lifesaving activities for statistical lives, the wording of the question is a very important issue. Consider an example outside the context of health care: If the government wants to help American companies with "incentives," 68 percent of the public favor the program; but if the government wants to provide "subsidies," then 60 percent are against it, even when the programs are exactly equivalent (Kinsley 1981). Economists have discovered a number of elegant techniques to elicit consumer WTP preferences, but such questionnaires have yet to be utilized for making substantial resource-allocation decisions. The most obvious practical problem with hypothetical WTP measures is that the questions could be considered too unreal to be treated seriously by some respondents. One way to avoid this problem is to present a plausible scenario that concerns a risky situation that has recently been reported on all news media.

Figure 13.1
Willingness-to-Pay Preference Questionnaire

Please think for a few minutes about the following five questions and then answer them as best you can. There are no right or wrong answers.

1. By attending class today you have been exposed to a rare, fatal form of Legionnaires disease. The disease has only been coming through the air vents for the past two hours. The probability that you have the disease is six in a thousand, .006. If you have the disease you will die a quick and painless death in one week. There is a cure for the disease that works 33.3% of the time but it has to be taken now. We do not know how much it will cost. You must say now the most you would pay for this cure. If the cure ends up costing more you won't get it. If it costs less, you will pay the stated price, not the maximum you stated.

   How much will you pay? _____

2. Same story as above *except* the risk of getting the disease is now .002 and the cure works 100 percent of the time.

   How much will you pay for the cure? _____

3. Same story as question one *except* the risk of getting the disease, thanks to the poor ventilation in this room, is now .250, and the newest cure works 100% of the time.

   How much will you pay for the cure now? _____

Assume for questions 4 and 5 that you have no prior exposure to the disease:

4. We are conducting experiments on the same disease for which we need subjects. A subject will just have to expose him or herself to the disease and risk a .002 chance of death. What is the minimum fee you would accept to become such a subject? _____

5. Same story as in question 4, except the risk of now getting the disease is .250. What is the minimum fee you would now accept to become such a subject? _____

The survey instruments should also be short. Figure 13.1 is an example of such a WTP questionnaire (Eastaugh 1983).

As with all surveys, the best WTP questionnaires would avoid the use of value-loaded wording. For example, one would not like to ask the question "How much is your grandfather worth?" More reasonable answers will be given if 1,000 people facing a 0.002 chance of dying next year are asked, "How much would you pay to reduce your risk by 0.001?" In other words, the 1,000 individuals are willing to pay the total sum of their responses to save the one statistical life, not to be identified until next year. It is common knowledge that society places very high values on identifiable lives facing a high probability of death or disfigurement. The media frequently report a high level of psychic benefit accruing to the population following a heroic rescue attempt or an attempt to aid an identified child. For example, individuals seem to experience more psychic benefits as a group in supporting the identifiable March of Dimes Poster Child than in supporting Medicaid for multi-institutional charity hospitals. Schelling (1968) was the first to observe that individuals jump to help one six-year-old identified life, but few shed a tear or write a check if a tax shortfall causes facilities to deteriorate, thereby causing a barely perceptible statistical increase in preventable deaths.

The most basic problem with WTP valuation is that the appropriate data base to make estimates with any adequate range of confidence does not exist. Three subsidiary problems concern (1) lack of physician input in identification of the subtle side effects that should go into the analysis, (2) lack of appropriate behavioral-science survey instruments, and (3) lack of an appropriate populace to survey in many cases. As an example of this last problem, in doing a WTP analysis of benzene cleanup activities, how are people to be selected for the survey—workers heavily exposed to benzene, all workers, or all those who bear the burden of the cleanup? Should people with a given disease be sampled while hospitalized, or should potential candidates for the disease be surveyed, or should all citizens be queried? How is the survey instrument to be written if researchers are unsure whether benzene starts to bring about significant increases in the incidence of leukemia by x percent at prolonged exposure levels of 40 parts per million, 20 parts, or 1 part?

Another problem with WTP consumer-preference surveys is that the results may not be very stable over time. The public may express a lower WTP for avoiding a relatively higher and familiar risk (like automobile fatality) than a lower but unfamiliar risk. Some individuals get alarmed over the prospect of a nuclear accident, yet tolerate much higher risks in their daily lives. Moreover, just because the public WTP to avoid uncertain risks is not in direct proportion to the nature and seriousness of some other risks does not mean that the public's preferences should be ignored.

ATTEMPTING TO IMPROVE APPLICATIONS OF WTP THEORY

The WTP preferences of healthy adults were tested on three groups of health professionals using the questionnaire in figure 13.1. The median results are presented in table 13.2 so as not to skew the results by overweighting the importance of the 4 to 8 percent of respondents who think that their life is worth somewhere between $1 billion and infinity. While there is nothing wrong with some people perceiving their value as infinite, it makes the mean response meaningless. The responses would undoubtedly vary across other professions. Within a given profession the median value of life probably varies with age, sex, and income. However, even more interesting than median results across groups is the difference in response for a given individual. First, a pairwise comparison of questions 1 and 2 provides support for the certainty effect. Under the postulated certainty effect, WTP is less for a reduction in probability from a small level (0.006) to an even smaller level (0.004) than WTP for an equivalent

Table 13.2
Imputed Median Willingness-to-Pay (WTP) Value of a Life for Three Groups of Health Professionals, 1990

Sample	Second Year Master's in Health Administration Students	Hospital Administrators in Summer HA Program	Third Year Medical Students
Age range	22-34	30-55	24-31
Sample size	25	23	29

A. Willingness to pay to gain life expectancy (prolong survival)

Q1, .333 cure rate	$250,000[a]	$375,000	$300,000
(.006 x .333)[b]	($500)[c]	($750)	($600)
Q2, perfect 1.0 cure rate	$500,000	$1,000,000	$1,250,000
(.002 x 1.0)	($1,000)	($2,000)	($2,500)
Q3, perfect cure rate	$600,000	$1,000,000	$1,400,000
(.25 x 1.0)	($150,000)	($250,000)	($350,000)

B. WTP to lose expected survival time by gambling as an experimental subject

Q4 (exposure to	$25 million	$50 million	$35 million
a .002 risk)	($50,000)	($100,000)	($70,000)
Q5 (exposure to	$4 million	$6 million	$4 million
a .25 risk)	($1 million)	($1.5 million)	($1 million)

[a]Median imputed value of a life (in this case, the actual median response divided by the .006 x .333 risk).
[b]Actual response situation in parentheses.
[c]Median response to the question on figure 13.1 in parentheses.

reduction in probability from 0.002 to zero. Of the three subject groups in table 13.2, 60 to 75 percent of the respondents in each group gave a lower answer for question 1 relative to question 2, even though the increase in survival probability was identical for each question.

Second, pairwise comparisons of questions 2 and 4 and of questions 3 and 5 lend support for the so-called endowment effect. Of the 77 respondents, 51 percent of the sample reported fivefold higher responses for question 5 than for question 3, and more dramatically, 92 percent of the sample reported fivefold higher responses for question 4 than for question 2. This supports the assertion that people must be paid a substantially higher WTP bribe to risk their endowment of remaining life than to reacquire the same endowment they had already lost due to bad luck.

A third interesting result of pairwise response comparisons is the lack of clear evidence for the von Neumann–Morgenstern game-theory axiom that a person should pay more per unit of risk reduction the higher the absolute level of risk (Luce and Raiffa 1957). A respondent with no bequest motives who obeys the conventional axiom would be expected to pay more per 0.001 of risk reduction the higher the absolute risk (0.25 risk versus 0.002). This axiom is intuitive if one considers the case of how much one is willing to pay to remove 1 bullet in a 500-bullet gun. In the extreme case, a person pays the maximum to remove the 500th bullet and have some chance for life. Analogously, it seems plausible that a 0.002 risk reduction might mean more to a 70-year-old with a 0.3 chance of dying than to a 40-year-old with a 0.01 chance of dying in the next year. However, the scenario in figure 13.1 may not be a fair test for this axiom, since the axiom might hold better in the high-risk section of the mortality probability curve (0.3–1.0) than in the flat of the curve (risks under 0.3). One could speculate that one of the reasons why middle-aged hospital administrators in column 2 of table 13.2 have somewhat higher WTP responses than their administration-student counterparts is that they are older (and therefore more subject to risk and more in touch with their mortality). An interesting ethical issue raised by these data is whether the results should be interpreted literally. Should those who value their lives the most be saved? Under such a WTP criterion, the life of a hospital manager in his forties would be saved before the life of a health administration student in his twenties, in contrast to the DFE higher relative valuation for the younger individual. Perhaps the WTP valuation is more indicative of the full value of individuals to their families, communities, and society (Eastaugh 1983).

In addition to valuing life, consumer-preference surveys can assist in the selection of an optimum therapy. Most progressive physicians have recognized, at least in theory, that treatment decisions should attempt to incorporate patient values into the decision. However, most clinicians are untrained in the disciplines of economics and behavioral decision theory and cannot scientifically survey patient preferences. The sensitive clinician attempts a "quick-and-dirty" approach to get some handle on patient values by asking, "Would you rather have short-term certain survival for say five years or gamble on an operation that has a low probability of death but offers an additional 20 years of life expectancy?" Physicians are increasingly coming to respect the value of asking such questions.

McNeil, Weichselbaum, and Pauker (1978) assessed patient preferences for certain near-term versus potential far-term years of life with a hypothetical gambling scenario. For example, the individual would be given a choice of a 50/50 gamble: (1) a quick death or full life expectancy (25 years) or (2) a guaranteed period of survival (x years). A risk-neutral individual would be indifferent to whether he or she received 12.5 years of guaranteed survival or 25 years times a 0.5 chance for survival. Individuals who select a value of x less than 12.5 are risk averse. A significant minority of patients (21 to 43 percent) are so highly risk averse that depending on their age, they would rather select radiation therapy with a far inferior five-year survival to the surgical alternative (McNeil, Weichselbaum, and Pauker 1978). Physicians are revising their clinical decisions as they discover that many of their patients are risk averse and have made rational internal utility judgments—that is, they prefer definitely surviving over the near term to possibly surviving over the far term (Eastaugh 1991).

Surgeons show a high degree of willingness to let their clients trade short-term survival for long-term survival. Is it fair of the surgeon, in the interest of maximizing professional income, to corner patients into having surgery when the gamble runs counter to patient preferences? Perhaps most surgeons are willing to accept the principle that the best treatment for a given patient is the one with the higher net expected personal utility for the patient. Alternatively, the American surgeon could believe that patients' individual preferences have no place and that the best treatment is the one that adds the most person-years of human capital to the economy (i.e., surgery). This last rule sounds more applicable to the ethos of a Soviet physician. American physicians and surgeons are much more interested in the individual quality of life for the patient after treatment.

Willingness-to-pay surveys are most critical in imperfect markets where the value of a service may exceed the price paid. Businessmen selling cars or strawberries do not need to do willingness-to-pay surveys. The price is the value to the buyer in the marketplace. Mitchell and Carson (1990) raised the interesting possibility of what would happen if businessmen operated in an insured marketplace requiring willingness-to-pay evaluation of value by survey. They offered the example of survey data on the value of strawberries compared to an estimated demand function from the marketplace. The two methods yielded amazingly similar results, suggesting that people pay and receive the equivalent value in the strawberry marketplace. It is probably less true that we are receiving benefits equivalent to expenses in the less perfect health care market. We can improve our valuation tools by doing a better job of estimating WTP of loved ones (surviving family; Cropper and Sussman 1988) and assessing risk (Matchar and Pauker 1987; Warner 1987). Moreover, the theoretical underpinnings of utility analysis can leave the intellectual minefields of the economics department and make the perilous jump to the real world of decision making (Kagel, MacDonald, and Battalio 1990; Safra, Segal, and Spirak 1990). We shall make one such jump to the real world with a survey of the value of disease-free, AIDS-free blood products.

WTP FOR SAFE BLOOD PRODUCTS

In the 1980s the quality of blood products, especially the issue of freedom from disease, created stress and opportunity to develop and market new, safer products and services. Hemoglobin solutions represent one such major new product coming to market in the 1990s. Purified stroma-free hemoglobin solutions were developed in the late 1980s thanks to scientific advances in polymerization, cross-linking technology, and purification/separation technologies. Risk-free hemoglobin solutions can be made from (1) human red cells as starting material, (2) bovine red cells (if the public and the physician community would accept such a product), and (3) perhaps from recombinant-DNA-derived hemoglobin.

According to the three companies that are marketing hemoglobin solutions in 1991, the expected American market demand should increase from 150,000 to 165,000 units (Eastaugh 1991) available in 1992 to 3 to 4 million units available in 1998. If the American demand for transfusions continues to grow at 1.0 percent per year, 13 million units will be needed in 1993 and 13.7 million units in 1998 (net demand after shunting blood outdates to manufacturers for the production of hemoglobin solutions). Hemoglobin solutions are not a perfect substitute for red blood cells, but they offer the following desirable product characteristics: prolonged biologic half life, oxygen binding/dissociation similar to that of red cells, no toxic or immunologic side effects, and stability when stored at room temperature for up to 200 days. This last characteristic is interesting because the product can sit in a vehicle or on the emergency-department shelf for months at room temperature.

A number of studies have suggested the high degree of public anxiety concerning transmissible diseases in the national blood supply (Surgenor et al. 1990). The public is concerned with cutting (or eliminating) the following risks of homologous transfusions: a 1:100 risk per unit of non-A non-B hepatitis, a 1:250 risk of hepatitis B, a 1:5,000 risk of human T-cell leukemia virus, and a 1:100,000 risk of human immunodeficiency virus. Individuals' valuation of risk is dependent on the nature of the risk; that is, the way of dying is important in addition to the estimated chance of dying (Fisher, Chestnut, and Violette 1989). For the purposes of this study a unit dosage of risk involves the four conditions listed above and the odds ratios as provided by the American Red Cross.

In the short run hemoglobin solutions are expected to be derived from human red cells (two units of human cells for every one unit of hemoglobin solution produced). Entrepreneurs have two basic concerns. First, will profits prove sufficient in the face of possible future competition from two substitute products in 7 to 15 years (engineered recombinant-DNA hemoglobin solution and nonhuman [bovine] hemoglobin)? Irrespective of this strategic concern, a second question can be answered by the willingness-to-pay economic technique for placing a value on benefits: Do informed consumers value the product more than (or equal to) the suggested retail price? This is a critical question for predicting the speed of technological diffusion (Urban and Hauser 1989). For example, hemoglobin solutions might experience the same slow growth path as that of intraoperative autologous transfusion (IAT) programs the past five years if they were priced as high as $500 to $600 per unit. The risks of receiving homologous transfusions (and infectious diseases) are the same risks avoided if the patient receives a unit of hemoglobin solution or a unit of his or her own IAT blood. IAT has remained a potential market (slow-growing) rather than a strong growth market because substantial consumer resistance exists at a price of $500 to $600. Payers and consumer groups need a valuation of how much the public would pay for a unit of hemoglobin solution.

The probabilistic nature of this willingness-to-pay survey (1:1,000 chance of being a patient in one of the hypothetical scenarios) is necessary in planning any health benefits plan or public service (see Mishan 1971 or Eastaugh 1983). Financing decisions are made in groups ex ante (up front) before it is known which members of the group have the chance of developing a new disease next year. If one surveys the generosity of 1,000 people to avoid a 0.001 risk of death next year, the resulting sum total represents the group's willingness to save one statistical life (not to be identified until next year). One cannot plan a rational public service on the basis of the preferences of respondents undergoing a catastrophe. Consider two examples of poorly written biased questions:

1. What is your willingness to pay for fire protection during a fire, given that you live on the currently unaffected half of the burning block?
2. What is your willingness to pay for new drug X if your chance of dying from AIDS in the next 12 months is currently 99 percent?

The second question is a classic example of the von Neumann–Morgenstern game-theory axiom that a person should pay more per unit of risk reduction the higher the absolute level of risk (see Eastaugh 1983 or Schelling 1968). In other words, one would pay more to reduce risks 0.01 from 99 to 98 percent than for an equal percentage-point reduction from 3.0 to 2.0 percent. If a gun were 100 percent loaded with bullets, in a game of Russian roulette most people would pay the maximum amount to take that first bullet out of the gun. However, in a gun with 999 empty chambers and only one bullet, most people would pay a risk-eradication premium (extra amount) to achieve zero risk (Eastaugh 1983; one pays more to cut risk from 0.001 to 0.0 than to cut risk from 0.002 to 0.001). Regulators and insurance executives make decisions based on probability estimates. If the average group member would pay $1,000 to avoid a 0.001 risk of death in 1992, then the group is acting as if the value of life equaled $1.0 million (or $1,000/0.001). However, one's estimates in such surveys include intangible benefits (not simple mortality reduction): pain reduction, time saved, and freedom from worry.

Some bias exists in any willingness-to-pay survey. For example, heterosexual nondrinkers express a lower willingness to pay for avoiding a relatively higher and familiar risk (automobile fatality) than a lower but unfamiliar risk (dying from AIDS or dying in a nuclear power plant meltdown). Just because the public willingness-to-pay response to avoid uncertain risks is not in direct proportion to the nature and seriousness of the risk does not mean that the public's pref-

erences should be ignored. Willingness to pay is less biased than the old traditional alternative: discounted future earnings (Schelling 1968). WTP methods
are not biased against the old, the handicapped, the AIDS patient, or any particular racial group. The discounted future earnings approach runs counter to the
emerging ethic that "health care is a right," not just a luxury good consumed
in proportion to the patient's ability to pay cash for better care.

A WTP survey was undertaken to assess the tangible and intangible (e.g.,
anxiety reduction) benefits to the public from this new product. An informed
population of 20 regional blood-bank managers and 50 health-services-
administration students was surveyed in 1990. Such a study was intended to
offer insight into two basic questions. The first question concerned coverage:
Should third-party payers cover this benefit (pay for hemoglobin solutions at
triple the price of packed red blood cells) and so assist the diffusion of this new
technology? The second question is the industrial marketing issue (Kotler 1991)
concerning whether there will be consumer price resistance for hemoglobin
solutions within the suggested price range of $225 to $300 per unit. Production
of hemoglobin solutions will involve $110 to $120 per unit of direct expense
and an estimated $40 to $60 of marketing and distribution expense. The entrepreneurs at Baxter Healthcare, Northfield Labs, and Biopure are targeting a 50
percent profit margin for this new product.

Five hypothetical patient scenarios were presented to a group of 20 regional
blood managers and 50 health-administration graduate students (Eastaugh 1991).
The five cases were shuffled and presented in random order so as not to bias the
results (e.g., scenario 1 was presented first 20 percent of the time). The five
scenarios can be summarized as follows:

Scenario 1: An elective surgery patient with no previous history of transfusions
has deposited (because of her fear of getting AIDS) two units of her autologous
blood for use during surgery. Bleeding is excessive, so two units of homologous
red cells are transfused along with autologous blood. With hemoglobin solutions,
two units of solution can be administered during surgery. The net risk reduction
is two units (from two to zero units of homologous blood being used).

Scenario 2: A helicopter arrives to transport an auto accident victim (bleeding
profusely from a crushed leg) to the nearest shock-trauma center. The patient is
stabilized and receives four units of homologous red cells. With hemoglobin
solutions, the patient would receive two units of hemoglobin solution in the
helicopter and a total of only two units of homologous blood at the trauma center.
The net risk reduction is two units (risk reduced from four units to two).

Scenario 3: An emergency-department (ED) patient vomits a large volume of
bright red blood. The blood bank is called, but compatibility testing is not
complete. The only option is to request six units of un-cross-matched O-negative
blood and infuse, risking a delayed transfusion reaction. With the new hemoglobin solutions, and with an adequate supply of solution on the ED shelf, ready
to use without any cross-matching, six units of solution will sustain the patient's

oxygen-transport needs for a few hours. The patient ends up receiving only three units of homologous blood components (rather than nine units). The net risk reduction is six units.

Scenario 4: A patient has been admitted for lifesaving liver transplant surgery. The patient requires 20 units of homologous blood products. With hemoglobin solutions, the first 10 units of red cells can be substituted by an equivalent concentration of solution. The net risk reduction is 10 units (from 20 to 10 units of homologous red cells).

Scenario 5: During a balloon angioplasty the patient has a balloon inserted in the coronary artery and inflated to open the occlusion. No provision is made to supply oxygen to tissue distal to the balloon during the procedure, so the probability of a fatal heart attack for this very sick patient is 3.0 percent. With hemoglobin solutions, the solution is perfused through the balloon during the procedure to deliver oxygen to the cardiac tissue distal to the balloon during the procedure, thus cutting the risk of death for this very sick individual to 1.5 percent. The net risk reduction is 1.5 percent (from 3.0 to 1.5 percent). (Note that this is an example of hemoglobin solutions offering a potentially improved procedure. However, for the bulk of less severely ill coronary artery disease cases the risk reduction from hemoglobin solution perfusion might be less significant, e.g., cutting the risk of fatal heart attacks from 0.21 percent to 0.19 percent and cutting the risk of nonfatal heart attacks from 2.5 to 2.45 percent, but the patient in scenario 5 is very sick.)

Each respondent was presented with these five scenarios and asked to consider a situation where he or she had a 1:1,000 chance of being that patient next year. The question was how much the respondents were willing to pay to have hemoglobin solutions available and reduce their level of risk (scenarios 2, 3, 4, and 5) or eliminate their risk (scenario 1). Survey results compared the responses to scenarios 1 and 2 in table 13.3, in which risk was cut by two units (from two to zero units in scenario 1 and from four to two units in scenario 2). Blood managers rationally attach a premium to the elimination of risk. That premium equals $1,000 for the median respondent ($2,000 in question 2 minus $1,000 in question 4). There exists a point where risk is so high that the measured marginal benefit from risk reduction offers only $100 of benefit (median response to question 4, units of risk cut from 20 to 10 units of homologous blood). This plateau of diminishing benefit or diminishing willingness to pay (WTP) is apparent in the declining median values for both samples (tables 13.3 and 13.4).

The results in table 13.4 for students confirm two previous findings (Eastaugh 1983) that young graduate students have WTP responses that are slightly lower than those of managers over the age of 40. One could speculate that blood managers are more educated in risk assessment and are also older and therefore more subject to risk and more in touch with their mortality. To this point the analysis has focused on the median individual, the 50th percentile. One should also consider subgroups. Judging by the results in table 13.3 for the 10th percentile, the least risk-averse older managers are most likely to admit a point of

Table 13.3
Imputed Willingness to Pay (WTP) for Valuation of a Unit of Risk-free Hemoglobin Solution and the Value of a Statistical Life Saved (Blood Distribution Managers)

	In Dollars		
		Tails of the Distribution	
Scenarios	Median	10th Percentile	90th Percentile
S₁ Risk reduction to avoid 2 units of risk[a] (2 cut to 0)	$4 (2,000)[b]	$2 (1,000)	$100 (5,000)
S₂ Risk reduction to avoid 2 units of risk (4 cut to 2)	$2 (1,000)	0 0	$4 (2,000)
S₃ Risk reduction to avoid 6 units of risk (9 cut to 3)	$5 (833)	$2 (333)	$10 (1,666)
S₄ Risk reduction to avoid 10 units of risk (20 cut to 10)	$1 (100)	0 0	$5 (250)
S₅ Reducing the risk of death from a required procedure from 3.0% to 1.5% with respondent given a 1:1,000 chance of being this patient	$100	$5	$200
Implicit value of life in S₅	$6.6 million	$330,000	$13.2 million

Source: Eastaugh (1991).
Note: Sample N = 20 blood distribution managers, mean age = 52.
[a]A unit of risk equals the risk of one unit of homologous blood, which in 1990, according to the American Red Cross, had a 1:100,000 chance of human immunodeficiency virus, a 1:5,000 chance of human T-cell leukemia virus, a 1:250 chance of hepatitis B, and a 1:100 chance of non-A non-B hepatitis.
[b]Dollar value per unit of solution in percentages.

Table 13.4
Imputed Willingness to Pay (WTP) for Valuation of a Unit of Risk-free
Hemoglobin Solution and the Value of a Statistical Life Saved (Health-
Administration Students)

| | In Dollars | | |
| | | Tails of the Distribution | |
Scenarios	Median	10th Percentile	90th Percentile
S_1 Risk reduction to avoid 2 units of risk (2 cut to 0)	$3 (1,500)[a]	$1 (500)	$8 (4,000)
S_2 Risk reduction to avoid 2 units of risk (4 cut to 2)	$2 (1,000)	$1 (500)	$3 (1,500)
S_3 Risk reduction to avoid 6 units of risk (9 cut to 3)	$4 (666)	$1 (167)	$7 (1,167)
S_4 Risk reduction to avoid 10 units of risk (20 cut to 10)	$1 (100)	$0.5 (50)	$5 (250)
S_5 Reducing the risk of death from a required procedure from 3.0% to 1.5% with respondent given a 1:1,000 chance of being this patient	$40	$5	$70
Implicit value of life in S_5	$2.64 million	$330,000	$4.62 million

Source: Eastaugh (1991).
Note: Sample N = 50 health-administration students, mean age = 27.
[a]Dollar value per unit of solution in parentheses.

diminishing returns and scarce resources and thus report a WTP value of zero under scenarios 2 and 4.

Irrespective of the reasons underlying the responses, the important thing is that people in their 20s and 50s exhibit a willingness to pay for a new product that is in excess of the minimum price needed by the manufacturer to make a target level of profit. Results for scenario 5 in table 13.3 for the value of a life, a median value of $6.6 million in 1990 dollars, are consistent with a number of studies in table 13.1. The future offers interesting challenges and opportunities for diversification into the hemoglobin solution business.

GOING BEYOND SURVIVAL: WEIGHTING THE QUALITY OF THE YEARS

We have been reviewing techniques to value life, but there are also important valuation questions concerning the quality of survival. In this context Stewart, Ware, and Johnston (1975) and Hadorn and Hays (1991) developed scales for measuring physical, social, psychiatric, and mobility limitations. The psycho-metric approach provided improvements over the 1948 Visick scales. Multiat-tribute utility theory has been applied to evaluate the benefits of treating sore throats (Giaque and Peebles 1976) and cleft lips in children (Krischer 1976). One of the best practical applications of these concepts was provided by Wein-stein, Pliskin, and Stason (1977) in their assessment of quality-of-life consid-erations after coronary artery bypass surgery. Quality-of-life outcome measures include pain at rest, pain with minimal activity, pain with mild activity, pain with strenuous activity, and no pain. Quite predictably, a potential surgical patient places a higher utility value on no pain if he avoids exercise. A utility function to value outcomes was specified as a function of life-style and life expectancy. The data are highly subjective, but reliance on imperfect analysis provides more insights than analytical nihilism.

The less tangible quality-of-life benefits comprise an increasing proportion of medical care benefits. For example, elective surgical expenditures are properly intended to achieve less tangible quality-of-life goals than mortality- or morbid-ity-rate reduction, such as relief of disability, pain, and disfigurement (Bunker, Barnes, and Mosteller 1977). Such quality-of-life factors are to be identified, then quantified in terms of their equivalent social costs by shadow-pricing, and finally balanced against commensurate shadow prices for quantity of life. Ad-vocates of the willingness-to-pay approach suggest the maximization of lives saved (Zeckhauser 1975) or, alternatively, quality-adjusted life years (QALYs) saved as the social objective. The decision sciences improved the traditional health-status indexes by multiplying life years by a weighting factor that reflects the quality of those years. The resulting QALY index was originally suggested by Fanshel and Bush (1970) and later developed by Torrance (1976) and Zeck-hauser and Shepard (1976), and Wagstaff (1991). QALY utility analysis pre-sumes risk neutrality, utility independence, and a constant proportional trade-off between life years and health status. Social issues of equity-efficiency trade-offs are familiar in acute medical care. A more general family of multiattribute utility functions that forgoes the risk-neutrality assumption has been applied to coronary bypass surgery (Pliskin, Shepard, and Weinstein, 1980).

Zeckhauser and Shepard (1976) made arbitrary assignments of QALYs saved. They assigned a QALY value of 0.8 to the year in which a nonfatal heart attack occurs and suggested a value of 0.95 for the second year because the patient's health has improved. If one dies, that year is given a QALY value of zero. One could speculate that even a coma patient experiencing psychosocial death before the inevitable biological death would place some low value on person-years of life spent in a coma (perhaps 0.02 of a QALY, plus or minus 0.02). A typical terminal cancer patient treated with the typical American level of narcotics to dull the pain might value a person-year at 0.10. The counterpart English patient provided with much higher doses of narcotics might value life at double that level because he or she feels less pain, and the high doses of narcotics, such as morphine, depress the respiratory function and shorten the painful dying process.

Research by McNeil, Weichselbaum, and Pauker (1981) indicated that 20 percent of cancer patients in the sample group were interested in trading off some quantity of life to acquire more quality of life. In this study one in five patients would forgo surgery and the resultant improved average longevity to preserve normal speech. The study group as a whole considered life without speech to be equal to 86 percent of life with it. The time-trade-off technique for scaling consumer preferences for states of health has been tried in other contexts. Sackett and Torrance (1978) reported lower values of utility for a wide range of chronic conditions (tuberculosis, 0.68; mastectomy, 0.48; long-term depression, 0.44; and hospital dialysis, 0.32 of a lifetime without the disability; perfect health equals 1, death equals 0). A sample response might help clarify the technique.

If a 40-year-old woman with a life expectancy of 33 years were willing to equate 23 years in perfect health with 33 years of life with tuberculosis, the relative value of a life with tuberculosis would be 23/33 or 0.70 for the individual. Temporary conditions were valued as less of a burden. A variation of this technique was applied by Card (1980). Card asked the respondents to specify a maximum surgical mortality they would accept to avoid blindness. He reported that the average medical professional was willing to undergo a 20 percent risk to avoid complete blindness. The value of life with blindness was projected to be 0.80. McNeil and Pauker (1982) reviewed the sources of bias in the two approaches. The time-trade-off approach seems to understate the positive utility of a person-year with a given condition—that is, it overstates the disutility of having a disease. In our tuberculosis example, the woman may understate the value of losing 10 years of life (years 63 to 73), and consequently the 0.70 estimate for tuberculosis may be an underestimate. The surgical mortality to avoid the disease gamble posed by Card (1980) has the opposite bias—overestimating the utility of a person-year with a given disease. Many respondents may overreact in favor of living with any condition to avoid the distasteful alternative, instant surgical death, hence overstating the value of having a condition (i.e., 0.8 for complete blindness seems high).

The standard method of QALY analysis is to run a Markov simulation (based on existing data points) comparing survival rates until all patients will have died and to add up all the quality-weighted years of life per capita for each alternative treatment group (Pauker and Kassirer 1987). For example, in a study of women with node-negative breast cancer, Hillner and Smith (1991) reported that adjuvant chemotherapy for an average 45-year-old woman added 5.1 quality months to life expectancy (at an average cost of $15,400 per quality year). For an average 60-year-old woman, chemotherapy added 4.0 quality months to life expectancy (at an average cost of $18,800 per quality year). Consequently, the chemotherapy was worth the expense for women in this age cohort with average health status. For women with poor health status, a small gain of 1.4 to 2.0 quality months of lifetime benefit might not justify chemotherapy.

Individual judgment of risk may be biased. On average, people in all risk strata may exhibit an optimistic bias about personal risks (Weinstein 1989). Weinstein speculated that most people, and especially young women with children, will overestimate their benefit gain and underestimate negative side effects (toxicity in chemotherapy). More research should be done concerning the topic of measurement error (Kirscht 1989). Smith, McKinlay, and McKinlay (1989) demonstrated that self-reporting in their risk-appraisal study was consistent for some items and highly inconsistent for other items (diet, physical activity, stress, and cholesterol).

One study suggested an interesting alternative to QALYs. Mehrez and Gafni (1991) suggested healthy-year equivalents (HYEs) as a measure of health status that combines the two attributes of interest, the quantity and quality of life. Unlike normative QALYs, HYEs fully represent patients' preferences, because they are calculated from each individual's utility using the standard gamble approach—that is, the approach uses a combination of lottery questions to assess the individuals' utility preference. More research is needed to measure the validity and reliability of the HYE concept. Mehrez and Gafni suggested that the reproducibility of the measures is satisfactory, in line with previous studies (Eastaugh 1991, 1983).

Doctors agree that patient preference is important in some circumstances, but if clinicians do not know how to quantitate the trade-off, they often overlook the issue of individual preference. A relatively unconventional, but rational, treatment, like wearing a truss for a hernia or trying radiation therapy for cancer of the larynx, is often ignored, downplayed, or misrepresented (relative to how ''wonderful'' surgery can be). Both society and the individual may not want to value all years of life equally. For example, a national artificial-heart program in 1993 (an unlikely possibility) may cost $300,000 to $900,000 per person-year of life saved (Lubeck 1982), and these person-years of life may only have a QALY value of 0.70 or 0.80. Alternatively, one might devote $1 billion to a nationwide cardiac disease prevention program like the Stanford Heart Disease Prevention Program's Three Community Study. The prevention alternative would be saving person-years of life with QALY values in excess of 0.95. Lubeck did not specifically take QALYs into account, but the issues of QALY weights may prove more critical in other cases (e.g., bone marrow transplants). The decision concerning a strategy to combat heart disease is a simpler case, since the benefit-to-cost ratio is somewhere between 20 to 200 times higher in the preventive program than in a heart implant program.

FUZZY REALITY AND THE RATIONALE FOR LISTENING TO JOHN Q. PUBLIC

Physicians and consumers typically deal with probabilities with a terminology that can best be described as fuzzy semantics: very likely, unlikely, very rare, and so on. The user of fuzzy probability statements often obscures the fact that the underlying uncertainty is possibilistic rather than probabilistic—that is, imprecise data lead to imprecise statements concerning possibilities. The concept of probability is based firmly on recorded outcomes (as a proportion or likelihood), and possibility is a more abstract concept to describe ''ease of compatibility.'' It is often said that a low possibility implies a low probability, but a high possibility need not imply a high probability (e.g., it is highly possible but not very probable that individual X has disease Y; Eastaugh 1991). Pathologists are unpopular with their fellow physicians for utilizing fuzzy language like ''cannot be ruled out'' or ''consistent with.'' This fuzzy language has been defended on the basis of the accuracy with which it describes the conditional possibilities (Legg 1981). This viewpoint is contrary to the statistical school of thought founded by Thomas Bayes. The Bayesian ''true-believer'' viewpoint is that all probability guesstimates are real numbers to be manipulated regardless of the imprecise nature of the limited data set.

Physicians do not like to be pinned down by patients on fuzzy issues such as ''What is the chance of improvement? Give me a number.'' Physicians who exhibit undue ex ante optimism concerning the prognosis for an individual patient are committing one of the most common human foibles. For example, economists have observed the phenomenom of overoptimism among poker players in overvaluing the chance of benefits (and prior winnings) and undervaluing the chance of losing (and understating prior losses). Adam Smith (1776) described this overoptimism in the context of health care: ''The overwhelming conceit which the greater part of men have of their own abilities is an ancient evil. . . . The chance of gain is by every man more or less over-valued . . . the chance of loss is undervalued, and by scarce any man in tolerable health (seldom) values loss more than it is worth.'' In considering WTP measures to value benefits, one should be cognizant of these potential respondent biases. However, that does not imply that we should ignore or downplay consumers' values, as some have suggested. Future research should address the question of whether the excessive faith the public has in new medical technology makes WTP surveys highly sensitive to misleading advertising campaigns or, alternatively, whether ''blind'' public faith in medicine is on the wane. The first position is supported by the Chicago Mount Sinai Medical Center 1977 market survey, which reported that area residents believed that medicine has future miracle techniques and spare parts to fix them no matter how they live their lives. The second position—

eroding faith in biomedical techniques and equipment—is supported by media reports concerning the frequency of malpractice. Public interest in medical problems and problems with the health-services delivery system is evidenced by the fact that over half of the stories in *Reader's Digest* and *National Enquirer* concern health issues. The coverage in these magazines and others is getting increasingly pessimistic about new medical techniques.

FIGHTING ANALYTICAL NIHILISM

One important motto that most politicians bear in mind is to "keep the experts on tap rather than on top." While it is good that we do not presently have a society run by technocrats, it seems reasonable to point out the shortcomings of our current political system. Politicians react to power rather than judiciously weighing all the facts and unquantifiable aspects of the issue. As a result, they have not been able to galvanize concern over the medical cost crisis to make simple benefit-coverage-limitation decisions. In this context, Blumenthal, Feldman, and Zeckhauser (1982) outlined a number of difficulties the government may face in making health insurance benefit-coverage decisions based on economic analysis. Given the rapidly expanding vista of new medical technology and the antiregulatory mood in Congress, it is hard to expect any one regulatory body to preempt the collective judgments of 6,000 hospitals and half a million clinicians.

The performance of the economics profession has not been without fault. There has been a high degree of public and political disenchantment with model builders who provide narrow definitions of direct benefits and ignore the limitations of their very crude data bases. Little theoretical work has been done to assess the degree to which workers weigh the price of risk taking and consider the probability of premature work-related death as a variable that is subject to their control.

The multiplicity of quality-of-life dimensions for weighting health benefits will always require the use of consensus decision making and value judgments. How else can society weigh the value of a 55-year-old's life saved against a 5-year-old's case of blindness prevented? Encapsulated in the classic quip that economists "know the price of everything and the value of nothing" is the realization that there are theoretical limitations to either market prices or willingness-to-pay prices in valuing benefits (Torrance 1986). Prices do not reflect the value of externalities and other assurances (of capacity if needed) enjoyed by nonusers of the service, and the imperfectly informed user of the service may fail to appreciate all the direct or indirect benefits accrued. If consumers valued health care as much as public health professionals, society could simply stop 52 million American smokers from puffing (Wasserman et al. 1991) and perhaps feed the tobacco plants to 5 million hungry livestock. The outcome of this scenario seems Pareto optimal to some health officials—that is, 350,000 individuals are prevented from dying annually and the world is fed with a few extra million cattle annually. Resources are distributed Pareto optimal if there is no alternative allocation that leaves everyone at least as well off and makes some people strictly better off. If a situation is *not* Pareto efficient, it means that there is some way to make somebody better off without hurting anyone else. This rather simplistic analysis overlooks one very important item. Consumers of hazardous chemicals report many intangible personal benefits that far outweigh the personal health and social costs to them.

Mishan (1971) pointed out that while our enlightened society can hardly avoid making WTP analytical efforts, shadow-pricing and value weighting present a multitude of difficulties for research. If consumers are provided with imperfect information, individuals' willingness to pay will sometimes be underestimated (e.g., vaccinations) and other times overestimated (e.g., laetrile). Unfortunately, prima facie evidence does not exist to suggest that every patient should have his or her own family decision analyst to perform risk analysis.

How much consumers are willing to pay for a specific therapy is highly dependent on their current health status. For example, Thompson (1986) estimated that persons without difficulty in climbing steps would pay roughly 19 percent of their income (or $5,160 annually) for a cure to their arthritis. This same figure almost doubled (to 35 percent) for those unable to climb steps. Willingness to pay, not surprisingly, is also correlated with pain (self-rated). Subjects without pain stated that they were willing to pay 15 percent, on average, of their income to be cured of arthritis, in contrast to 32 percent for those with the highest-rated pain levels. Thompson reported reasonable, consistent, and rational patterns of response to the WTP survey for over 84 percent of the 247 patients with rheumatoid arthritis. This pattern of plausibility reflects a good questionnaire design, in contrast to some earlier studies (Muller and Reutzel 1984).

WTP INCLUSION OF INTANGIBLE BENEFITS: DEFENDING AIDS RESEARCH

Congress in 1991 criticized the cost of AIDS research in normative terms, relative to the lower cost of cancer clinical trials. While it is true that AIDS research programs are five times as expensive per patient as cancer clinical trials, the reasons for this differential are manifold and complex (e.g., varying levels of private insurance coverage subsidizing patient care and research expenses). Future health care managers should be well prepared in four disciplines to justify biomedical research: accounting, health economics (joint costing of multiple products—care, research, and education), finance (e.g., start-up costs of initiating a research team and the annual fixed and variable costs of operation), and medicine (impact of patient severity and longevity on costs). With correct tools drawn from these four disciplines, health care managers can work with policy makers to enhance efficiency, protect the public health, and improve the biomedical capacity of the nation. This management-science approach may call into question the conventional wisdom that AIDS trials are grossly inefficient or mismanaged.

In 1991 acquired immune deficiency syndrome (AIDS) ranked as the fifth leading cause of premature mortality in the nation. The federal government is investing an increasingly larger share of the National Institutes of Health (NIH) budget in AIDS research ($1.74 billion FY 1992), and analysis of the cost of research clinical trials is of considerable interest to Congress, payers, and providers. A recent estimate (Hellinger, 1991) suggests that the lifetime medical care cost of a person with AIDS is $85,333. An estimated $10.4 billion will be spent treating all Americans with AIDS in 1994. The NIH AIDS research program will increasingly compete with other health programs in the budget process. AIDS research may have resulted in only a 10 percent reduction in the National Cancer Institute (NCI) budget for 1991, but just one-fourth of cancer grant applications approved by review committees on the basis of scientific merit received funding in 1991 (compared to a 46 percent NCI funding rate for FY 1980). One in every six comprehensive specialty cancer centers nationwide is scheduled to receive no NCI support over the next two years. In macroeconomic terms, the federal Office of Management and Budget (OMB) appears to think that the nation should make cancer facilities pay for AIDS research and patient care (Eastaugh 1991, 1989).

Hospital-based medical research is caught between a rock and the proverbial hard place. The "rock" comes in the form of nonfederal payers for health services: They are increasingly labeling "research" or "experimental" as a synonym for "payment denied." After two decades of ignoring their written regulations, insurance companies are enforcing out-of-date clauses that claim that they do not pay for experimental drugs or high-tech biologicals. In such cases, must providers decrease service to patients with nonstandard conditions like AIDS and cancer? The unintended consequence of the 1980s' cost-control movement is that the constraints forced insurance companies and state Medicaid programs to take a minimalist approach to paying for severely ill AIDS patients.

The centrality of clinical trials to enhance the delivery of state-of-the-art patient care is an axiom of American medicine. The incentives for the school and the hospital to participate are obvious. A clinical trial guarantees reimbursement and therefore subsidizes patient-care revenues for the hospital. Research grants subsidize faculty salaries and indirect costs of the medical school. Three basic policy research questions should be considered. First, what factors explain the variations in costs between AIDS programs? For example, there may be a wide variation in social-service costs and special medical needs of AIDS patients that place higher (or lower) burdens on their research units. Some facilities are less expensive because they have more volunteer "free" labor or more generous reimbursement from city, local, or state governments to pay for costs that would otherwise be underwritten by the National Institute for Allergy and Infectious Diseases (NIAID) grant. The patient mix will differ between facilities (Turner, Kelly, and Ball 1989), so the evaluation will have to consider a measure of patient severity (with four stages of illness; stage one is the least expensive; Kaposi's sarcoma cases cost less than stage-three complex infectious disease cases, which in turn cost less than a stage-four Pneumocystis carinii pneumonia case). One must adjust for patient severity and external subsidies (free labor or a more generous reimbursement climate) to answer the first research question concerning relative efficiency of clinical trial AIDS programs.

The second question is normative. Why do AIDS trials cost NIH 2 to 10 times as much as cancer trials in the same institutional context, in the same hospital? Some of the added cost of AIDS trials, in comparison to cancer trials, is undoubtedly related to the fixed costs of initiating a new research team, the inefficiency implicit in rushing the effort to fight this new plague as quickly as possible, and the lower generosity of third-party payers to finance AIDS costs in comparison to cancer patient/research costs. AIDS patients have social-service needs and special medical costs that place greater burdens on their research units, burdens that are not experienced in clinical trials of other diseases (e.g., oat-cell cancer of the lung, a subset of DRG 82, certain lymphomas in DRG 404, or Hodgkin's disease within DRG 403). A suggested 1993 federal study on AIDS-fund allocation will identify routine medical care items that third-party payers reimburse for cancer patients but avoid or underpay for AIDS patients. Underpaying for AIDS cases is not a conspiracy, but can often result from insufficient cost-accounting information on-site, especially in public hospitals. Cost-accounting expertise varies widely among hospitals and medical schools. AIDS patients require much more intensive nursing care than cancer patients, including special isolation techniques, but the third-party payers cannot pay a nursing differential if the hospitals do not document the increased minutes of nursing time for AIDS patient care. The indirect benefits of extra nursing care must also be measured.

The third question is how to identify lean (efficient) quality research programs and low-cost (but not so efficient) research units in a generous environment (thanks to third-party payers) or a nurturing environment from a critical mass of research support. To address this last research question, a fund-flow analysis on a case-study basis must be performed to identify sources of cross-subsidy. AIDS clinical/research costs will be compared to cancer trial costs within the same facility. If the hospital under study has an insufficient number of oat-cell lung cancer cases or Hodgkin's cases, three other types may be selected from DRGs 402, 403, and 404.

The cancers selected were selected by physicians because the multimodel therapy for each is primarily nonsurgical (as with AIDS). Oat-cell cancer as a comparative analog to AIDS has the advantage of similar mortality statistics to AIDS and more innovation in treatment modalities (recently) than Hodgkin's disease. Hodgkin's disease has the advantage of a generally younger patient population compared to the age distribution for AIDS cases. Congress should fund econometric studies to provide a precise estimate of the multiple factors that determine the cost of AIDS care and the cost of research. The effect that one variable alone might exert on research costs (or relative costs of AIDS versus oncology) could be determined while controlling for all the other confounding factors.

AIDS is a very expensive condition, and other sources of financial support should not go underutilized. In May 1988 the National Center for Health Services Research and Health Care Technology Assessment (now the Agency for Health Care Policy and Research [AHCPR]) estimated the cumulative lifetime costs for AIDS patients by 1991 at $61,800 per person, more than $30,000 less than previous forecasts. The inclusion of azidothymidine (AZT) in this forecast and the expectation of new coordinated systems for managed care (alternative settings, hospices, and home health care) were the two critical factors in this $61,800 estimate. Lifetime costs for other conditions range from $68,700 for paraplegia due to auto accidents to $67,000 for middle-age heart attacks, and $44,000 to $47,500 for gastrointestinal cancer or oat-cell cancer of the lung or Hodgkin's disease. These estimates for the cost of treating AIDS are now in the ballpark compared to the cost of treating other serious illnesses. The intangible benefits that certain AIDS social programs offer must be shadow priced by WTP surveys.

AIDS care and clinical research is expensive for a number of reasons. Some research teams attempted to collect far too much data per patient. The clinical intensity and dollar expense of required monitoring of AIDS patients is clearly a more substantial cost item in explaining the high cost of research. Immunoassays involved in AIDS research can cost $200,000 to $600,000 per year, including costs for 12 to 36 laboratory technicians, 1 to 3 research associates, and a full-time immunologist involved in AIDS research. There are substantial problems in separating research costs from patient-care costs and educational costs. Shared service arrangements back and forth between medical school and hospital have significant monetary value, but because of the generally informal nature of the affiliation the shared items are not captured by the accounting systems. Therefore, in the process of site visits accountants should identify the resource flows and shadow-price a monetary value on items utilized in the process of delivering the joint products of care, research, and education. Such fund flows will seldom act as a perfect offset (balance zero); the hospital will feel undercompensated from the school, but this cost imbalance may be offset by the services that faculty and doctors in training render to the hospital (see Chapter 8).

Once a uniform national data base is compiled, researchers in 1993 will employ a statistical method called multiple linear regression to explain the variation in AIDS and cancer costs for research and patient care as a function of a number of independent variables:

1. Patient severity level (four levels)

2. Five patient age groupings (10 percent are children)

3. Fraction of total labor cost that is free (volunteer)

4. Intern and resident full-time equivalents per bed

5. Patient eligibility for reimbursement through a private insurance company

6. The federal wage index for national area wage differences for hospital employees

Four independent variables as an index for infrastructure or research capacity will be included:

1. Number of principal investigators with active NIH grants

2. Other research dollars (in millions)

3. Age of research program (years)

4. A dichotomous variable for whether the program administrator is an oncologist or infectious-diseases specialist

AIDS reimbursement and research funding is a rapidly changing field. A principal investigator trained in infectious diseases may be unfamiliar with the concept of billing routine inpatient costs to the patient's insurance company and thus overutilize a NIH grant to subsidize patient care. Both oncologists and infectious-diseases specialists may be inexperienced with alternative channels for cost recovery. On the other hand, the high cost of AIDS trials may be closer to the true cost of clinical research; that is, it may be the case that AIDS is not overpaid, but that cancer is underpaid in normative terms.

A continuum-of-care San Francisco managed-care model has been emulated in a number of cities, but the supply of volunteer workers varies widely across the nation. Of the total AIDS patient resource dollars going to health care services, the percentage of costs going to hospitals ranges as high as 60 percent at UCLA and George Washington University and 80 percent for three New York City hospitals. The hospital need not get such a high percentage of the AIDS patient dollar (from all sources, not just federal and state government). But without an ample supply of volunteers, managed care may only reduce the amount of total AIDS patient costs going to hospitals to the 40 to 50 percent range. With the San Francisco supply of volunteers this figure can be driven down to 25 percent of the AIDS dollars going to hospital care. In the context of low historic occupancy figures of teaching hospitals (outside New York City), private teaching hospitals may continue to view insured AIDS patients as a source of cash flow to replace "cold sheets" with some marginal revenue. Hospitals with a commendable business office and an oncologist in charge of the AIDS grant can work to hold down the amount of patient-care costs billed on the NIH grant by billing private insurance firms.

Patient-care costs billed to the NIAID research grant can run between 0 and 41 percent of the grant. Hospitals run by infectious-diseases specialists report a certain timidity toward billing the patient's insurance company because of (1) the stigma of AIDS and (2) the ease with which such costs can be charged to NIH. Economists refer to this second attitude as the "free-rider" approach to grant management. All charges associated with the protocols, such as clinical laboratory tests, X-rays, and scans, are charged to the NIH grant; however, additional nursing costs can be charged to the NIH grant; however, additional nursing costs can be charged off to the patient's private insurance plan in some states. Immunology and virology tests are charged to the grant. (Those tests charged to the NIH grant are subject to the indirect-cost-rate payment negotiated between the federal government and the university.) Typically, economists are unfamiliar with issues concerning fund accounting and charge/billing policies. Hospitals are increasingly specialized, and these skills are necessary for full recovery of direct costs. In addition to recovery of fixed costs, we need to educate policy makers and insurance executives that payment of indirect costs is not a bonus or profit to the hospital or university. Indirect costs ranging from 25–65 percent are the expenses necessary to maintain the infrastructure necessary for any research to go on. Research institutions with older physical plants incur heavier costs (maintenance, utilities) and receive higher percentage indirect cost rates (Eastaugh 1992).

CONCLUSIONS

This chapter has summarized some of the reasons for the less than total enthusiasm for expanding the application of cost-benefit techniques. Cost-benefit analysis, despite all its shortcomings, can improve the quality of micro- and macrolevel resource decisions. No one wishes to appear to be, or intends to be, callous concerning the selection of a price level for valuing a human life. One could suggest that a more realistic projection of the future for cost-benefit analysis would surely involve cyclic periods of boom and bust. When the economy is in a boom period, cost-benefit will be in a bust period, and vice versa. In economic boom periods, society will reject the arbitrary and capricious irrational decisions of leaders who call for increased prudent use of cost-benefit techniques. In other words, society will be revulsed by the heartless cold decisions of those cost-benefiters in cyclic economic boom periods, but will support increased reliance on a benefit-cost calculus in the bust periods. In time, a stable pattern of decision making will evolve, and progress in treating disease will not depend solely on one political lobby against another (e.g., hemophiliacs versus AIDS research). There are no quick and easy answers to a number of technical problems raised in this chapter, and whether reasonable satisfactory solutions can be found remains unclear.

Members of humanitarian professions often provide outrageous reactions to what they describe as utilitarian econometric pyrotechnics for valuing life. The need for candor, consumerism, and a free flow of information to consumers has been implicit in the analysis. Contrary views predominate in many political science departments. For example, Rhoades (1978) argued that ''absence of total candor leaves the way open for the periodic appearance of ambitious reporters and politicians who expose the Dr. Strangelove–like analysts at the heart of the bureaucracy." However, an alternative plan of action invoking total candor, frequent consumer-preference surveys, and open communication between the bureaucracy and the public might provide better prospects for the health economy in the 1990s. To label economists simply as Dr. Strangeloves and hope that Congress will operate in the name of "doing good" is a highly suspect way of assuring that the health economy can compete with the defense economy.

In summary, the willingness-to-pay approach to cost-benefit analysis is one elixir that will not make decision making any easier, but at least the process could increase consumer input and illuminate the assumptions that currently prevail. The Institute of Medicine (1989) review of the valuation question concluded that the "measurements" are better described as illustrations of methodology than as serious attempts to derive representative answers. The true role of cost-benefit valuation of life resides somewhere between the pessimism of the Institute of Medicine and the naive optimism of many in the economics profession. Analysis becomes critical as the cost of new biomedical technology skyrockets beyond any recent projections (Doolittle 1991).

REFERENCES

Acton, J. (1973). *Evaluating Public Programs to Save Lives: The Case of Heart Attacks*. Rand Corporation Report R–950-RC. Santa Monica, Calif.: Rand Corporation.

Annas, G. (1977). "Allocation of Artificial Hearts in the Year 2002: Minerva v. National Health Agency." *American Journal of Law and Medicine* 3 (Spring), 59–76.

Appel, L., Steinberg, E., Powe, N., Anderson, G., and Dwyer, S. (1990). "Risk Reduction from Low Osmolality Contrast Media: What Do Patients Think It Is Worth?" *Medical Care* 28:4 (April), 324–337.

Arrow, K. (1978). "Risk Allocation and Information: Some Recent Theoretical Developments." *Geneva Papers on Risk and Insurance, Conference Proceedings* 8:1 (May). Geneva, Switzerland.

Bailey, M. (1989). *Measuring the Benefits of Life-Saving*. Washington, D.C.: American Enterprise Institute.

Banta, H., and Thacker, S. (1990). "The Case for Reassessment of Health Care Technology: Once Is Not Enough." *Journal of the American Medical Association* 264:3 (July 17), 235–240.

Barry, M., Mulley, A., Fowler, F., and Wennberg, J. (1988). "Watchful Waiting vs. Immediate Transurethral Resection for Symptomatic Prostatism: The Importance of Patients Preferences." *Journal of the American Medical Association* 259:24 (June), 3010–3017.

Basu, A., and Hastak, M. (1990). "Multiattribute Judgements under Uncertainty: A Conjoint Measurement Approach." *Advances in Consumer Research* 17 (Spring), 454–460.

Beery, W., Schoenbach, V., and Wagner, E. (1988). *Health Risk Appraisal: Methods and Programs*. Department of Health and Human Services Publication PHS–88–3396. Washington, D.C.: U.S. Government Printing Office.

Blomquist, G. (1979). "Value of Life Saving: Implications of Consumption Activity." *Journal of Political Economy* 87:3 (June), 540–558.

Blumenthal, D., Feldman, P., and Zeckhauser, R. (1982). "Misuse of Technology: A Symptom, Not the Disease." In B. McNeil and E. Cravalho (eds.), *Critical Issues in Medical Technology*, 163–174. Dover, Mass.: Auburn House.

Bovbjerg, R., Sloan, F., and Blumstein, J. (1989). "Valuing Life and Limb in Tort: Scheduling Pain and Suffering." *Northwestern University Law Review* 83:4 (Summer), 908–976.

Boyd, N., Sutherland, H., and Heasman, K. (1990). "Whose Utilities for Decision Analysis?" *Medical Decision Making* 10:1 (January–March), 58–67.

Brody, B., Wray, N., and Bame, S. (1991). "Impact of Economic Considerations on Clinical Decisionmaking: The Case of Thrombolytic Therapy." *Medical Care* 29:9 (September), 899–910.

Brookshire, D., Thayer, M., Schulze, W., and Arge, R. (1982). "Valuing Public Goods: A Comparison of Survey and Hedonic Approaches." *American Economic Review* 72:1 (March), 165–177.

Bunker, J., Barnes, B., and Mosteller, F. (eds.). (1977). *Costs, Risks, and Benefits of Surgery*. New York: Oxford University Press.

Callahan, D. (1990). *What Kind of Life: The Limits of Medical Progress*. New York: Simon and Schuster.

Card, W. (1980). "Rational Justification of Therapeutic Decisions." *Metamedicine* 1, 11–28.

Catlin, R. (1981). "Does the Doctor Understand What I Am Asking?" *American Journal of Public Health* 71:2 (February), 123–124.

Cooper, B., and Rice, D. (1976). "The Economic Cost of Illness Revisited." *Social Security Bulletin* 39:1 (February), 21–36.

Cropper, M., and Sussman, F. (1988). "Families and the Economics of Risks to Life." *American Economic Review* 78:1 (March), 255–260.

Dardis, R. (1980). "The Value of Life: New Evidence from the Marketplace." *American Economic Review* 70:5 (December), 1077–1082.

Diamond, G. (1992). "Off Bayes: Effect of Verification Bias on Posterior Probabilities Calculated Using Bayes' Theorem." *Medical Decision Making* 12:1 (January-March), 22–31.

Dickie, M., and Gerking, S. (1991). "Valuing Reduced Morbidity: A Household Production Approach." *Southern Economic Journal* 57:3 (January), 690–702.

Dickinson, G., and Klimas, N. (1991). "Automated Severity Classification of AIDS Hospitalizations." *Medical Decision Making* 11:4 (October-December), S41–S45.

Dillingham, A. (1979). "The Injury Risk Structure of Occupations and Wages." Ph.D. diss. Department of Industrial and Labor Relations, Cornell University.

Donaldson, C. (1990). "Willingness to Pay for Publicly-provided Goods." *Journal of Health Economics* 9:1 (June), 103–118.

Doolittle, R. (1991). "Biotechnology: The Enormous Cost of Success." *New England Journal of Medicine* 324:19 (May 9), 1360–1362.

Eastaugh, S. (1992) "Economic Issues in Defining Stable Funding Levels for AIDS Research." *Journal of Health Administration Education* 10:1 (Winter) 139–150.

———. (1991). "Valuation of the Benefits of Risk-free Blood: Willingness to Pay for Hemoglobin Solutions." *International Journal of Technology Assessment in Health Care* 7:1 (Winter) 51–59.

———. (1990). "Resource Usage in AIDS Research at 35 Medical Centers." Final Report 89–311 to NIH, NIAID office, Bethesda, Md. (January).

————. (1989). "Cost of Hospital-based AIDS Research." *Hospital Topics* 18:6 (November–December), 18–22.

————. (1983). "Placing a Value on Life and Limb: The Role of the Informed Consumer." *Health Matrix* 1:1 (Spring), 5–21.

Eastaugh, S., and Hatcher, M. (1982). "Improving Compliance among Hypertensives: A Triage Criterion and Cost-Benefit Implications." *Medical Care* 20:8 (August), 1001–1017.

Fanshel, S., and Bush, J. (1970). "A Health-Status Index and Its Application to Health-Services Outcomes." *Operations Research* 18:6, 1021–1066.

Fein, R. (1971). "On Measuring Economic Benefits of Health Programs." In *Medical History and Medical Care*, 181–217. London: Nuffield Provincial Hospitals Trust.

Feinberg, H., and Hiatt, H. (1979). "Evaluation of Medical Practices." *New England Journal of Medicine* 300:18, 1086–1090.

Fisher, A., Chestnut, L., and Violette, D. (1989). "The Value of Reducing Risk of Death." *Journal of Policy Analysis and Management* 8:1 (January) 88–100.

Fuchs, V., and Zeckhauser, R. (1987). "Valuing Health—A 'Priceless' Commodity." *American Economic Review* 77:2 (May), 264–268.

Giaque, W., and Peebles, T. (1976). "Application of Multidimensional Utility Theory in Determining Optimal Test-Treatment Strategies for Streptococcal Sore Throat and Rheumatic Fever." *Operations Research* 24:5 (September–October), 933–950.

Glass, N. (1973). "Cost Benefit Analysis and Health Services." *Health Trends* 5:1 (January), 51–60.

Hadorn, D., and Hays, R. (1991). "Multitrait-multimethod Analysis of Health-related Quality-of-life Measures." *Medical Care* 29:9 (September), 829–840.

Hapgood, F. (1980). "Risk-Benefit Analysis: Putting a Price on Life." In S. Rhoads (ed.), *Valuing Life: Public Policy Dilemmas*. Boulder, Colo.: Westview.

Harris, P. (1980). Press Release, Office of the Secretary, Department of Health and Human Services, June 12, Washington, D.C.

Hartunian, N., Smart, C., and Thompson, M. (1981). *The Incidence and Economic Costs of Major Health Impairments*. Lexington, Mass.: D.C. Heath.

Hellinger, F. (1991). "Forecasting the Medical Care Costs of the HIV Epidemic: 1991–94." *Inquiry* 28:3 (Fall), 213–224.

Hilden, J., Glasziou, P., and Habbema, J. (1992). "A Pitfall in Utility Assessment: Patients' Undisclosed Investment Decisions." *Medical Decision Making* 12:1 (January-March), 39–43.

Hillner, B., and Smith, T. (1991). "Efficacy and Cost Effectiveness of Adjuvant Chemotherapy in Women with Node-negative Breast Cancer." *New England Journal of Medicine* 324:3 (January 17), 160–168.

Himmelstein, D., and Woolhandler, S. (1984). "Free Care, Cholestyramine, and Health Policy." *New England Journal of Medicine* 311:23 (December 6), 1511–1514.

Hirshleifer, J., Bergstrom, T., and Rappaport, E. (1984). *Applying Cost-Benefit Concepts to Projects Which Alter Human Mortality*. Los Angeles: UCLA.

Institute of Medicine. (1989). *Costs of Environment-related Health Effects: A Plan for Continuing Study*. Washington, D.C.: National Academy of Sciences.

Jones, E., Densen, P., and McNitt, B. (1979). "An Approach to the Assessment of Long Term Care." In W. Holland, J. Ipsen, and J. Kostrzewski (eds.), *Mea-

surement of Levels of Health, 299–311. Copenhagen: World Health Organization, Regional Office, Europe.

Jones, J., Clough, J., Klinenberg, J., and Davis, P. (1981). "The Role of Therapeutic Plasmapheresis in the Rheumatic Diseases." *Journal of Laboratory Clinical Medicine* 97, 589–598.

Kagel, J., MacDonald, D., and Battalio, R. (1990). "Tests of Fanning Out of Indifference Curves: Results from Experiments." *American Economic Review* 80:4 (September), 912–921.

Kaplan, R., Anderson, J., and Wu, A. (1989). "Quality of Well-being Scale—Applications in AIDS, Cystic Fibrosis, and Arthritis." *Medical Care* 27:3 (March), S27–S43.

Kass, L. (1975). "Regarding the End of Medicine and the Pursuit of Health." *Public Interest* 40 (Summer), 11–42.

Kinsley, M. (1981). "Polls and People's Opinion of Hazards." *New Republic* (June 20), 15–19.

Kirscht, J. (1989). "Process and Measurement Issues in Health Risk Appraisal." *American Journal of Public Health* 79:12 (December), 1598–1599.

Klarman, H. (1965). "Syphilis Control Programs." In R. Dorfman (ed.), *Measuring Benefits of Government Investments*, 367–410. Washington, D.C.: Brookings Institution.

Klema, E., Travis, C., Richter, S., Crouch, E., and Wilson, R. (1989). "The $2 Million Value of a Life." Joint monograph, Oak Ridge National Laboratory, Tennessee.

Kotler, P. (1991). *Marketing for Nonprofit Organizations*. 3d ed. Englewood Cliffs, N.J.: Prentice-Hall.

Krischer, J. (1976). "The Mathematics of Cleft Lip and Palate Treatment Evaluation: Measuring the Desirability of Treatment Outcomes." *Cleft Palate Journal* 13:4 (April), 165–180.

Landefeld, J., and Seskin, E. (1982). "The Economic Value of Life: Linking Theory to Practice." *American Journal of Public Health* 72:6 (June), 555–566.

Legg, M. (1981). "What Role for the Diagnostic Pathologist?" *New England Journal of Medicine* 305:16 (October 15), 950–951.

Leigh, J., and Fries, J. (1992). "Health Habits, Health Care Use and Costs." *Inquiry* 29:1 (Spring), 44–53.

Lipscomb, J. (1990). *Multiattribute Evaluation of Health Outcomes: Theory and Evidence*. Durham, N.C.: Duke University Press, Institute of Policy Sciences and Public Affairs.

Littenberg, B., Garber, A., and Sox, H. (1990). "Screening for Hypertension." *Annals of Internal Medicine* 112:2 (February), 192–202.

Lomas, J., Anderson, G., Domnick-Pierre, K., Vayda, E., Enkin, M., and Hannah, W. (1989). "Do Practice Guidelines Guide Practice?" *New England Journal of Medicine* 321:21 (November 22), 1306–1311.

Lubeck, D. (1982). "A Cost-Effectiveness Analysis of Treatment and Prevention of Heart Disease." Working paper, Stanford University Medical Center and the Data Bank Network, Palo Alto, Calif.

Luce, R., and Raiffa, H. (1957). *Games and Decisions*. New York: John Wiley.

Matchar, D., and Pauker, S. (1987). "Endarterectomy in Carotid Artery Disease: A Decision Analysis." *Journal of the American Medical Association* 258:6 (August 14), 793–798.

McCarty, D. (1981). "Treating Intractable Rheumatoid Arthritis." *New England Journal of Medicine* 305:17 (October 22), 1009–1011.

McNeil, B., and Pauker, S. (1982). "Incorporation of Patient Values in Medical Decision Making." In B. McNeil and E. Cravalho (eds.), *Critical Issues in Medical Technology.* Dover, Mass.: Auburn House.

McNeil, B., Weichselbaum, R., and Pauker, S. (1981). "Tradeoffs between Quality and Quantity of Life in Laryngeal Cancer." *New England Journal of Medicine* 305:17 (October 22), 982–987.

———. (1978). "Fallacy of the Five-Year Survival Rate in Lung Cancer." *New England Journal of Medicine* 299:24 (December 10) 1397–1401.

Mehrez, A., and Gafni, A. (1991) "Healthy-Year Equivalents (HYE): How to Measure Them Using the Standard Gamble Approach." *Medical Decision Making* 11:2 (April–June), 140–146.

Mishan, E. (1971). "Evaluation of Life and Limb: A Theoretical Approach." *Journal of Political Economy* 79:4 (July–August), 687–705.

Mitchell, R., and Carson, R. (1990). *Using Surveys to Value Public Goods: The Contingent Valuation Method.* Washington, D.C.: Resources for the Future.

Moore, M., and Viscusi, K. (1988). "Doubling the Estimated Value of Life: Results Using New Occupational Fatality Data." *Journal of Policy Analysis and Management* 7:4 (Fall), 476–490.

Muller, A., and Reutzel, T. (1984). "Willingness to Pay for Reduction in Fatality Risk: An Exploratory Study." *American Journal of Public Health* 74:8 (August), 808–812.

Mushkin, S. (1962). "Health as an Investment." *Journal of Political Economy* 70:5 (October), 129–157.

Nordhaus, W. (1990). "Greenhouse Economics: Count before You Leap." *Economist,* July 7, 21–22.

Olson, C. (1981). "An Analysis of Wage Differentials Received by Workers on Dangerous Jobs." *Journal of Human Resources* 16:2 (Spring), 167–186.

Pauker, S., and Kassirer, J. (1987). "Decision Analysis." *New England Journal of Medicine* 316:5 (January 29), 250–258.

Pearlman, R., and Uhlmann, R. (1988). "Quality of Life in Chronic Diseases: Perceptions of Elderly Patients." *Journal of Gerontology* 43:2 (March, Medical Sciences supplement), M25–M30.

Pliskin, J., Shepard, D., and Weinstein, M. (1980). "Utility Functions for Life Years and Health Status." *Operations Research* 28:1 (January-February) 206–224.

Portney, P. (1981). "Housing Prices, Health Effects, and Value Reductions in Risk of Death." *Journal of Environment Economics and Management* 8:1 (March), 72–78.

Ramsey, S., and Nettleman, M. (1992). "Cost-effectiveness of Prophylactic AZT Following Needlestick." *Medical Decision Making* 12:2 (April-June), 142–148.

Rhoads, S. (1978). "How Much Should We Spend to Save a Life?" *Public Interest* 51 (Spring), 74–92.

Rice, D. (1966). *Estimating the Cost of Illness.* Health Economics Series no. 6. Washington, D.C.: U.S. Government Printing Office.

Rifkin, M., Zerhouni, E., and Gatsonis, C. (1990). "Comparison of MRI and Ultrasonography in Staging Early Prostate Cancer: Results of a Multi-institutional

Cooperative Trial.'' *New England Journal of Medicine* 323:10 (September 6), 621–626.

Sackett, D., and Torrance, G. (1978). ''The Utility of Different Health States as Perceived by the General Public.'' *Journal of Chronic Disease* 31, 697–704.

Safra, Z., Segal, U., and Spivak, A. (1990). ''Preference Reversal and Nonexpected Utility Behavior.'' *American Economic Review* 80:4 (September), 922–930.

Schelling, T. (1968). ''The Life You Save May Be Your Own.'' In S. Chase (ed.), *Problems in Public Expenditure Analysis*, 127–162. Washington, D.C.: Brookings Institution.

Shattuck, L. (1850). *Report of the Sanitary Commission of Massachusetts, 1850*. Cambridge, Mass.: Harvard University Press.

Smith, A. (1776). *The Wealth of Nations*. London: London Press.

Smith, K., McKinlay, S., and McKinlay, J. (1989). ''Reliability of Health Risk Appraisals: A Field Trial of Four Instruments.'' *American Journal of Public Health* 79:12 (December), 1603–1607.

Smith, P., Keyes, N., and Forman, E. (1982). ''Socioeconomic Evaluation of a State-funded Comprehensive Hemophilia Care Program.'' *New England Journal of Medicine* 306:10 (March 11), 575–579.

Smith, R. (1976). *The Occupational Safety and Health Act*. Washington, D.C.: American Enterprise Institute.

Spilker, B. (1990). *Quality of Life Assessments in Clinical Trials*. New York: Raven Press.

Stewart, A., Ware, J., and Johnston, S. (1975). ''Construction of Scales Measuring Health and Health-related Concepts from the Dayton Medical History Questionnaire.'' In *The Conceptualization and Measurement of Health in the Health Insurance Study*. Santa Monica, Calif.: Rand Corporation.

Surgenor, D., Wallace, E., Hao, S., and Chapman, R. (1990). ''Collection and Transfusion of Blood in the USA.'' *New England Journal of Medicine*, 322:23 (June), 1646–1651.

Thaler, R., and Gould, W. (1982). ''Public Policy toward Life Saving: Should Consumer Preference Rule?'' *Journal of Policy Analysis and Management* 1:2 (Winter), 223–242.

Thaler, R., and Rosen, S. (1976). ''The Value of Saving a Life: Evidence from the Labor Market.'' *National Bureau of Economic Research* 40, 265–298.

Thompson, M. (1986). ''Willingness to Pay and Accept Risks to Cure Chronic Disease.'' *American Journal of Public Health* 76:4 (April), 392–396.

Thurow, L. (1984). ''Learning to Say No.'' *New England Journal of Medicine* 311:24 (December 13), 1569–1572.

Torrance, G. (1986). ''Measurement of Health State Utilities for Economic Appraisal: A Review.'' *Journal of Health Economics* 5:1 (March), 1–30.

———. (1976). ''Health Status Index Models: A Unified Mathematical View. *Management Science* 22:9, 990–1001.

Turnbull, A., Graziano, C., Baron, R., Sichel, W., Young, C., and Howland, W. (1979). ''The Inverse Relationship between Cost and Survival in the Critically Ill Cancer Patient.'' *Critical Care Medicine* 7:1 (January), 20–23.

Turner, B., Kelly, J., and Ball, J. (1989). ''A Severity Classification System for AIDS Hospitalizations.'' *Medical Care* 27:4 (April), 423–437.

Urban, G., and Hauser, J. (1989). *Design and Marketing of New Products*. Englewood Cliffs, N.J.: Prentice-Hall.

Viscusi, W. (1978). "Wealth Effects and Earnings Premiums for Job Hazards." *Review of Economics and Statistics* 60:3 (August), 408–416.

Wagstaff, A. (1991). "QALYs and the Equity-efficiency Trade-off." *Journal of Health Economics* 10:1 (May) 43–64.

Warner, K. (1987). "Health and Economic Implications of a Tobacco-free Society." *Journal of the American Medical Association* 258:15 (October 16), 2080–2086.

Wasserman, J., Manning, W., Newhouse, J., and Winkler, J. (1991) "Effects of Excise Taxes and Regulations on Cigarette Smoking." *Journal of Health Economics* 10:1 (May) 43–64.

Weinstein, M., Pliskin, J., and Stason, W. (1977). "Coronary Artery Bypass Surgery: Decision and Policy Analysis." In J. Bunker, B. Barnes, and F. Mosteller (eds.), *Costs, Risks, and Benefits of Surgery*, 342–371. New York: Oxford University Press.

Weinstein, N. (1989). "Optimistic Biases about Personal Risk." *Science* 246:22 (June 18), 1232–1233.

Zeckhauser, R. (1975). "Procedures for Valuing Lives." *Public Policy* 23:4 (Fall), 419–464.

Zeckhauser, R., and Shepard, D. (1976). "Where Now for Saving Lives?" *Law and Contemporary Problems* 40:4 (Autumn), 5–45.

VII FUTURE POLICY TRENDS

14 Capitation, Consolidation, and Universal Entitlement

Our current problems are past solutions.

—John D. Thompson

Think in terms of health status of the entire population. Most of us who are health care providers are principally preoccupied with the effort to deliver more personal health services, which, unfortunately solves acute problems but returns patients to the same environment.

—Gail L. Warden

Quality is a matter of survival. Sometimes people get caught up with all kinds of fuzzy, abstract "quality is a warm puppy" notions. That is wrong. Quality is profit and productivity and market share. And that's no warm puppy.

—John Guaspari

Americans want incompatible goals: unlimited access to the best care at an affordable cost. Compared with other countries, America has a schizophrenic attitude concerning the production and financing of medical services. The American tradition is to seldom support the classic externalities argument for supporting medical services as a public good. There are few services where one can demonstrate that the society as a whole earns more if the coworkers are kept healthy through preventive medicine (Eastaugh 1981). Most medical dollars go to curing and caring, not prevention. Some liberals would go so far as to argue that medical services are a merit good, so crucial to preserving the general welfare of society that the services should be financed by government even if they are not cost-beneficial. Such an attitude is maintained in the Netherlands and the United Kingdom, where medical care is produced and financed as if it were a public good—a social service too important to be rationed on market principles. The Netherlands has the highest medical cost-inflation rate of any OECD member

(Organization for Economic Cooperation and Development [OECD] 1991). By contrast, England takes the viewpoint that certain medical services are not cost-beneficial and should not be included in the National Health Service. Other countries, like Japan, Korea, France, and Switzerland, produce and finance medical services as if they were normal consumer goods. Insurance is available for expensive medical services, but the coinsurance rates range as high as 30 to 50 percent.

However, the United States has one of the most inconsistent policies toward medical service: We produce it as a consumer good, finance it as a public good, and complain when providers react in a rational way, promoting excess demand and behaving in an inflationary "quality is all important" style of care for the subsidized service. A decade ago American health care providers were best described as a fragmented group of fiercely independent organizations. Over 90 percent of the physicians were independent operators in private practice, and hospitals engaged in cost-increasing fierce competition for prestige and the newest capital equipment. Now physicians and hospitals are being subjected to a cost-decreasing mode of competition that is both consumer driven and payer driven. The nature of health-services delivery is changing. We can no longer deny that health care is a blend of art, business, life-style, and science. Providers' traditional objectives have been expanded to include consumer-sensitive service in a more economical style, advocating patient compliance and health promotion while offering the best technical quality of care. Overemphasis on any one aspect may spell disaster for the provider. Providers who pursue only business interests will be no more protected or respected than a used-car dealership. Likewise, those who disrespect business skills, marketing, and consumers' shifting tastes may face an early retirement in the 1990s. Changes in payment systems occur so rapidly that providers and medical suppliers are hard put to keep pace and react, much less plan proactively. There is still room for improved efficiency in a health sector that spends $1 billion every 19 hours. Some of the resources do little good, but the majority of the care averts death, pain, and erosion of functional health status. However, we must be careful not to discount quality or access in the name of economic efficiency. There is a delicate balance to maintain between health care as a social good and health care as a consumer good.

INNOVATION OR STAGNATION AND UNBALANCED GROWTH

The health economy should not be viewed as completely independent from the general economy. The health sector is in some sense a microcosm of Baumol's model of unbalanced growth for the economy (Baumol, Blackman, and Wolfe 1985). An oversimplified health economy might divide into three productivity-growth sectors, one "stagnant" (inpatient) and two "progressive" (ambulatory care and long-term care). The share of the gross national product devoted to inpatient care may rise to above 5 percent. We will spend more on the "miracles of modern medical technology,'' but the hospital census may remain in a permanent recession relative to 1980–83 levels. The share of health expenditures invested on the stagnant inpatient sector may increase in the long run as our appetite for transplants and high-tech medicine expands. However, the progressive sectors' share of the labor force might increase with the aging of the population and the decline in hospital workers. Productivity improvements may have to underwrite the volume expansion in numbers of services within the two progressive sectors. The progressive ambulatory-care clinics are already innovating themselves out of their cost-dominating market position. If shoddy-quality operators tarnish the service reputation of certain market segments, interest in universal entitlement and regulatory solutions may experience a rebirth (Herzlinger 1992).

This book has presented a number of basic themes. Preferred practice patterns (PPPs) are needed as clinical guidelines for the practice of cost-effective clinical decision making (chapters 11 and 12). PPPs, including workload-driven staffing, gainsharing incentive pay to employees, and increased reliance on nurse extender/technicians, are necessary for enhanced productivity. PPPs are also necessary for better investment decisions, financing decisions, and capital-structure decisions. With regard to these issues, some recent texts have suggested substantial recent improvement in the state of the practice (Kovner and Neuhauser 1991), while other texts have documented major shortfalls in management performance (Gapenski 1992).

A number of analysts, lead by Woolhandler and Himmelstein (1991) argue for the Canadian model to achieve the twin goals of cost containment and universal entitlement. The argument is simply presented as follows: Because Canada spends under 9.2 percent of gross national product (GNP) on health care, it must be superior to the United States in cost containment. This same sort of flawed logic was presented to the author when he was an economist at the National Academy of Sciences. When Canadian spending on health care as a percentage of gross domestic product (GDP) declined from 7.47 percent in 1971 to 6.88 percent in 1974, officials promoting the ''efficiency gain'' were quick to label Canada as a superior example of cost containment. However, any economist worth his weight in oil knows that it is necessary to look for both currency shifts and real resource shifts. If the Canadian health care system improved its efficiency, it would be using less inputs (e.g., fewer nurses). Unfortunately for the cheerleaders quick to jump to a conclusion, nurses as a percentage of the work force increased from 1.766 percent to 1.834 percent in the relevant period 1973–74. From the point of view of technical efficiency, the ''efficiency gain'' was nonexistent. Moreover, it is easy to demonstrate that the efficiency differential between Canada and the United States is equally illusionary.

If we update the Canadian example to the current context, we find that from 1970 to 1990 Canada's real inflation-adjusted per capita GNP increased 72.1 percent, while the real growth in the American GNP per capita was only 35.6

percent. In the 1960s the two nations had equal average annual growth rates. A higher relative GNP gain explains why Canada spends less of its GNP on health care. If one factors out currency exchange rates, utilizes per capita spending in constant dollars in each nation's own currency (factoring out population-growth differences and currency shifts), and adjusts for inflation by the local GNP deflator, one finds that Canada and the United States had the exact same rate of cost inflation from 1970 to 1990, and each nation has dedicated a cumulative increase of 2.55 percent in real health care spending per capita. Abel-Smith (1985) was incorrect in the observation that a health care system relying more on some overall control of spending (like Canada) has better control of health care costs than those relying on a more decentralized mechanism of control (the United States).

THE CANADIAN MODEL

Advocates of a one-payer national health care system like Canada frequently claim that the transition can be self-financing. That is, the cut in administrative waste can more than make up for the additional dollars needed to cover uninsured Americans. For example, Woolhandler and Himmelstein (1991) offer the inflated claim that in 1987 dollars the U.S. health care system could save $69–$83.2 billion by attaining the Canadian level of administrative efficiency. Two-thirds of the assumptions in this article are based upon personal communications that no reader can independently verify. The authors assume that administrative costs are overhead costs, so they count supplies, rent, equipment, and professional liability insurance as if they were administrative expenses that would disappear under their advocated one-payer national health insurance scheme. The appropriate method of cost analysis is marginal cost analysis, or what an accountant calls differential cost analysis. Even if one could accept that American physicians spent 43 percent of office expenses on administrative costs, the expected savings in moving to a universal one-payer system would not be $30 billion. The cost of operating a physician's office, utilities, supplies, and rent cannot be counted as administrative waste in the American health care system. The authors self-select for their comparison Quebec, because this province has the lowest physician fees, and thus the lowest ability to employ enough clerical personnel. The Canadian health care system might be eroding productivity and economic efficiency by having physicians do too many clerical tasks. Woolhandler and Himmelstein also utilize 1972–73 data from Quebec for their analysis.

The American figures on physicians' administrative expense in the Woolhandler and Himmelstein (1991) study are overstated because the data is self-reported to the AMA by individual physicians. Physicians have a reporting bias to overstate administrative time, to in turn pressure government and other third-party payers to trim red tape. No provider reports there is too little paperwork and not enough administrative duties. Woolhandler and Himmelstein (1991) also double count time spent on medical records and claims, by adding an additional $4.5

billion of opportunity cost (6 minutes per patient) to their already bloated estimate. Rather than spending $170,000 per physician office in administrative tasks,
a more careful range of estimates would peg the potential savings in moving to
a one-payer system at between $10,000–$27,000. The Canadian figures on doctor
offices are more valid and reliable because they are drawn from tax records.

The Woolhandler and Himmelstein (1991) analysis is an even worse comparison between apples and oranges for the hospital sector. It is a surprise that
these two New England-based authors select California hospitals for their yardstick of hospital administrative expense in the United States (this entire ad hoc
article is designed to make Canada look efficient and the U.S. look bad). With
more commercial insurance carriers doing business, and competitive bidding
programs, California has higher administrative costs per average than the typical
American hospital. California has 30 more employees per 100 beds than the
average American hospital. The figures for the Canadian health care system are
low-ball estimates because: the education department pays for teaching hospital
expenses not included in the health budget; Canadian government officials do
not record the administrative indirect expenses like processing claims; and the
additional costs of collecting more revenue through the tax system are not considered in the Woolhandler and Himmelstein article. The administrative benefit
of going to a one-payer national system in the U.S. is an open question for future
analysis. This article is an example of advocacy posing as evidence. Gray (1991)
provides the better example by balancing evidence and advocacy, presenting the
numbers (the Dragnet "just the facts" approach), and then advocating the policy
positions favored by the particular analysts. The process of health policy making
can be viewed through a variety of prisms, but we do not need more studies
offering biased evidence in the name of advocacy.

The American experience with rate setting involves less consensus building
activities and less concern for efficiency than most industrial nations. Our nonfederal payers rarely have the resources to evaluate economic and operational
efficiency of their health care providers even within systems such as PPOs
designed to enhance such economic goals. State and regional reimbursement
methodologies have generally been static in nature, concentrating on arraying
the costs of health care providers by some definition of allowable costs, and
setting the reimbursement rate at a prescribed percentile based on the array.
Some states sort providers into "peer groups," but these groupings often ignore
quantitative indicators of provider efficiency, and instead focus on size, general
care levels or geographical location. In addition, these groupings tend to be static
over time and do not allow the changing dynamics of both the provider and its
beneficiaries to influence future reimbursements.

GLOBAL BUDGETING—LIKE GERMANY?

A "Federal Reserve Board" for setting health care spending caps as done in
Germany is not "a socialist system for planned payment" or a form of rigid

price controls. It is a fundamentally different organism in both structure and intent than the Economic Stabilization Program (ESP) in effect from August 1971 to April 1974. An ideal Global Budgeting Board (GBB) for health care should have the consensus building focus that ESP lacked, and the real power that American health planners always lacked. The GBB need not encroach on the economic integrity of successful semi-competitive market participants. The efficient provider need not feel any pressure from GBB activities. By allocating capital and operating funds the local GBBs will provide incentives for enhanced efficiency. Quantitative measurements of relative provider efficiency could include measures that are:

1. directly included in the rate setting methodology;
2. used retroactively to measure the effects of any year's plan;
3. used retroactively to reward efficient providers with a reimbursement adjustment (or penalize with an inefficiency penalty);
4. used by rate setters to measure the ongoing trends in provider efficiency, by segregating relatively efficient and inefficient costs incurred by health care providers.

How would such a GBB process work in the American context? Should the national specialty societies have input to a national body (a Federal Reserve board for health care) that sets spending caps? Should state boards be set up to implement local caps? To what extent should state boards allow the state medical society or hospital association to have input? Should the local boards be multistate in character, like our monetary Federal Reserve, covering up to 20 million Americans in each region (large states could have their own board)? The caps on spending must be allocated to each sector and each region, and locally apportioned to individual hospitals and other providers. The process of resource allocation must reward efficiency; i.e. not underpay efficient HMOs or hospitals. Therefore the system must pay for outputs, case mix adjusted with some consideration for severity (e.g. refined DRGs, RDRGs), and not pay on the basis of historical cost reports (high cost may simply indicate higher inefficiency). The idea behind the GBB is to assist progress towards a more equitable health care system, and promote the law of comparative advantage: as more service volume is supplied by the most efficient providers, all in society will be richer—accomplishing this will require both attention to operational detail and broad consensus. The German roundtable on GBB was one decade in the making (Schneider 1991; Iglehart 1991).

The GBB process would establish fees and total annual expenditures for physicians, nonphysician providers, hospitals, and freestanding centers through a formal negotiating structure. Providers cannot set their own fees due to the obvious conflict of interest, but their input is vital because they understand their work product better than the typical civilian. However, the decision to implement a GBB or pass a national health plan rests in the hands of a larger political community. That larger political community should have a place on the national

GB board and on local GB boards. The nature of the GBB at some level may be corporatist: closed to all but the principal players. But at a national level and at periodical local GBB meetings the process must be public. A consensus building process cannot be secretive.

Will the passage of a German style GBB promote social cooperation and aid the eventual passage of a national health plan? Is GBB a *quid pro quo* for reducing administrative expense incurred by providers? With one payment process nationally there will be less administrative expense. Is GBB expected to make national health care affordable? Can GBB discern the public interest and promote good economic and good quality health care? In the spirit of democracy and pluralism the GBB will subject each interest group to public scrutiny. Four years of experience with the Physician Payment Review Commission (Chapter 4) suggests the potential benefits of public scrutiny. The hope is that this process will yield a more efficient, effective, and equitable health care system.

One final caveat should be considered. The consensus building for GBB is a bit more difficult in the American context of separation of powers. By contrast, GBB is more easily created in parliamentary systems with inherent consensus between legislative and executive branches. However, just because a GBB is more difficult to initiate does not mean that the GBB will be any less effective at cost control once created. All nations with GBB spend one-third less a proportion of GNP on health care than the United States. Moreover, creation of a GBB might be the catalyst that breaks the gridlock against national health care reform for the 34 million uninsured Americans and those otherwise squeezed by the current approaches. Implementation of GBB will not cause the United States to spend 4.0 percent of Gross National Product (GNP) less on health care, but it will free up the resources necessary to make health care coverage more affordable. GBB can reduce the need for explicit rationing (e.g. the Oregon Medicaid program). The distributional impact of GBB may yield more funding for long-term care.

SUPPLY OF NURSING HOME BEDS

Does the nation need a markedly higher supply of nursing home beds per 1,000 aged Americans? It may be true that certain states have an insufficient supply of nursing home beds, but we do not wish to treat health care problems of an aging population mainly by institutionalization. For example, it is better economics and leads to a better quality of life to channel patients into low-cost sites of service distribution (e.g., low-tech and high-tech home health care). High-tech home health care workers distribute drugs and intravenous (IV) treatments without "chaining" the patient to a nursing home bed. In 1992 the cost of home health care is predicted to exceed $7.1 billion (financed 45 percent from Medicare and 35 percent from Medicaid). More growth in care modalities will be needed to keep pace with the aging of the population. From 1971 to 1991 the nursing home bed supply increased at an annual rate of 2.26 percent, reaching an estimated 1.74 million nursing home beds by 1992. Bed supply has not kept pace with the aging of the population. Since 1971 the prime nursing home population cohort, the elderly 85 years of age or over, has increased in number by 4.22 percent annually, resulting in a 1.93 percent per year average decline in nursing home beds per 1,000 elderly aged. A number of states with less than three-fourths the national average of beds per 1,000 elderly aged are considering major expansion programs in nursing home construction (including Florida, Alabama, South Carolina, West Virginia, and New Jersey). In each state it will be difficult to find an appropriate balance between regulation and competition (Young 1991).

The American Association of Homes for the Aging (AAHA 1992) predicts that by the year 2010 the nation will need 1.65 million additional nursing home beds to achieve the target ratio of 55 beds per 1,000 aged. Also by the year 2010 the nation will need 150,000 life-care facility (LCF) beds, 200,000 other continuing-care retirement center (CCRC) beds, and 750,000 congregate housing beds to achieve a target ratio of 65 alternative-living-arrangement beds per 1,000 aged in 2010. There will probably be a disequilibrium between these estimates of "need" and bed supply created because of insufficient reimbursement rates, local health planners' restrictions on new building, poor financial planning, and insufficient external financing (debt and equity). However, a sufficient expansion of long-term-care beds would help reduce the discharge delays at hospitals located in areas with few such beds and in states with tight prospective Medicaid nursing home payment rates (Kenney and Holahan 1990; Nyman 1989). Technology may reduce the need for chronic services for certain demographic segments, such as those with Alzheimer's disease. Evans (1990) estimated that without any technological breakthrough the number of elderly Americans with "probable Alzheimer's disease" will increase from 3.8 million to 10.3 million in the year 2050.

An interesting comparison can be drawn between the United States and two other decentralized health care systems with superior economic growth: Japan and Korea. Comparisons between the three countries are offered in table 14.1. The United States spends the highest fraction of resources on the elderly (table 14.1, line 13). However, because Japan has the most rapidly aging population in the world, it will exceed the U.S. figure during the 1990s. Japan spends only 7.7 percent of GNP on health care, offers no apparent surgical queues or other forms of rationing (unlike Canada; Rachlis and Kushner 1990; Fuchs and Hahn 1990), and leads the world in life expectancy and low infant mortality (Powell and Anesaki 1991). The Japanese staffing ratio per bed (table 14.1, line 5) is superior to the American figure for all types of hospitals because of superior labor productivity and because Japanese (and Korean) patients receive feeding and some basic nursing care from family members in large hospital wards. The Japanese fraction of GNP going to health care is probably underestimated by 2.4 percentage points of GNP because official government statistics exclude personal expenditures for medical care and preventive medicine (Powell and

Table 14.1
Health Care Statistics in the United States, Japan, and Korea, 1991

	United States	Japan	Korea
1. Life expectancy at birth			
Male	72	77	68
Female	79	83	73
Manpower ratios			
2. Physicians per 100,000 population	230	161	89
3. Surgeons per 100,000 population	60	39	22
4. Dentists per 100,000 population	16	55	62
5. Hospital personnel per occupied bed	2.9	1.0	0.8
Hospital sector			
6. Acute-care beds per 1,000 population	4.1	5.5	2.3
7. Hospital costs as percentage of GNP	4.7	2.8	1.6
8. Percentage of beds that are for-profit	16	64	74
9. Annual admissions per 1,000 population	114	82	69
Total health care spending			
10. Spending per capita ($)	2,634	1,320	315
11. Health as a percentage of GNP	12.2	7.7	5.8
Service allocation (percentage of total health spending going to a given age group)			
12. Ages 0-14	19.8	21.2	19.0
13. Ages 65+	42.4	39.3	33.0

Sources: OECD Data Bank, 1991; Eastaugh (1991); World Bank, *World Development Report, 1991*, Washington, D.C.: World Bank.

Anesaki 1991; this is also true for the Korean statistics; Eastaugh 1990). Korea finished the decade-long process of implementing national health insurance by signing up the last uninsured market segment, one in six citizens, during 1989. Japan has had universal entitlement for three decades (Ikegami 1991). However, if we factor out the higher rate of economic growth in the two Asian countries, both nations would spend over 11.5 percent of GNP on health care if they had experienced the sluggish American growth rate during the period 1970–90. The critical point is that health care cost inflation is a worldwide problem. No nation, including Canada, offers a magic formula to resolve the worldwide problems of access and cost control. It is easy to put down the American medical care system with glib lines like "We have no health care system; rather, we have a disjointed sickness-care nonsystem." A disjointed American delivery system experiences as much health care cost inflation as a ''jointed'' government planned delivery system like those in Canada or the Netherlands.

COMPETITION AND SERVICE DELIVERY

Mandatory employer-based health insurance, as outlined in chapter 7, will not cover all uninsured Americans and will introduce a new set of problems (a classic example of John Thompson's rule: Our current problems are past solutions). Korea mandated health insurance by employer group, phased in over 12 years (1977–89), and has the most rapid rate of medical cost escalation. Germany has 11 decades of experience with social insurance, but its health care system appeared to be in severe trouble even prior to German reunification in 1990 (Iglehart 1991). The German economy is concentrating high-risk patient groups in local sickness funds, many of which are in severe economic trouble. Wysong and Abel (1990) reported that the growing segmentation of risk groups in Germany threatens the concept of solidarity on which the system is founded.

The concept of solidarity has already experienced a meltdown in a number of countries, including New Zealand (Coney 1991), where the government is dismantling the health and welfare systems. Sweden now suffers from the same queues for surgery and inadequate continuity of care that many other victims of national health insurance have experienced. To expand patient choice, county councils in Sweden have begun a program of ''comparative competition'' between private and public providers, linking consumer-choice decisions to providers' salaries and institutional budgets. Sweden still wants to maintain a publicly operated health system ''with a planned/market approach'' (Saltman 1990). The phrase ''planned/market approach'' may be a classic oxymoron, two words that do not go together, like ''postal service.'' If one wants to spend a little extra and have more consumer choice, one can adopt the Japanese model of universal entitlement. The premiums are kept affordable in Japan because the law requires that the premium be based on a percentage of income rather than on actuarial risks. However, if people want their doctors and nurses to serve them like postal workers, a planned government-run national health insurance system will suffice. Americans prefer a quality service and a health care delivery system that is more than adequate, that does more than suffice. A nationalized system offers bureaucrats to whom the consumer can appeal and from whom consumers can experience inaction, insensitivity, and occasionally relief. To hope that government can be reformed by idealists replacing insensitive bureaucrats is to root for the Christians to have a big fourth quarter against the lions. Nice idea, but the bureaucrats are as effective as the lions at capturing or killing idealists.

From a macroeconomic viewpoint the key issue is how much the health economy grows as a multiple of general economic growth. For example, in table 14.2 Korea has the highest rate of health-sector economic growth for two primary reasons: the ''catch-up phenomenon'' of a large volume of unmet health care

Table 14.2
Elasticity of per Capita Health Expenditures Relative to per Capita Gross Domestic Product, 1975–1990

Nation	Nominal Elasticity	Real[a] Elasticity
Korea	1.58	1.61
Japan	1.29	1.41
United States	1.29	1.15
Netherlands	1.22	1.09
Switzerland	1.18	1.04
Canada	1.16	.94
Iceland	1.14	1.45
Sweden	1.10	1.03
United Kingdom	1.08	1.02
Australia	1.08	.94
Germany[b]	1.06	.93

Source: Government of Republic of Korea (1990), OECD (1991).

[a]Health-price-deflated per capita health spending relative to GDP-deflator-adjusted per capita GDP.

[b]Germany has the lowest growth rate in health expenses, and spends 4.3 percent less of GDP on health care compared to the United States.

needs, and a doctor-dominated monopolist/laissez-faire delivery system that tightly restricts nonphysician providers (e.g., there is only one small home health care agency in the nation; Eastaugh 1990). The nominal elasticity of 1.29 for Japan and the United States in table 14.2 indicates that for every 10 percent increase in nominal per capita GDP since 1975 the nation experienced a 12.9 percent increase in nominal per capita health care spending.

The Japanese economy expects that continued high economic growth will finance more health care spending, but the American policy makers tend to talk of rationing services (Ginzberg 1991). Americans witness the anomaly of increased discussion of rationing while the number of empty hospital beds exceeds 300,000. Rationing in a market with much excess capacity is an anomaly discussed in chapters 1, 7, and 11. Some excess capacity is going out of business. American policy makers should begin to realize that (1) hospital closure is a lagged function of local economic activity (many hospitals closed in Texas and Michigan four to eight years after downturns in economic activity), and (2) health care spending follows an adapted expectations model (blips up in health spending track with an exponential-smoothed average of the last six years of economic growth; Getzen 1990; Rublee and Schneider 1991).

EQUITY DEMANDS

The preceding sections might appear insufficiently critical of the American health care system. In the spirit that half a loaf of reform is better than having no reform in the American health care system, this author supports the Ginzberg (1991) list of four priorities:

1. All persons below the poverty line should be covered by Medicaid, a proposal that has the support of both the American Medical Association and the Health Insurance Association of America.

2. States should experiment with buying into Medicaid for persons with incomes between 100 and 200 percent of the poverty level.

3. Private insurance companies, after amendment of the Employee Retirement Income Security Act, should offer stripped-down policies for catastrophic care at an affordable price, around $1,000 per year, to younger employed persons with incomes above 200 percent of the poverty level, who represent a sizable proportion of the uninsured.

4. States should develop a funding pool for reimbursing providers, particularly in the public sector, who take care of large numbers of indigent patients; revenues could be generated through sin taxes and other levies.

Long-time advocates of national health insurance will seize on any prediction of major disruptions in the industry as a rationale for passing just such a universal program. In the near future their hopes and dreams may come to fruition if the clamor for quality care and indigent care peaks. The attention cycle in support of universal health insurance coverage has gone up and down. National health insurance has appeared forever imminent on a number of occasions between 1933 and 1979 (Fein 1986). If the current push for competition results in too many scandals of poor quality or poor access, the politicians might pass a national program.

A fifth reform idea, which is already being implemented by the Agency for Health Care Policy and Research (AHCPR; chapter 11) is the development of practice guidelines for providers. Physician education, if given sufficient time and funding, can assist the provider community in developing a cost-effective clinical decision-making mindset. Even if all American physicians practiced in salaried HMO settings, guidelines would still be as helpful as fiscal incentives in achieving the elusive goal of cost containment. The lack of clear clinical guidelines for efficient quality medical care, as defined by Ott (1991) and others, is one major reason why industrial nations are all plagued with the cost-containment problem. Canadian physicians could profit from these guidelines, especially in view of their longer lengths of stay and higher hospitalization rates in Canada relative to the United States (Anderson et al. 1990). Having visited with clinicians and managers from dozens of such countries, this author can verify that the physicians of the world will be the consumers of these future AHCPR guidelines (cooks everywhere need a good cookbook as a guide). The "invisible hand" of financial incentives is typically all thumbs, but clinical guidelines offer a light touch: the chance to distinguish necessary tests and procedures from discretionary or inappropriate care. When directed by the willingness-to-pay valuation technique, the guidelines can offer the humanistic quality-adjusted-life-year metric into our resource allocation decisions.

CAPITATION: THE MEDICINE TO CURE UNBUNDLING

Many employers and government regulators fear that unbundling of services has co-opted attempts at stringent price controls, discount purchasing, and rate regulation. Capitation payment is the·ultimate defense against unbundling. Without capitation, when payers squeeze down on one end of the cost-inflation problem, the balloon pops up on the other end in the form of increased quantity of different transitional-care services. The problem may not be solved through invention of a better regulatory control system. For example, tinkering with the DRGs by adding a severity measure may only open a trapdoor to bottomless grief. The price system may be made more equitable, but does this substantially reduce the incentive to game the system? Capitation can cure the potential for gaming the system through inflated transitional care and can leave the health-system partners the discretion for dividing fair payment rates between institutions and individuals (especially if payers use the Anderson-Steinberg PACS methodology described in chapter 5).

Enthoven (1989) outlined the economics of a system for competing medical plans. Noneconomists incorrectly understand "competition" to be present if there are multiple suppliers in the marketplace (Jones 1990). By that definition the insurance marketplace is competitive in Virginia if there are 363 suppliers. However, the marketplace is not competitive in the economic (price-competition) sense if most employers pay 80 to 90 percent of the premium dollar. Employers should pay a fixed dollar amount for health care, equal to 100 percent of the premium for the lowest-cost local health plan, and employees should pay the excess if they want to sign up with a more expensive insurance plan. As premium expenses rise for the Cadillac health care plans, if employees are paying 100 percent of the added expense (rather than only 10 to 20 percent), they will make a more cost-conscious consumer choice. Ginzberg (1990) pointed out that reform has been slow in this marketplace, but Enthoven (1990) counterargued that the blame rests with employers and the federal government. Employers should get tough and set the company contribution at a fixed amount. Moreover, employers should pressure Congress to advocate limits on tax-free employer contributions to health care premiums. The employers are currently sensitive to the employee wishes that premiums be paid in "cheaper" tax-free dollars (rather than after-tax dollars). If we want more poor people to get insurance coverage, we should stop subsidizing extra expensive health care premiums. A minimum tax subsidy should be offered, and the underlying tax collections could be channeled to expanded Medicaid coverage.

If risk selection forced sicker employees to purchase the more expensive health plans (Jones 1990), one might suggest special risk pools run by employers or the federal government to underwrite certain individuals (e.g., for AIDS or sickle cell). A better alternative, with less administrative expense, might involve the Japanese approach of requiring that the premium be based on a percentage of income rather than on actuarial risks. More healthy individuals should not be allowed to act as free riders and sign up with the least-cost health plans to avoid subsidizing their sicker peers. A third approach, which has been tried in Norway and North Dakota, is to set the per capita annual payments to reflect the likely higher use of services by certain chronic-disease risk groups, thus forcing an implicit subsidy of the sick by the healthy. However, we should not scrap the idea of competition between health plans and thus place no pressure on insurers to be cost-effective just because there is wide variation in health status within the population.

CAPITATION FEVER FROM NORWAY TO NORTH DAKOTA

Employers may have an easier time of deriving per capita rates for employed populations with lower coefficients of variation in health status per person compared to the elderly population. A crude morbidity adjustment in the aggregate for nonelderly groups may be sufficient to set capitation rates in an adjusted average per capita cost (AAPCC) formula. The current American climate of enthusiasm for substantial payment reform may follow the path in the 1990s that Norway followed in 1980. After eight years of a prospective payment price system, Norway initiated a population-based morbidity-adjusted capitation formula in 1980 (Crane 1985). This capitation approach achieved a more equitable distribution of resources among the 89 hospitals and redistributed more resources to chronic-long-term-care services. A 1991 Office of Technology Assessment report on physician payment systems singled out capitation as the best long-term solution to paying for care. However, in the fall of 1991 less than four percent of Medicare enrollees were paid on a per capita basis. In the American spirit of piecemeal movement toward a major policy shift, we may move state by state and employer by employer to a fully capitated health care system sometime in the 1990s. Gradualist policies will not bring the majority of public patients under capitation in the near future, but future success with private managed-care systems might prompt all payers to push for capitation.

Some regions already have experience with capitation payments. Two rural hospitals in Maryland are paid on a per capita basis by the state rate-setting commission. Blue Cross and the Hartford Foundation have financed a number of additional capitation experiments. A capitation experiment for rural inpatient care was initiated in North Dakota (five hospitals within the state and a sixth hospital over the state line in Minnesota) and in Massachusetts (four hospitals) in 1981. Mangion (1986) reported on the results from one hospital. Significant savings were produced in the first three years, with the hospital retaining 75 percent of the savings and Blue Cross retaining the balance. Employer-based managed-care systems will undoubtedly be less generous than Blue Cross in setting the rates, but the hospital would be fully at risk to retain 100 percent of the savings (or losses). The per capita fixed-payment programs provide hospitals with obvious incentives to economize. GBB may stimulate the growth of capitation systems. In any context, it would be beneficial to link the payment formulae to quality of care; the better get paid better.

QUALITY-ENHANCING BIDDING

Some analysts have suggested patching up the system of hospital price controls (DRGs) by including a severity-adjustment factor (see chapter 8) and operating the system on refined DRGs (RDRGs). This new and improved prospective payment system (PPS) would make for a fair "prudent buyer" and help preserve the biomedical capacity of the nation. In theory this approach could save money, and the savings could be redistributed to finance the rising demand for long-term care. One should consider ways to design a PPS scheme that better protects the four basic dimensions of equity:

1. Vertical equity, ensuring that different types of hospitals, such as specialty hospitals or teaching facilities, are treated equally
2. Horizontal equity, ensuring that within a peer category, the facilities with equivalent case mixes are paid equally
3. Financial equity, ensuring that pay is for performance, considering service quality and volume, and not just in proportion to the number of cases
4. Geographic equity, ensuring that national DRG rates do not let "windfall profits" accrue beyond what is judged fair, given operating efficiency and effectiveness

Quality of service is the one major element missing in the analysis.

Ideally, one would want a payment system that fosters improvement in quality of care, pays less than average price for less than average quality, and stimulates closure of unnecessary low-quality hospitals. A reform in the current PPS should offer incentives for low-quality performers to improve and should provide punishment for those who do not improve their quality and efficiency. A quality-enhancing bidding (QEB) system could achieve these stated goals, minimize extra administrative costs, and address the issues of geographic inequity and windfall profits. Under a QEB system, Medicare could receive annual sealed competitive bids along the lines of the California MediCal system (Johns, Anderson, and Derzon 1985; Christianson 1985). QEB would differ from MediCal contracting in three crucial ways:

1. The sealed bids would not involve catchall per diems, but rather average payment per DRG with a cost weight equal to 1 (e.g., if the bid were $4,000 and the DRG weight for that condition equaled 1.25, the payment would be $5,000).

2. Hospitals would be required to bid if they were judged to have below-average quality by their local PRO, and in the pilot-test phase of QEB if they existed in a windfall-profit state.

3. Retrospective incentive compensation for quality improvements would be offered one to two years later (e.g., if a hospital bid $4,100 in a market where the national price would have been $4,900 and it improved its quality rating by 10 percent relative to the PRO moving average, the hospital would receive a retrospective 10 percent kicker bonus for quality improvement). The total payment would not exceed national DRG prices, so this proviso is budget neutral.

Some representatives of the hospital industry are likely to object to QEBs by claiming that "capping the most costly institutions always erodes quality," based on the false premise that the "most costly hospitals are the best and serve the most severely ill." However, equitable compensation for severity can be incorporated into the bidding system either (1) directly, by continuous measurement of severity as a new sixth digit code, or (2) indirectly, on a sampling basis by factoring a reasonable incidence of retrospectively measured case severity into each class of hospital (university medical center, major teaching, moderate teaching, minor teaching, and nonteaching). Quality does not increase cost as a general rule, but rather decreases cost: The skilled and adroit are more cost-efficient than the slow and clumsy users of excess procedures or inappropriate therapeutic adjuvants. It is necessary to invest in quality by designing a bidding system that constrains costs and encourages better service and convenience. The quality-oriented PPOs and HMOs already aggressively seek competitive bids for referral hospital care based on the cost/quality/convenience mix their enrollees desire. The elderly and poor should be equally protected, with PROs defining a floor on quality and HCFA managing the bidding process.

Quality-enhancement payments would give physicians more leverage to go to trustees and management and say, "Do not forgo this quality-improvement investment." If it helps patient care, the facility will get paid for it. To avoid the liar's dice dilemma, QEB would encourage the development of quality and efficiency in tandem. Restricting QEB to low-quality hospitals is important because these hospitals have the greatest potential for improvement, much as the worst-run companies are often the easiest to turn around. At least until QEB is judged cost-beneficial (Eastaugh and Eastaugh 1986), incentive pay to improve quality should be restricted to those hospitals where the investment is most likely to change behavior. Wringing the windfall profits out of suboptimal hospitals—and redistributing the resources to more efficient, quality-enhancing providers—represents financial equity at its best. A QEB program would help inject the Smith-Barney slogan into medicine: "We earn patients the old-fashioned way: We treat them better."

OLIGOPOLY OF MINISYSTEMS OR DUOPOLY?

Paul Elwood's "supermed" theory predicted that rapid consolidation should soon produce eight major health corporations providing and insuring 80 to 90 percent of the health services in the nation by 1995 (Elwood 1986). Elwood suggested that only one of these eight firms would be nonprofit. His theory failed, and big systems retrenched (Eastaugh 1992). A nonbeliever in both the supermed theory and the conventional wisdom should consider past examples of markets where the experts predicted rapid consolidation. In 1960 the experts predicted that we would have only two auto companies worldwide by 1968; yet we now have six dozen. In 1968 the experts predicted that we would have 90 percent fewer microchip firms by 1975; yet we now have 1,200 percent more in 1991. Experts like to predict consolidation in the name of a well-ordered world, but the world continues to be a messy, complex place.

Single freestanding hospitals are much like the mom-and-pop grocery stores of old; many survived by banding together. The strategy typically goes beyond simple horizontal integration of like institutions and usually involves vertical integration through common ownership or control of multiple (nonequivalent) enterprises, one of which can use as its input the output of another. Some analysts have argued that informal networking and formal systems development can provide small and costly rural and urban hospitals with the only opportunity to retain local community control (Grim 1986). High-cost medical centers increasingly seize the opportunity to sell their expertise in alternative care services to lower-cost local hospitals and facilitate formal referral patterns for easy cases out of the medical center (so their managed-care contracts can remain cost competitive). This builds a minisystem strong enough to withstand pressures to sell or close. Autonomous hospitals can band together locally, go it alone, or become a franchise in a national firm. In either of the last two cases hospitals should avoid going so heavily into debt that their survival is unlikely. Johns Hopkins Hospital, Northwestern, Rush-Presbyterian-St. Luke's Medical Center, and the Mayo Clinic expanded into small hospital groups in their respective cities during the late 1980s. But few hospitals have such access to capital. Avenues for capital include insurance companies interested in regional or local health systems, ex-partners of failed supermed ventures, nursing home chains, local dominant employers in the city, and ultimately the individual hospital's medical staff. As to this last possibility, the marketing points to the physician community could include the following: "You don't want to become an AMI or Humana physician? Then make a financial investment in your local hospitals."

Experts are nearly united in predicting substantial increases in multihospital systems' market share. In this era of rapid change, there is so much written about what "will be" that it is easy to forget current market conditions. In times of stress we often "circle the wagons" and join together in groups, but the circle need not be too large. One should question whether economics suggests that consolidations favor large over small groups of hospitals. Consider the contrast to another market, the toaster industry. Quality in health care is more heterogeneous and costs are more labor-intensive. Unlike the kitchen toaster market, the product/service in health care varies widely in quality across geographic regions of the country—that is, the Humana brand of quality service varies more widely than the GE brand of toaster. Unlike a stockpiled manufactured good, health services are produced and consumed locally. The postulated economies of scale in running a big chain are likely due to the fact that the principal cost input is locally sourced labor. Consequently, if a small hospital reaps purchase discounts through membership in a group buying agreement, the facility need not experience scale economies inferior to those of a 50,000-bed hospital chain (Zuckerman and Kaluzny 1991). The first generation of alliances born in the 1970s involved shared services and multihospital systems (Eastaugh 1981), but the second generation of alliances involves continuity of care, HMOs, and PPOs—a new challenge of cooperation in the 1990s.

In the context of hospital care, local hospitals need not always join a for-profit chain or the nonprofit group with 600 member hospitals if they can find a local market niche. This point is doubly true in a local service-delivery industry like health care, in contrast to microchips and automobiles where there is less concern for distance between the firm and the customer. By 1995 some 20 megasystems may control 50 percent of the market, but 200 to 400 local minisystems may control 60 to 80 percent of their local market shares with a locally developed and controlled insurance product. Consolidation begins to offer few advantages when the service cannot be stockpiled as inventory and the central office becomes too removed from the local community. Minisystems should be capable of out-competing against the megasystems if they remain flexible, adaptive, and non-bureaucratic in response to their market (Shortell 1991; Fein 1991).

The principal disadvantage of small hospital minisystems is the aforementioned reduced access to low-cost capital. However, this is counterbalanced in that local control and small size offer the ability to be quick and flexible in adapting to changing community needs (Peters and Austin 1985). Flexibility often beats size, and size often breeds rigidity and bureaucracy. The investor-owned megasystems are beginning to respond to this last point and are attempting to trim corporate staff and lone (single) hospitals with poor profitability. Local hospitals must sacrifice a little autonomy, initiate master limited partnerships, and band together as minisystems. Enhanced productivity will trim staff-obese institutions with excess overhead. In the 1990s one cannot ignore the productivity/quality challenge.

The rate of hospital mergers may increase in the 1990s. Mergers are like human relationships; they can range from love and marriage to courtship followed by friendship or fast pillage and one-night stands. Employees often experience turmoil and confusion in merging companies, which often undermine the most careful financial and strategic plans. Financial managers do a good job by avoiding the ''Noah's Ark'' syndrome and cutting administrative fat rather than keeping two of every job position following a merger. Morrisey, Sloan, and Valrona's (1989) study of hospital markets suggested that mergers are not likely to harm competition. Neither urban nor rural markets are that highly concentrated. With the exception of one California chain that had to divest one of a town's three hospitals because of an 81 percent market share, mergers are no antitrust threat to competition.

Under perfect competition a large number of buyers and sellers will drive the producers to outprice, outvalue, and outmaneuver each other to the benefit of all consumers (with the ability to pay). Under an oligopoly the market is composed of a handful of producers whose pricing decisions are interdependent and thus higher than purely competitive market prices (Eastaugh 1981). If a chain has a monopoly on the area market due to a natural monopoly (e.g., a one-hospital town) or because antitrust enforcement is weakened, it has no competitors to dissuade it from charging higher prices and reaping classic monopoly profits. In the case of a duopoly, the two firms can better collude to reap more profits than in an oligopoly situation. Consolidation of the health sector into a few supermeds may have some advantages for large corporations (reaping super discounts), but competition is not among them. Minisystems and the preservation of the freestanding autonomous hospital will best assure a competitive market if and only if such facilities fight hard to trim excess costs and invest in quality-enhancing activities. The aforementioned quality-enhancing bidding schemes (QEBs) may support this more competitive marketplace.

RETURNS FROM BETTER INFORMATION

Quality has been a major subplot in this text. One hospital used its severity-adjusted fatality data to convince the medical staff to standardize orders for antibiotics and blood cultures in the emergency department (where 92 percent of pneumonia fatality cases originated). Within three months the severity-adjusted fatality rates had declined 45 percent to the average level for teaching hospitals in that city.

Some health policy makers have tended to reduce health economics to the level of a forensic science, full of rhetoric and devoid of research results. A main objective of this book has been to engage the interests of policy makers and managers in the research results of academicians. Policy makers, like institutional managers, are too occupied with putting out daily brush fires and reacting to symptomatology to adequately keep abreast of the health-services research literature.

The health industry and the regulators have taken a largely defensive stand. Each party has become preoccupied with the actions and expectations of the other. However, an internal cost-containment ethos and fair reimbursement of total institutional financial requirements are necessary if we are to develop a more rational national health policy; rhetoric concerning "fat" providers and mindless "bureaucrats" is counterproductive. Will the 1990s be a period of uncontrolled growth and expansion of the health economy? Can the recent record of poor performance and sluggish productivity be reversed? The public has come to recognize that the key problems for health policy are cost containment and

access to care. The solution to containing costs may be found in better implementation of management strategies and better research in the areas of finance
and health economics. In our pluralistic society, better information is a necessary,
but not sufficient, condition for achieving a healthier health economy.

The quality of discharge data should improve in 1993 with implementation
of the new ICD–10 diagnosis coding system. The new system is responsive to
calls for greater specificity and differentiation between services and illnesses.
The new "Z codes" offer an expanded category of codes for asymptomatic HIV
status, required administrative medical exams, antenatal screening, contraceptive
management, drug use, and housing status (homelessness and inadequate insurance). All nations will not utilize every code field; for example, Korea currently
only codes three digits (resulting in 340 Korean DRGs, not 490).

PHYSICIAN REACTION TO "TOO MUCH CHANGE"

Many conservative clinicians dislike guidelines and fear that they will be
stripped of admitting privileges if their practice profile exhibits an inability to
adjust to the "new medicine" of decision analysis, PPS, PPOs, and HMOs.
These clinicians argue that "personal care" gets lost in the shuffle as DRG trees,
software, outliers, economic grand rounds, and "think-adjustment" sessions
force professionals toward "cookbook medicine." Carrying their case to the
extreme, conservative physicians often make four points:

1. If the practice profile is too expensive relative to excessively low government or third-
   party payment rates, the doctor is labeled "a dyscodic outlier heterogenicist" and
   faces loss of admitting privileges.
2. "True" doctors cannot join a PPO or a system because they are "neither providers
   nor preferred" (medicine is a "calling," not a commercial enterprise, and should be
   preferred for quality caring, not price discounts).
3. Doctors are forced to provide only the admissions that are profitable to the hospital
   and jettison the nonprofitable services (Fallon 1991).
4. Doctors are forced to abide by market analysis and selling strategies (Ashmos and
   McDaniel 1991).

Hospital managers and medical-staff leaders should develop a cogent response
to each of these four points of misunderstanding.

First, data-based "credentialing" for membership on the medical staff is a
negotiated process. If the chief of medical staff can build a reasonable case for
retaining an individual whose practice habits are more expensive for uncontrollable reasons (for receiving more severely ill cases than evidenced simply by
the DRG or for specializing in treatment of intrinsically unprofitable DRGs the
trustees want admitted), then the doctor should be retained on the medical staff
and not declared a "shameless statistical deviate." As to the second point,
patients do value economic attributes, such as lower out-of-pocket payments for

health care, lower premiums, and higher wages because costs are more under control (i.e., so the employer does not have to pay much of the wage increase to health care providers; because they have less funds for wage hikes if they spend more and more on health care costs).

In response to the third point, hospital executives should point out that cost accounting is required to financially plan the institution's future. Moreover, clinicians should rid themselves of the myth that hospital charges are highly correlated with actual resource costs. All parties concerned need accurate standard cost accounting. The hospital is never required to make a profit on each service product line. However, trustees need to know how much they lose on certain product lines so they can expand or initiate money makers such that the final bottom line is sufficient to maintain a quality hospital. If clinicians do not trust the dollar figures derived from accounting or the CFO, the data can be presented in opportunity-cost terms. A nonphysician manager should never say the "unthinkable" and claim that a given product line is a $500,000 example of "economic malpractice." Instead, the clinicians working in this inefficient service area can be told that the "opportunity costs of this service require that we fire 20 people hospitalwide plus your postgraduate fellow to underwrite the cost of this money-losing product line."

As to the fourth point, physician disdain for marketing is both archaic and antipatient. Health marketing places the consumers as kings and asks how best to meet their medical needs with quality service at an affordable cost. Marketing is simply doing right by the patients, channeling them to the service mode of delivery that is most appropriate. Effective marketing is not "hucksterism" or selling. Good marketing involves open communication, development of trust, and instilling in the public the differential advantages and abilities offered by a given provider. Social marketing programs determine what consumers need, tailor services to meet those needs, and suggest that patients utilize services in a timely preventive manner—that is, before something more serious develops.

SUPPORT FROM THE MEDICAL STAFF

Offering stock in a firm or franchise was an unusual financing arrangement until passage of tax reform in October 1986. Even well-known firms, such as the Boston Celtics professional basketball team, were selling up to a 40 to 49 percent stake in the franchise under a master limited partnership. Most hospitals do not have the national marketability of the Boston Celtics or the Mayo Clinic, but they have a local captive group of potential investors—their physicians. The master limited partnership could be presented to the medical staff in general terms—that is, if you do not invest in this facility, the workshop where you perform patient care will erode (i.e., plant and equipment will become obsolete). In addition, one could appeal to clinicians' specific (individual) self-interest with various "perks." For example, physicians who invest in the partnership would be provided the best operative time slots, the best work schedules, and relief from bureaucratic burdens. Financially distressed facilities may have to charge those who do not invest in the master limited partnership a monthly "rent" for the right to admit their private-pay patients to the hospital. At the extreme, those doctors not wishing to invest cash in their workshop/hospital would have to pay with their time for the right to be on the medical staff and have admitting privileges. The shift from a field dominated by doctors as nonpaying "partners" (keeping the hospital at financial risk) to one where they must invest their funds to keep the facility state-of-the-art destroys the obsolete philosophy of professional dominance. Moreover, the organizations that employ or rent admitting rights to physicians will demand that managers share in decisions regarding professional roles and dominate decisions involving capital acquisitions. In a world where the climate for dialogue between payers and providers has never been worse, the opportunity for joint deals between hospitals and physicians has never been better (Herzlinger 1992; Williams and Coolidge 1991).

One would hope that most hospitals could still base medical-staff membership decisions on the professional input and not the financial input of the individual doctor. However, in a basic economic sense, if the hospital and the doctor are involved in joint production, and the hospital is under severe financial pressure, the institution may have to demand financial resources from the producer group experiencing higher rates of return—the physician community. Lower physician investment will lead to more hospital closings, to longer travel time to reach the workshop/hospital, or perhaps even to many physicians lacking admitting privileges at any hospital.

THE ROAD AHEAD

Some members of organized medicine express fear that prepaid Medicare is an invitation to create medical ghettos for the elderly. One noted economist argued that we may soon turn to a false form of national health insurance—one offering a voucher for minimum coverage but leaving the individual to fend for a large share of medical costs (Ginzberg, 1991). Politicians frequently seek headlines by claiming that the bulk of the medical cost problem is caused by the fraud and abuse of a few providers. This contributes to piecemeal attention being given to such infrequent problems as Medicaid kickbacks and HMO scandals, rather than the more insidious problem of inflationary or quality-eroding incentive structures. A quality-enhancing bidding system would go a long way toward promoting good medicine and good economics.

In visiting Chinese hospitals and medical schools in 1980, I was interested to discover that the ancient proverb, "May you live in interesting times," was often misinterpreted by Caucasian visitors as a curse. The opportunity for substantial reform is best in just such times of stress and strain. In fact, the Chinese term *wei ji* has a simultaneous dual interpretation: opportunity and danger. Over the next five years our health system faces immense opportunity and danger in a reformation on four fronts: access, efficiency, effectiveness, and quality of

Figure 14.1
Financial Typology for International Health Delivery Systems (GBB = global budget board for setting hospital budgets)

Patient Cost Gov Sharing Control	Effective GBB for Hospitals	Fees Kept Low For Procedures	Fee-For-Service/ No GBB	Total
High (above 25%)	XX	--	S. Korea	ZZ
Moderate	USA in 1999? France Chile	USA 1996	USA	New Zealand
Low (under 10%)	Australia Norway Germany*	Japan Holland	YY	United Kingdom

*Germany also has GBB for meeting physician fees and a global budget. Holland tried this approach for one month in 1987 before physician strikes.

life. The challenge for providers and managers during this period of unparalleled opportunity is to win a clear victory on all four fronts and not erode either access or quality in the name of efficiency. This is a clear challenge for both managers and policy makers. The job is doubly tough for our physicians. The challenge to physicians will be to carry on one shoulder lifesaving technology and the concomitant financial burden and, on the other shoulder, the will and imagination to apply modern management techniques.

How well the physicians and managers work together will determine whether we experience the bad or good side of the "invisible hand." Bad competition will result in overemphasis on a narrow business focus and an attempt to avoid providers' social obligations. This dark side of competition attacks the special moral importance of health care in society. Warden (1990) argued that health care derives its moral importance from its impact on the normal range of opportunities in society; and opportunity is reduced when illness impairs functioning. However, any balanced view of health care should consider it as both a social good and a consumer good. Good competition will invoke a broader business focus and health-delivery orientation. Good competition can stimulate neighboring providers to offer better services at more reasonable expense through specialization, economies of scale, and quality assurance. This process can improve, and not erode, patient access to quality services throughout all market segments. However, given the recent passage of a Minnesota statewide universal health insurance program for 1992, we may be headed down the regulatory road. In which case, the German model of GBB (see figure 14.1) is the most effective approach.

REFERENCES

Abel-Smith, B. (1985). "Who Is the Odd Man Out? The Experience of Western Europe in Containing the Costs of Health Care." *Milbank Quarterly* 63:1 (Spring), 1–17.

American Association of Homes for the Aging. (1992). *Continuing Care Retirement Communities*. Washington, D.C.: AAHA.

Anderson, M., Pulcins, I., Barer, M., and Evans, R. (1990). "Acute Care Hospital Utilization under Canadian National Health Insurance: British Columbia Experience." *Inquiry* 27:4 (Winter), 352–358.

Ashmos, D., and McDaniel, R. (1991). "Physician Participation in Hospital Strategic Decision Making: The Effect of Hospital Strategy and Decision Content." *Health Services Research* 26:3 (August), 375–401.

Baumol, W., Blackman, S., and Wolfe, E. (1985). "Unbalanced Growth Revisited: Asymptotic Stagnancy and New Evidence." *American Economic Review* 75:4 (September), 806–817.

Brownson, R., Smith, C., and Jorge, N. (1992). "Role of Data-driven Planning and Coalition Development in Prevention." *Public Health Reports* 107:1 (January–February), 32–36.

Christianson, J. (1985). "Competitive Bidding: The Challenge for Health Care Managers." *Health Care Management Review* 10:2 (Spring), 39–53.

Coney, S. (1991). "New Zealand Dismantles Its Health and Welfare System." *Lancet* 2:8371 (January 12), 101–102.

Crane, T. (1985). "Hospital Cost Control in Norway: A Decade's Experience with Prospective Payment." *Public Health Reports* 100:4 (July/August), 406–417.

Eastaugh, S. (1992). *Health Care Finance: Economic Incentives and Productivity Enhancement*. Westport, Conn.: Greenwood.

———. (1990). "Impact of National Health Insurance on Korean Health Care Expenditures." Consultant report, World Bank, Washington, D.C.

———. (1981). *Medical Economics and Health Finance*. Dover, Mass.: Auburn House, 318–322.

Eastaugh, S., and Eastaugh, J. (1986). "Prospective Payment Systems: Further Steps to Enhance Quality, Efficiency, and Regionalization." *Health Care Management Review* 11:4 (Fall), 37–52.

Eddy, D. (1991). "Oregon's Methods: Did Cost-effectiveness Analysis Fail?" *Journal of the American Medical Association* 266:15 (October 16), 2135–2141

Elwood, P. (1986). "Supermed Concept Gaining Ground." *Federation of American Executives Review* 19:2 (March/April), 69–71.

Elwood, P., and Paul, B. (1984). *Here Come the SuperMeds*. Excelsior, Minn.: Interstudy.

Enthoven, A. (1990). "Multiple Choice Health Insurance: The Lessons and Challenge to Employers." *Inquiry* 27:4 (Winter), 368–373.

————. (1989). *Theory and Practice of Managed Competition in Health Care Finance*. Amsterdam: North-Holland.

Evans, D. (1990). "Estimated Prevalence of Alzheimer's Disease in the United States." *Milbank Quarterly* 68:2 (Summer), 267–289.

Fallon, R. (1991). "Not-for-profit Is Not No Profit: Profitability Planning in Not-for-profit Organizations." *Health Care Management Review* 16:3 (Summer), 47–61.

Fein, O. (1991). "Restructuring Services in the Academic Medical Center: One Approach to Primary Care Services for the Urban Poor." *Bulletin of the New York Academy of Medicine* 67:1 (January–February), 59–65.

Fein, R. (1986). *Medical Care, Medical Costs: The Search for a Health Insurance Policy*. Cambridge, Mass.: Harvard University Press.

Fuchs, V., and Hahn, J. (1990). "How Does Canada Do It? A Comparison of Expenditures for Physician Services in the U.S. and Canada." *New England Journal of Medicine* 323:13 (September 27), 884–890.

Gapenski, L. (1992). *Healthcare Financial Management*. Ann Arbor, Mich.: Health Administration Press.

Getzen, T. (1992). "Forecasting International Health Expenditures." *Public Budgeting and Financial Management* 4:1 (Spring), 149–170.

————. (1990). "Macro Forecasting of National Health Expenditures." In *Advances in Health Economics and Health Services Research*, edited by R. Scheffler, Greenwich, Conn.: JAI Press, 27–47.

Ginzberg, E. (1991). *The Contribution of Health Services Research to National Health Policy*. Cambridge, Mass.: Harvard University Press.

————. (1990). "Health Care Reform: Why So Slow?" *New England Journal of Medicine* 322:20 (May 17), 1464–1466.

Gray, B. (1991). *The Profit Motive and Patient Care: The Changing Accountability of Doctors and Hospitals*. Cambridge: Harvard University Press.

Grim, S. (1986). "Win/Win: Urban and Rural Hospitals Network for Survival." *Hospital and Health Services Administration* 31:1 (January–February), 34–42.

Herzlinger, R. (1992). *Creating New Health Care Ventures: The Role of Management*. Gaithersburg, Md.: Aspen.

Hollingsworth, J., Hage, J., and Hanneman, R. (1991). *State Intervention in Medical Care: Consequences for Britain, France, Sweden, and the United States*. Ithaca, N.Y.: Cornell University Press.

Holoweiko, M. (1992) "Health Care Reform in Hawaii." *Medical Economics* 69:3 (February 3), 158–174.

Iglehart, J. (1991). "Germany's Health Care System." *New England Journal of Medicine* 324:7 (February 14), 503–508.

Ikegami, N. (1991) "Japanese Health Care: Low Cost Through Regulated Fees." *Health Affairs* 10:3 (Fall), 87–108.

Johns, L., Anderson, M., and Derzon, R. (1985). "Selective Contracting in California." *Inquiry* 22:4 (Winter), 335–347.

Jones, S. (1990). "Multiple Choice Health Insurance: The Lessons and Challenge to Private Insurers." *Inquiry* 27:2 (Summer), 161–166.

Kauer, R., and Silvers, J. (1991). "Hospital Free Cash Flow." *Health Care Management Review* 16:4 (Fall), 67–78.

Kenney, G., and Holahan, J. (1990). "The Nursing Home Market and Hospital Discharge Delays." *Inquiry* 27:1 (Spring), 73–85.

Kirkman-Liff, B., and van de Ven, W. (1989). "Improving Efficiency in the Dutch Health Care System: Current Innovations and Future Options." *Health Policy* 13:4 (October), 35–53.

Kovner, A., and Neuhauser, D. (1991). *Health Services Management: Readings and Commentary*. 4th ed. Ann Arbor, Mich.: Health Administration Press.

Krasny, J., and Ferrier, I. (1991). *The Canadian Healthcare System in Perspective*. Toronto: Bogart Delafield Ferrier.

Kuhn, E., Hartz, A., Gottlieb, M., Rimm, A. (1991). "Relationship of Hospital Characteristics and Peer Review in Six Large States." *Medical Care* 29:10 (October), 1028–1038.

Linder, J. (1991). "Outcomes Measurement: Compliance Tool or Strategic Initiative." *Health Care Management Review* 16:4 (Fall), 21–33.

Lister, J. (1986). "The Politics of Medicine in Britain and the United States." *New England Journal of Medicine* 315:3 (July 17), 168–173.

Mangion, R. (1986). "Capitation Reimbursement: A Progress Report." *Hospital and Health Services Administration* 31:1 (January–February), 99–110.

Marmor, T. (1992). *The Politics of Medicare*. Hawthorne, N.Y.: Aldine.

McDonough, J. (1992). "The Demise of Massachusetts Hospital Rate Regulation." *American Health Policy* 2:2 (March/April), 40–44.

Moore, F., and Priebe, C. (1991). "Board-certified Physicians in the United States, 1971–1986. *New England Journal of Medicine* 324:8 (February 21), 536–543.

Morrisey, M., Sloan, F., and Valvona, J. (1989). *Cost of Capital and Capital Structure in U.S. Hospitals*. Washington, D.C.: National Center for HSR and Technology Assessment, report 209903.

Nemes, J. (1991). "Hospitals Signaling Distress." *Modern Healthcare* 21:9 (March 4), 37–40.

Neuschler, E. (1990). *Canadian Health Care: Implications of Public Health Insurance*. Washington, D.C.: Health Insurance Association of America.

Nyman, J. (1989). "Analysis of Nursing Home Bed Supply." *Health Services Research* 24:4 (October), 511–537.

Organization for Economic Cooperation and Development. (1991). *National Accounts of OECD Countries*, 1950–1990. Paris: OECD.

Ott, J. (1991). "Competitive Medical Organizations: A View of the Future." In J. Moreno (ed.), *Paying the Doctor*, 83–92. Westport, Conn.: Auburn House.

Peters, T., and Austin, N. (1985). *A Passion for Excellence*. New York: Random House.

Powell, M., and Anesaki, M. (1991). *Health Care in Japan*. New York: Routledge, Chapman, and Hall.

Rachlis, M., and Kushner, C. (1990). *Second Opinion: What's Wrong with Canada's Health-Care System and How to Fix It*. Toronto, Ontario: Collins.

Rakich, J. (1991). "The Canadian and U.S. Health Care Systems: Profiles and Policies." *Hospital and Health Services Administration* 36:1 (Spring), 525–542.

Rockefeller, J. (1991). "A Call to Action." *Journal of the American Medical Association* 265:19 (May 15), 2507–2511.

Rublee, D., and Schneider, M. (1991). "International Health Spending Comparisons." *Health Affairs* 10:3 (Fall), 187–197.

Saltman, R. (1990). "Competition and Reform in the Swedish Health System." *Milbank Quarterly* 68:4 (December), 597–617.

Schneider, M. (1991). "Health Care Cost Containment in the Republic of Germany." *Health Care Financing Review* 12:3 (Spring), 87–101.

Shortell, S. (1991). *Effective Hospital-Physician Relationships*. Ann Arbor, Mich.: Health Administration Press.

Skarupa, J., and Matherlee, T. (1989). *The Hospital Medical Staff: Closed Medical Staffs Are Not Inevitable*. Chicago, Ill.: American Hospital Publishing.

Smith, D. (1992) *Paying For Medicare: The Politics of Reform*. Hawthorne, N.Y.: Aldine.

Sullivan, L. (1992). "Bush's Comprehensive Health Reform Package." *American Health Policy* 2:2 (March/April), 15–18.

Thompson, R. (1991). "Total Quality Management." *Healthcare Executive* 6:2 (March–April), 26–27.

Todd, J., Seekins, J., Krichbaum, J., and Harvey, L. (1991). "Health Access America: Strengthening the U.S. Health Care System." *Journal of the American Medical Association* 265:19 (May 15), 2503–2507.

Warden, G. (1990). "Future Directions for Urban Health Care." *Henry Ford Hospital Medical Journal* 38:3 (Fall), 178–183.

Williams, J., and Coolidge, R. (1991). "Annual Hay Compensation Survey: Incentive Plans on the Upswing." *Trustee* 44:10 (October), 7–10.

Woolhandler, S., and Himmelstein, D. (1991). "Deteriorating Administrative Efficiency of the U.S. Health Care System." *New England Journal of Medicine* 324:18 (May 2) 1253–1258.

Wysong, J., and Abel, T. (1990). "Universal Health Insurance and High-Risk Groups in West Germany: Implications for U.S. Health Policy." *Milbank Quarterly* 68:4 (December), 527–560.

Young, D. (1991). "Planning and Controlling Health Capital: Attaining a Balance between Regulation and Competition." *Medical Care Review* 48:3 (Fall), 261–93.

Zuckerman, H., and Kaluzny, A. (1991). "Strategic Alliances in Health Care: The Challenges of Cooperation." *Frontiers of Health Services Management* 7:3 (Winter), 3–22.

Author Index

Note: Page numbers followed by n refer to full bibliographic references.

Subject Index